Developing the Athlete

An Applied Sport Science Roadmap for Optimizing Performance

William J. Kraemer, PhD
The Ohio State University
Columbus, OH, USA
University of Connecticut
Storrs, CT, USA
Edith Cowan University
Perth, AU

Nicholas A. Ratamess, PhD
The College of New Jersey
Ewing, NJ, USA

Thomas H. Newman, MS
Mass General Brigham
Boston, MA, USA

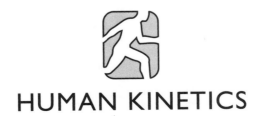

Library of Congress Cataloging-in-Publication Data

Names: Kraemer, William J., 1953- author. | Ratamess, Nicholas A., author. | Newman, Thomas H., 1985- author.
Title: Developing the athlete : an applied sport science roadmap for optimizing performance / William J. Kraemer, Nicholas A. Ratamess, Thomas H. Newman.
Description: Champaign, IL : Human Kinetics, 2025. | Includes bibliographical references and index.
Identifiers: LCCN 2023024570 (print) | LCCN 2023024571 (ebook) | ISBN 9781718218574 (paperback) | ISBN 9781718218581 (epub) | ISBN 9781718218598 (pdf)
Subjects: LCSH: Physical education and training. | Athletes--Training of. | Physical fitness--Physiological aspects. | Sports sciences. | BISAC: HEALTH & FITNESS / Exercise / Strength Training | SPORTS & RECREATION / Bodybuilding & Weightlifting
Classification: LCC GV711.5 .K73 2024 (print) | LCC GV711.5 (ebook) | DDC 796.071--dc23/eng/20230711
LC record available at https://lccn.loc.gov/2023024570
LC ebook record available at https://lccn.loc.gov/2023024571

ISBN: 978-1-7182-1857-4 (paperback)
ISBN: 978-1-7182-1860-4 (loose-leaf)

Copyright © 2025 by William J. Kraemer, Nicholas A. Ratamess, and Thomas H. Newman

Human Kinetics supports copyright. Copyright fuels scientific and artistic endeavor, encourages authors to create new works, and promotes free speech. Thank you for buying an authorized edition of this work and for complying with copyright laws by not reproducing, scanning, or distributing any part of it in any form without written permission from the publisher. You are supporting authors and allowing Human Kinetics to continue to publish works that increase the knowledge, enhance the performance, and improve the lives of people all over the world.

To report suspected copyright infringement of content published by Human Kinetics, contact us at **permissions@hkusa.com**. To request permission to legally reuse content published by Human Kinetics, please refer to the information at **https://US.Human Kinetics.com/pages/permissions-information**.

This publication is written and published to provide accurate and authoritative information relevant to the subject matter presented. Care has been taken to confirm the accuracy of the information and to describe generally accepted practices. However, the authors, editor, and publisher are not responsible for errors or omissions or for any consequences from application of the information in this publication and make no warranty, expressed or implied, with respect to the currency, completeness, or accuracy of the contents of the publication. It is published and sold with the understanding that the authors, editor, and publisher are not engaged in rendering legal, medical, or other professional services by reason of their authorship or publication of this work. If medical or other assistance is required, it is the responsibility of the reader or user to obtain the services of a doctor or other appropriate, competent professional. Application of this information in an educational or any other situation remains the professional responsibility of the practitioner; the clinical treatments described and recommended may not be considered absolute and universal recommendations.

The web addresses cited in this text were current as of June 2023, unless otherwise noted.

Senior Acquisitions Editor: Roger Earle; **Managing Editor:** Kevin Matz; **Copyeditor:** Sean Tommasi; **Proofreader:** Joyce Li; **Indexer:** Karla Walsh; **Permissions Manager:** Laurel Mitchell; **Graphic Designer:** Dawn Sills; **Cover Designer:** Keri Evans; **Cover Design Specialist:** Susan Rothermel Allen; **Photographs (cover):** skynesher/E+/Getty Images, Yellow Dog Productions/The Image Bank/Getty Images, and Human Kinetics, Inc.; **Photographs (interior):** © Human Kinetics, unless otherwise noted; **Photo Production Manager:** Jason Allen; **Senior Art Manager:** Kelly Hendren; **Illustrations:** © Human Kinetics, unless otherwise noted; **Printer:** Sheridan Books

The authors would like to thank Mr. Oluseun Omonije, MRPH.AI Company, New York, NY, 10007, USA for creating the artwork used in the Looking in the Rearview Mirror and Looking at the Road Ahead boxes.

Human Kinetics books are available at special discounts for bulk purchase. Special editions or book excerpts can also be created to specification. For details, contact the Special Sales Manager at Human Kinetics.

Printed in the United States of America   10 9 8 7 6 5 4 3 2 1

The paper in this book is certified under a sustainable forestry program.

Human Kinetics
1607 N. Market Street
Champaign, IL 61820
USA

United States and International
Website: **US.HumanKinetics.com**
Email: info@hkusa.com
Phone: 1-800-747-4457

Canada
Website: **Canada.HumanKinetics.com**
Email: info@hkcanada.com

E8977 (paperback) / E8978 (loose-leaf)

To my wife, Joan; my three children, Daniel, Anna, and Maria;
my daughter-in-law, Amie; my granddaughters, Olivia and Catherine;
and my sister, Judith Kraemer for their love and support.
—William J. Kraemer

This book is dedicated to my wife, Alison; my children, Jessica, Vinnie, and Nicole;
and my parents, Nick and Veronica, for their love and support.
—Nicholas A. Ratamess

I dedicate this book to Maureen Newman, PhD. You are my strength
when I am weak, and you are my light when it is dark. Always and forever.
—Thomas H. Newman

Contents

Preface vii • Acknowledgments ix

1 Developing the Human Machine — 1
The Human Machine 3
The Athlete Composite 4
Factors Influencing Player Development and Performance 4
Alignment in the Player Development Program 6
Factors Affecting Sport Performance 8
The Developmental Pathways 9
Development of the Athlete from Youth to Adulthood 11

2 Player Profiles, Sport Matching, and the Player Development Team — 21
Program Alignment 25
The Player Development Team Model 27
Units in the Player Development Team 28
Level of Competition 31
Determining Sport Demands 37
Impact of Athlete to Sport to Position Matching 52

3 Testing and Assessments in Player Development — 55
Setting the Standards for Testing and Assessments 56
Preparing for the Testing Sessions 58
Testing Protocols 58
Testing Organization 61
Choice of Tests for the Player Composite 64
Development of the Player Composite 65
Testing Athletes 65

4 Understanding the Workout Stimuli: Impact on the Athlete Composite — 101
Size Principle: Understanding Is Crucial to Practice 101
The Exercise Stimuli Create an Exercise Drug 102
Safety for the Athlete Is Priority One 102
The Stimulus–Response–Adaptation Cycle 103
Logistical Comfort and Peak Performance: A Symbiosis 104
Program Variables in Training Program Design 104
Variation in Training Programs Mediating Recovery and Performance 106
The Acute Exercise Response 108
The Role of Genes in Exercise and Adaptation 111
Chronic Training Adaptations 112

5 Monitoring and Accounting in Player Development — 125

The Importance of Proper Monitoring 125
Skill Sets Needed 130
Responsibilities of the Athlete 135
Decisions on What Data Need to Be Entered 139
Data Input and Quality Entry 143
Reports to Coaches and Athletes 148

6 Interpreting and Evaluating Testing Results of the Athlete Composite — 151

Roles of Player Development Team 151
Sources of Knowledge 152
Understanding Context of Training Steps and Target Goals 155
Organizing the Database 156
Looking to Analyze the Data 157
Interpreting the Results 158

7 Training and Recovery Approaches in Player Development — 183

Importance of Individualization 183
Training Program Variation 184
Understanding the Exercise Stimuli Variables in Workout Design 184
Programming in Athlete Development 184
Rest and Recovery 190
Training Approaches for Different Elements in Player Development 200
Methods of Program Variation 224

8 Looking Back and Ahead at the Road for Player Development — 229

The Conceptual Model of Player Development 229
Historical Models Can Provide Object Lessons for Implementation 230
Academic and Research Influences 231
Influence of the Strength and Conditioning Coach 232
Player Development Models in the United States 232
Sport Analytics and Technology: The Good, the Bad, and the Ugly 238
Historically Proven Programs to Fit Any Paradigm 239
Future Challenges for Strength and Conditioning and Sport Performance Professionals 242
Flexible Nonlinear Programming—Another Historical Look 244
The Post-Competitive Career 245

References and Suggested Readings 249 • Index 263
• About the Authors 269 • Earn Continuing Education Credits/Units 270

Preface

Over the past decade, the complexity of player or athlete development has increased, and sport science has become obsessed with metrics and genetics since the movie *Moneyball* and the publication of *The Sports Gene*. However, there is a lack of practical guidance on how to integrate this information with existing fields to optimize performance. The abundance of tangential information confuses the sequential path to understanding how things work to influence athlete development.

Navigating athlete development becomes complex when there are internal and external disruptors. These can stem from disagreements within the athlete development team itself or from external administrators overseeing the team. Alignment of everyone working with the athlete is vital for optimal progress over time. Such challenges can hinder interventions and slow progress. In today's sports landscape, numerous professionals vie for an athlete's attention. This competition can dilute efficiency and create confusion for the athlete. It's vital to maintain clear, quality communication and interventions with each athlete to prevent these challenges from derailing their optimal development. Sport science and analytics need a foundation of evidence-based facts, and streamlined programs must be in place to integrate optimal development to a reasonable extent. The three Cs of credentials, competence, and commitment need to be intact to ensure each professional can contribute evidence-based practices in their lane of expertise as well as their own perspectives on each issue.

Sport coaches and professionals in the field of strength and conditioning and sport performance need a better understanding of how other disciplines can contribute to their worlds and help them win. No book has been written that provides a model and explains the dimensions of a player development process rooted in the individual athlete without being cumbersome in its interventions and analyses; thus, there is a need for a book that develops a basic and proven roadmap for success.

Success in this process involves evaluating the potential for an individual to compete at a given level of a sport and optimizing their physical and psychological development to take on the demands of the sport. Understanding the factors that influence development will then allow sport science professionals, sport scientists, and sport coaches to understand the athlete development process.

Practitioners in applied sport sciences must tap into the known scientific principles and practices that help the process of athlete development. Individualization is paramount, and understanding how to test, evaluate, monitor, and archive data is a vital skill set needed for optimizing each athlete's journey.

Ultimately, a proven roadmap can frame the process and demonstrate how other fields can be applied to day-to-day athlete development. This book is the first to provide such a view on this concept from the multiple perspectives that must be taken into consideration when evaluating, assessing, and developing athletes to compete and succeed at every level of competition.

Acknowledgments

It takes a team of professionals to put together any book in the world of publishing. Because we have had experience with writing books, we know that there are many people to thank for this opportunity to contribute to our field. First, we want to thank Roger Earle, our acquisition editor, who carefully listened to our pleas that such a book is needed to add more dimensions to this aspect of sport science and performance. Roger's support was paramount to being successfully published by Human Kinetics. We also appreciate all of the work Human Kinetics and its professionals have done on this book's production. Thank you to Kevin Matz, our managing editor, for his careful work and help in this process. We all feel, as authors, that it was enjoyable to work on this project together and interact with the various insights arising from both the practical and scientific aspects of this book's topic.

Dr. Ratamess would like to give special thanks to Dr. Avery Faigenbaum for his insights on youth fitness and Dr. Tamara Rial Rebullido for their assistance with some of the figures. Lastly, he would like to thank Jenna Ingui and Justin Dominique for modeling some exercises in this book.

Coach Tom Newman would like to thank the many people who have contributed to his growth as a professional, from his years as a strength and conditioning coach to his time in the world of business and athlete development.

I, WJK, stand at a juncture where I am compelled to reflect on the myriad interactions, both fleeting and enduring, that have shaped my professional evolution over the years. From my early days in coaching to my scholarly pursuits in science, the tapestry of my career is woven from the insights, guidance, and inspiration bestowed upon me by countless colleagues, students, mentors, and peers. The breadth and depth of these connections, spanning many decades, defy a mere enumeration. Indeed, the very attempt to delineate every individual would belittle the profound and unique imprint each has left on my development. Whether through casual conversation or lifelong collaboration, the collective wisdom and encouragement I have received have not merely influenced my trajectory but have, in fact, become the very essence of who I am as a professional. In recognizing the impossibility of extending individual gratitude to all who have contributed to my growth, I find solace in the realization that each person's impact transcends mere acknowledgment. Their influence resonates in my work, my philosophies, and my continued pursuit of excellence within my field. To all who have walked this path with me, guiding me with wisdom, challenging me with questions, and supporting me with steadfast belief, I extend a heartfelt thank you. Your contributions are indelibly etched into my career, and I carry forward the legacy of your impact with profound respect and gratitude. May this work stand as a testament to our shared journey and a tribute to the interconnectedness of human endeavor that transcends titles, disciplines, and time. It is a vivid reminder that we are, each and every one of us, products of our interactions and experiences, forever shaped by those who believe in us and invest in our potential.

We thank everyone for helping these interactions and experiences come to life in writing this book on athlete development and the importance of a unified TEAM approach in this process.

Developing the Human Machine

This book examines the concept of player development and provides a roadmap for its success. As noted in the preface, we use the terms *player* and *athlete* interchangeably. The development of a player or athlete is tied to the desire to win in a competition; therefore, the player development process has evolved as a multifocal and multivariate effort to enhance a player's potential for success in a sport.

Unfortunately, there have been instances where athletes, from high school and beyond, are doomed to failure from the start just by placing them in a position in the sport that, while they may perform adequately, would never excel at higher levels. Sports coaches can be some of the biggest violators and disruptors of optimal player development due to power and control. Historically this is why there has been a cry for more sports coaching education, especially in the United States. The others surrounding the athlete can fail in many cases saying this task is overwhelming and just give up on, in statistics this is called "regression to the mean," or in coaching words, "it is good enough" or "how can I do that" or "it is above my pay grade" or "we do not have the funding," but this is code-speak for I do not have the energy, time or commitment to do this the right way and in essences the athlete is left to their circumstances. This problem persists at all levels of sports, primarily due to the absence of one or more of the three critical elements: credentials, competence, and commitment you will read about in this book. My father (WJK) once told me, "I can understand ignorance, but it is stupidity I cannot tolerate when you know better". Usually, that means you must do things to remove your ignorance. Such is the challenge for each professional in sports. I (WJK) always remember back now, over three decades ago, the late great Strength and Conditioning Head Coach at the University of Connecticut, Coach Jerry Martin, sending his assistants to the library (that place you use to have to go to find articles and books) to search out answers and bring it back to meetings on the different questions. Such is the demand for sports professionals today.

It's crucial to establish well-structured athlete development teams, catering to athletes' individual needs and enabling them to train, compete, and recuperate efficiently. Currently, despite numerous efforts, the sports community is falling short in achieving this across varying levels of competition. This support is vital, not just for those aiming for Olympic gold or a professional career, but for anyone striving to excel in their chosen sport and position at any level. Being the best they can be enables players to compete effectively, which in turn fuels their personal growth and self-esteem.

Furthermore, the popular notion that "anyone can be a champion" demands redefinition. Being a champion should mean maximizing one's innate abilities through dedication and relentless effort. However, this can't be accomplished in isolation; athletes need guidance and the right conditions to thrive. Cutting-edge information and guidance are needed each step of the way. This is where an efficiently structured player development team becomes indispensable. It creates an environment conducive to excellence, guiding athletes in unlocking their full potential.

A player development team is also important because sports participation does not equal health and wellness. Every athlete will get injured, and while young athletes recover quickly, those injuries are paid for later in life (e.g., arthritis, osteoarthritis), Additionally, if post-career transition programs for fitness, nutrition, and health promotion are not instituted from high school onward other life threatening conditions can be observed (e.g., obesity, type 2 diabetes, high blood pressure, and osteoporosis). An optimal player development program with cutting edge, evidence-based programs arising from the influence of each unit limits the potential for the number and magnitude of injuries and post-career medical complications.

As the field of sport science becomes increasingly dependent on technology and analytics, it is crucial to understand that the "gut instincts" of the individuals on the player development team are essential to modulate the decisions that are made. As the Nobel laureate Daniel Kahneman said, "life is unpredictable." Algorithms and machine learning have blind spots, but evidence-based practice allows for the direction to be set; then, with care and insight, individual decisions and the processes of sport science can optimize player development. It is apparent that prediction equations have blind spots and prejudices in their approaches. As such, in many sports, pure analytics without context and interpretation can oversimplify complex problems that are dynamic and not static in nature. While sports analytics can provide insights, it must be viewed in context of the needed interpretation for proper use as a tool.

Sports analytics has become an increasingly vital component in the modern sports landscape, providing insights that can guide decision-making in areas such as player performance, injury prevention, game strategy, and team management. However, the integration and reliance on sports analytics have raised several issues and challenges that need to be considered, especially for the coach and sports performance professional:

1. *Data quality and integrity*: Collecting accurate and meaningful data is fundamental. Any inconsistencies, inaccuracies, or biases in the data can lead to incorrect conclusions, potentially affecting decisions on training, recruitment, and strategy.

2. *Overemphasis on quantitative analysis*: While data-driven decisions are crucial, there may be an overreliance on quantitative metrics at the expense of qualitative insights. The human element, including personal observations, experience, and intuition, still plays a vital role in sports and should not be overshadowed by numbers alone.

3. *Privacy concerns*: With the collection of detailed biometric, physiological, and psychological data on athletes, privacy issues can arise. Proper handling and securing of this sensitive information are paramount.

4. *Interpretation and application*: Interpreting complex data and translating it into practical and actionable insights can be challenging. Without a clear understanding, data can be misused or misinterpreted, leading to suboptimal decisions.

5. *Accessibility and cost*: Advanced analytics often require specialized software, hardware, and expertise. These resources might be out of reach for smaller organizations, creating a competitive imbalance and limiting the broader application of analytics in sports.

6. *Integration with existing practices*: Merging analytics with traditional coaching and performance assessment practices may meet resistance or lack of understanding from the coaching staff or athletes, requiring education and clear communication.

7. *Ethical considerations*: How the data is used, who has access to it, and what decisions are made from it can lead to ethical dilemmas. Transparency and ethical guidelines must be established and adhered to.

8. *Potential for over-analysis*: The abundance of data can lead to paralysis by analysis, where constant scrutiny and overemphasis on minor details can overshadow broader strategies and intuition.

9. *Individualized approach*: Generalizing data or applying the same analytics across different athletes without considering individual differences in physiology, psychology, and other factors can lead to ineffective or even detrimental strategies.
10. *Long-term consequences*: Focus on immediate performance gains using analytics may overlook potential long-term health and well-being consequences for athletes.

In conclusion, while sports analytics offers unprecedented opportunities to enhance performance, its application must be carried out with caution, understanding, and a multifaceted approach that integrates various domains, including physiology, biochemistry, biomechanics, motor learning and neuromuscular science. A balance between the technology-driven approach and traditional human intuition, coupled with ethical consideration and a focus on individualized needs, will likely yield the most effective utilization of sports analytics.

The Human Machine

The adaptive ability of the human machine is the foundation for the development of each player. The *genotype* (i.e., the genetic composition of an individual) provides the starting point for the expression of the *phenotype* (i.e., the observable characteristics of an individual). Upon maturity, some phenotypes are able to change (i.e., they are mutable) while others are not (i.e., they are largely nonmutable). Understanding these factors is vital for optimal player development and affects many decisions, from recruiting to the type of conditioning program implemented.

As you forge ahead in the ever-evolving landscape of player development, it's crucial to sharpen your study habits as a professional. Staying on the cutting-edge is non-negotiable; immerse yourself in the latest evidence-based discoveries in sports and exercise science. But don't just look ahead—look back with a discerning eye. Delve into and keep the established theories, concepts, principles, and laws fresh in your mind, while rigorously evaluating them. This balance of old and new can be the catalyst for groundbreaking insights and applications in your player development endeavors.

In the field of athletic development, certain steadfast principles prevail. A prime example of this is the concept of maximal one repetition maximum (1RM) strength, which serves as the bedrock of all programs aimed at enhancing an athlete's physical prowess. This principle applies to whole-body kinetic exercises (e.g., squats, deadlifts, power cleans), upper-body bench press, and seated row. If not, the sport (e.g., powerlifting, Olympic weightlifting) strength hits the needed level (e.g., men 2 × body mass, women 1.8 × body mass in the squat), and maintenance then becomes the priority, and training time is redistributed to other important metrics that are mutable and not in a maintenance mode (e.g., speed, power, other angular hypertrophic development of muscles needed for dimensional hypertrophy around a body part like the shoulders). In today's college sports, it has become evident that athletes are not strong enough to take on the rigors of collegiate athletics, and "strength" as the primary construct of the athlete, has not been appropriately addressed at the secondary school levels due to many reasons, especially in the USA. Thus, for many athletes this takes time and careful progression of programs over time at the collegiate level are needed to get the athlete on track as to the base of athletic fitness "strength."

The integral role of strength training in the foundational development of athletes is an essential component that underpins all other athletic capabilities. Regrettably, contemporary training paradigms have sometimes lost sight of the crucial nature of one-repetition maximum (1RM) strength, particularly in the principal lifts. The 1970s trend of pursuing the 300-pound bench press club's status overshadowed the vital importance of relative strength to body mass, as well as the acknowledgment of other significant whole-body kinetic lifts like the squat and power clean.

It is important to clarify that the primary objective of strength training within this context is not to cultivate athletes into powerlifters or weightlifters per se, but to enhance maximal strength to a level that serves as a platform for the further development of power, speed, agility, and movement skills. Upon reaching the predetermined benchmarks, the focus then shifts to maintenance, as exceeding these levels into the territory specific to weightlifting or powerlifting sports would yield diminishing returns. The strength levels required for those sports constitute a separate domain and necessitate a distinct approach to programming.

In summary, the systematic development and subsequent maintenance of strength in athletes is an essential and multifaceted process that, when conducted properly, enables the advancement of a wide array of athletic capabilities. The holistic approach to strength training transcends mere lifting benchmarks and considers the broader application of strength as a foundational element for overall athletic development. By understanding and implementing these principles, coaches and athletes can more effectively target their training, fostering not only physical robustness but also a more balanced and efficient athlete.

The Athlete Composite

Ultimately, it is the *athlete composite* we are concerned with. The composite dictates the level at which an athlete can ultimately compete. The athlete composite is constantly changing due to daily positive influences (e.g., proper training and nutrition) and negative influences (e.g., injury and fatigue). We compete with the athlete composite in a game against ourselves (e.g., golf or gymnastics) or against an opponent (e.g., soccer, tennis, American football, or wrestling).

There is a moral imperative to understand the athlete composite to have honest conversations with each athlete about where they are, what can be done, and what sport and position they are most compatible with. Placing the athlete in the best position to be ready to compete is the moral responsibility of the sport coaches and all of the player development team members. This presents a major challenge in sports today due to the extraordinary financial implications of player recruitment.

Factors Influencing Player Development and Performance

While it starts with the athlete, player development continues in various fields that can affect optimal performance. As we make our way through the player development process in this book, we will see that addressing the ever-growing needs of the modern athlete is becoming more complex. The availability of professionals with experience and expertise in each field will affect the success of a program. In many situations, especially for young athletes (e.g., high school or younger), coaches are asked to take on responsibilities beyond their skill sets. As Clint Eastwood says in *Magnum Force*, "A man's got to know his limitations"; we will add to that: A woman must know as well. Knowing one's limits is key to understanding where one's expertise starts and ends in a field. The need for professional staff members—or at least input from professionals who are not on staff—is essential to success. Failure to achieve this is often due to budget constraints or athletic administrators and sport coaches not understanding what skill sets are needed for a player development program.

Figure 1.1 shows the model we propose needs to exist and be represented by a professional in each of the areas to address all of the needs of the modern athlete. However, the influences on athletic performance are extensive, and many topics fall within the expertise areas noted. The different areas we call units must be integrated and aligned in order for the paradigm to effectively and efficiently get cutting-edge programs and interventions to the athletes in each sport.

Creating a cohesive player development team presents an array of challenges that emerge at different stages of an athlete's career. In the early stages, specifically during youth development and high school, establishing a team dedicated to an athlete's consistent care is particularly challenging. This situation changes in the professional stages, where union regulations or player associations can restrict interactions during specific parts of the training cycle. These regulations often drive athletes to commercial training facilities, causing a disruption in their training continuity.

A model solution for early phase development could be the adoption of a system similar to that found in U.S. high school athletics, where an effort was made by the Korey Stringer Institute at the University of Connecticut to promote having each school employ a certified athletic trainer. Similarly, every high school should engage a certified strength and conditioning and a sports scientist professional. These experts could then act as the starting point for the development of the team that could be constructed around them whether

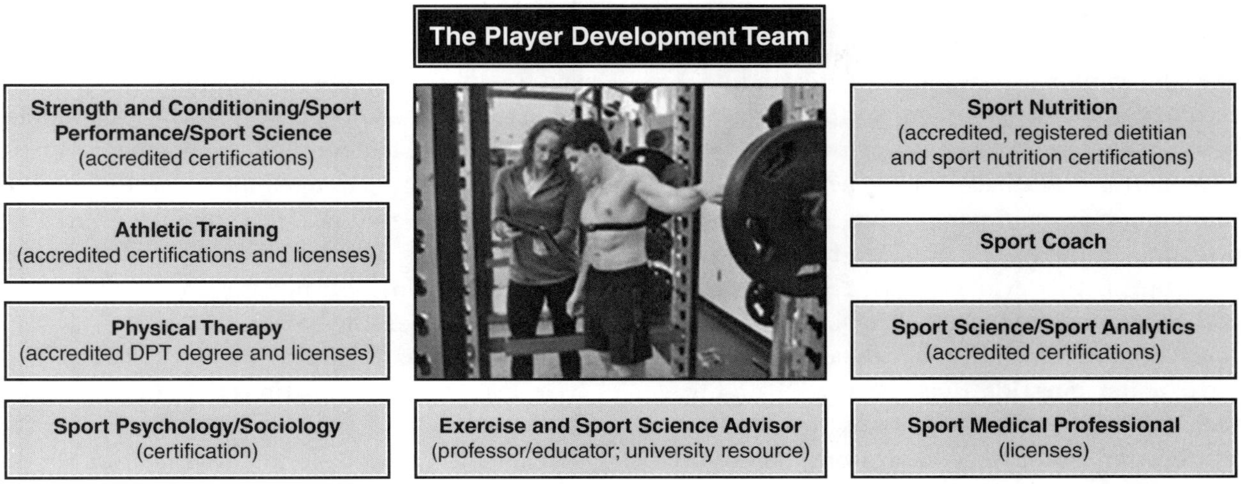

The Player Development Team

- **Strength and Conditioning/Sport Performance/Sport Science** (accredited certifications)
- **Athletic Training** (accredited certifications and licenses)
- **Physical Therapy** (accredited DPT degree and licenses)
- **Sport Psychology/Sociology** (certification)
- **Exercise and Sport Science Advisor** (professor/educator; university resource)
- **Sport Nutrition** (accredited, registered dietitian and sport nutrition certifications)
- **Sport Coach**
- **Sport Science/Sport Analytics** (accredited certifications)
- **Sport Medical Professional** (licenses)

FIGURE 1.1 Different areas of expertise that must be tapped into and used as the domains for a successful player development program. With the use of evidence-based practice approaches and the alignment of the team of professionals, the optimal program can be designed and implemented. Some certifications are accredited by independent accreditation organizations and others are not.

from a proximal location or virtually. This would then provide the necessary care for athletes and ensure evidence-based program progressions and interventions.

However, in some professional ranks, the problem of continuity remains a hurdle. The high rate of change in locations and variability over the yearly macrocycle create overwhelming challenges often handled by the athletes themselves. Furthermore, seasonal care is often hampered by a plethora of meetings and injury treatments, leaving little time or attention to address issues of tissue detraining, which can lead to injury vulnerability.

In essence, both the early and later stages of a player's career pose unique challenges to the effective organization and implementation of player development teams. Overcoming these challenges is critical for optimizing an athlete's training and overall development of the athlete composite.

A major challenge is understanding the competencies of each of the professionals involved in a player development program. Appropriate academic preparation and degrees are part of this competency basis, as are practice licenses typically regulated by the government. The number of certifications has increased in every area, and they may contribute to experience, but they are not always reliable indicators of competency. Evaluating a certification program depends on the field being covered and the organization that provides the program and testing. Some certifications have valid testing programs, but others only require attendance. Some are now online with little or no quality control. The first question to ask is whether the program is accredited by an independent national body (e.g., the National Commission for Certifying Agencies). However, certifications only legally stipulate minimal competence. Professionals should also have experience with the types of athletes they want to work with. Working with high school athletes is very different from working in a fitness gym with adults. While it is possible that someone who only has experience in a gym could also work with high school athletes—many contracted companies perform both roles—there could be blind spots. Top professional, medical, and scientific organizations have published professional standards that can be referred to (NSCA 2017). These are especially important for athletic administrators who set out to hire professional staff in the different areas of expertise needed for the player development program noted in figure 1.1.

A seminal book on evidence-based practices demonstrates that it takes a team of professionals to evaluate information and scientific findings for accuracy, and context is required for the questions being asked in a player development program (Amonette, English, and Kraemer 2016). Thus, the interactions and perspectives of coaches and everyone on the team are valued for their area of expertise in this evidence-based process, which will be discussed in detail later in this book. It is essential to remember that the core experts on a particular question must be valued highly in such a process. Often, sport coaches or athletic administrators, for whatever reasons, do not heed the expert's recommendations and make poor decisions that are not in the athletes' best interests (e.g., deciding against an in-season resistance training program or not hiring an athletic trainer or strength and conditioning professional on staff in a high school). This can be due to little or limited understanding of the player development process. Sport coaches are responsible for making many decisions outside their skill sets. Without understanding the different areas, as well as from a fear of not being perceived as a leader, they may fall back on personal experience, the Internet, and friends for help. At best, this is less than optimal in most situations! Optimal programming depends on accurate information and professional competencies. However, we will see that each decision in a player development program has its own context that must be understood to find the right answer. Here lies the art of practice or the so-called rub in player development.

Alignment in the Player Development Program

One of the most important conditions of a player development program is that all the influences and people who control the athlete's time understand the goals and objectives of each phase. The professionals involved need to have meetings as part of the evidence-based team approach and come to an agreement—especially if a conflict exists—through an evidence-based process. Thus, communication and evidence-based practices must be used to address questions, controversies, and arguments to eliminate program disruptors.

A lack of communication among the athlete, the support personnel around them, parents, family, and friends can disrupt the program's progression. Athletes need to know how and why the program will help them achieve their developmental goals. Educating the athlete about the purpose of method of working out and training cannot be overlooked by the strength and conditioning professional in this process. Goal setting over time is vital, as we will learn later in the book.

There are various physiological systems that have structures and functions that, in part, determine success in a sport. These, along with the psychological aspects, form a *sport composite* of the athlete. This individual composite is brought to the sport's competition at any point during a career. Developing the athlete's composite is essential to enhancing a player's potential for success. It is only the *mutable* characteristics that are targeted for significant improvement. Yet the gain potential of a mutable characteristic has limitations depending upon the target characteristic. In twin studies, one observes a range of about 5% to 45% improvement from the starting point of the genotype. This brings up an old saying from back on the farm in my Wisconsin days (WJK): "One cannot make a silk purse out of a pig's ear." The *nonmutable* characteristics, therefore, are even more critical and are used to optimize selections for player positions or the sport itself. Some nonmutable characteristics are mutable during growth and development, while others may be mutable during injury, disease, surgery, or potentially with some drugs (i.e., human growth hormone). We use the phrase "largely or mostly nonmutable" to reflect that genetic attributes still have some malleability under certain circumstances. For example, a strongly genetic variable such as vertical height still has some plasticity. Studies have shown that genetics may explain up to 80% of the variance (and not 100%!) in height between individuals (Tucker and Collins 2012). Epigenetic factors such as health or nutrition may affect height during maturation, showing that even a largely nonmutable characteristic may be malleable under certain circumstances. The mutable characteristics are primarily targeted through athletic training development programs. Studies on athletes have shown that genetics may account for 30% to 80% of the variance between individuals (Issurin 2017). Attributes with lower percentages tend to be more trainable. Although genetics plays a critical role in essentially all elements of sports, the level of improvement brought about through training could be the tipping point that allows an athlete to reach full potential. As the demands of a sport increase at higher levels of competition, the composites of some athletes will not be successful. There are limitations on what sport and level of competition each athlete can succeed in. Player development programs must keep this in mind to better frame an athlete's expectations and assist in optimizing self-esteem and enjoyment of the sport.

Mutable and largely nonmutable characteristics are discussed throughout this book. Taken from various player analytics from different sports, what follows are some examples of primary, post maturation, largely nonmutable characteristics, at full maturity of the athlete, that can only change by a small percentage (< 3%) due to external factors (e.g., injury, surgery, or hyperplasia) that can affect performance potential:

- Height
- Limb lengths and ratios
- Hand size
- Foot size
- Arm wingspan
- Tendon and ligament lengths
- Origin and insertion points of tendons and ligaments
- Number of skeletal muscle fibers
- Type of skeletal muscle fibers (slow- versus fast-twitch)

The human machine is a function of the interplay of the different physiological systems, which have all been examined in extraordinary detail in books and papers over many years. This type of knowledge is an essential part of the base of professional expertise in any given area. Continued education and digging deeper into a topic are also vital to professionals in the player development program, from coaches to experts. As I (WJK) noted in one of the early national meetings of the National Strength and Conditioning Association, "We have to go back and open up the books again!" The massive amount of information must be evaluated using an evidence-based approach. One of the basic skill sets needed by professionals in player development today is the ability to evaluate information as well as its sources, efficacy, and relevance to the context of the decisions that need to be made for an individual athlete.

There are up to 11 divisions of systems involved in the human-machine makeup and functions that frame the potential for successful participation in a specific sport but also determine the readiness of an athlete to train or compete on a given day. The primary systems of the human body are:

- Nervous
- Muscular
- Cardiovascular
- Digestive
- Endocrine
- Skeletal
- Integumentary and exocrine
- Immune and lymphatic
- Renal and urinary
- Reproductive
- Respiratory

Let us build a primary human machine with several different systems to review some of the essential functions and see their potential roles as we address player development. We can do this in layers to provide a conceptual model for examining the vast array of needs and programs to enhance the athlete.

To start, we can build the human machine with a skeletal system that includes all the connective tissue. This provides the structural girders or latticework upon which movement is achieved. At maturity, the skeletal system contains both mutable and largely nonmutable elements. For example, bone length is largely nonmutable because bone lengths and sizes are set by age 25 (and earlier for several appendicular skeleton bones). However, the density of the bone is mutable with training. Connective tissues are also set in their origins and insertion positions, but their densities are mutable with training.

Continuing to build the human machine, we add all the skeletal muscles that provide for the body's movement. Here again, we see mutable versus mostly nonmutable characteristics because the number of muscle fibers at maturity is thought to be fixed. However, hyperplasia (i.e., an increase in the number of muscle fibers) has been a topic of discussion, especially with large or extreme levels of hypertrophy, but it only contributes less than 1% to 3% to the increased size of muscle in such situations. However, the size, density, and metabolic capabilities of muscles are mutable and can be improved with training.

Let us next integrate the nervous system, which controls all our human-machine functions. We live in the era of the brain and are learning more each day about its functions and ability to change and cope with the external demands of the environment, from exercise to aging. A baby's 100 to 200 billion neurons are about what an adult brain has, but not all the interneuron connections are made yet. The total number of neurons may be set, but how they are connected and how different hubs in the brain interact are a function of growth and development. These concepts will come into play in connection with the nervous system when we address the developmental phases of young athletes later in this chapter.

Human movement is based on a highly specific sequence and combination of skeletal muscle motor unit activations. In 1925, Nobel Laureate Sir Charles Sherrington came up with this crucial idea and introduced the *motor unit* (Liddell and Sherrington 1925). The motor unit consisted of an alpha motor neuron and its associated fibers that are activated and produce force. Dr. Elwood Henneman (1915 to 1996) later developed a more specific way to look at motor unit activation called the *size principle*. For those of us in sports and conditioning, this was a seminal principle, and we will repeatedly refer to it throughout the book. In brief, the type and amount of muscle activated are based on the external demands of the exercise or sport skill. As the external demands (e.g., weight on the barbell or speed of the run) for force and power increase, more motor units are recruited in a progressive manner based on sizing factors (e.g., the number of motor units, whether the fibers are fast- or slow-twitch, and the number of fibers in the motor unit) to meet the demands (Bawa, Jones, and Stein 2014; Duchateau and Enoka 2011; Raikova et al. 2021). From this work, it is important to remember that the magnitude of the amount of muscle activated (e.g., biceps curl versus a squat) will dictate the extent to which the other physiological systems will be involved. For example, the increase in heart rate and involvement of the cardiorespiratory system will be lower when performing an arm curl versus a squat exercise at the same percentage of maximum strength. Similarly, while the acute stress and recovery processes may be the same, the magnitude of the endocrine response would also be lower. Finally, only the motor units that are repeatedly activated and the other physiological systems needed for support will experience adaptations or a training effect, which brings the concept of *training specificity* into play.

The cardiovascular and respiratory systems are now integrated into our human machine. Its integrated functions of pumping blood and moving oxygen in and carbon dioxide out of the body provide the basis for life itself. This system's functionality is measurable and related to aerobic endurance performance and recovery capabilities.

We now integrate the endocrine system, which plays an important role in regulating all the other physiological systems. It is a primary system that supports the activation of muscle tissue for its repair and anabolic (building) remodeling processes. It is also involved in the catabolic (breaking down) processes during overreaching or when overtraining is detrimental to recovery. Sports and conditioning programs affect the structure of these glands positively and negatively depending on whether stressors are correctly managed in the player development program. Finally, the interactions of the digestive, urinary, reproductive, integumentary, renal, and lymphatic and immune systems interact at several levels for normal body function. The composite human machine can now set up many types of demands for performance and player development (for review, see Kraemer, Fleck, and Deschenes 2021; Ratamess 2022).

Factors Affecting Sport Performance

It has become apparent that many factors dictate sport performance at a given time and over a career (see figure 1.2). Each can play a positive role in a

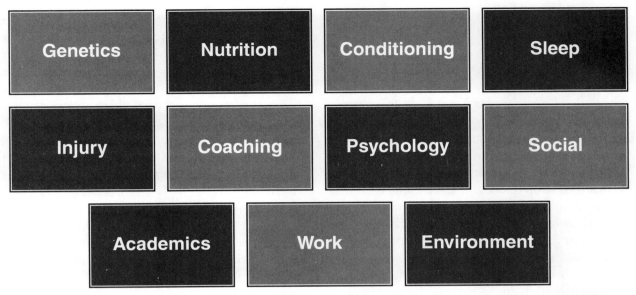

FIGURE 1.2 A general paradigm for factors that affect performance. Performance is related to both growth and development over time and is also bounded by the inherent genetic endowment of the individual. Furthermore, performance has an acute temporal element: On a given day in a competition, the individual can bring all the elements of player development together to win the race, make the winning shot, or throw the winning pass in a game.

player development program or, conversely, have negative influences and become what we call a *disruptor*. Each of these influences must be managed. Throughout the book, to address why this is so important, we will discuss topics such as evidence-based practice and the alignment of the professionals involved in the process.

These influences can affect performance in a particular play, on a given day, or over a whole career if not appropriately managed. Management involves understanding, assessing, and implementing the best practices for that individual athlete. What has become apparent is that the process of player development is not general but rather individual. We often think of player development as being like the management of health by a physician: While there are approaches to preventing and treating any disease, choices must be made regarding the individual approach used. This has led to pushback from many administrators who might not want to recognize the need for more staff, such as for athletic training or strength and conditioning, due to budget constraints. This in turn has led to burnout in these professions from extraordinarily long hours and low pay. The individual is not optimally managed in this player development process. This is comparable, in the medical field, to the difference between routine and "concierge" medical care. Regardless of the reasons, in player development it is the individual athlete that must be managed. While appropriate general approaches are valid, slight deviations in program progression are needed to fine-tune a response or adaptation to an intervention.

The Developmental Pathways

With the popularity of the book *The Sports Gene*, it became evident that genetics provides a basis for extraordinary athletic performances (Epstein 2014). As we have discussed, each athlete brings a composite of mutable and largely nonmutable characteristics to a sport. Player development programs can start at a young age in youth sports. Based on physical development, each athlete will progress up to their genetic potential. The composite state of that athlete is dynamic and affected by the various influences noted in figure 1.2.

The developmental time course differs from youth to adult maturity for men and women. With the many outmoded ideas about women in sports and intense conditioning (e.g., heavy resistance training), many women often miss important developmental windows for achieving optimal gains within a time frame of maturation (e.g., bone development). Nevertheless, total conditioning is needed no matter when one starts to engage in developing the mutable characteristics in conditioning programs.

In figure 1.3, we see a continual aggregation of the genetic expressions until the full maturity of an adult. This entire expression and the influence of various interventions over time will dictate the absolute performance potential of an athlete in a sport on a given timeline of the age progression. As athlete composite increases for each age range, plateaus develop and the interventions used in a player development program (e.g., strength and conditioning, nutrition, sleep, and skills coaching) allow the athlete composite to track upward to the genetic potential for that age. Thus, the composites of athletes may differ, despite having the same genetic potential, due to external interventions.

Therefore, due to successful interventions at certain ages, performance may be higher in some than in others with the same genetic potential who still need to optimize their athlete composites. A study by Blimkie demonstrates a critical concept: the need for training to stay above peers at the same age and the risk of strength advantages disappearing due to normal adolescent growth and development (Blimkie 1989). This was the case when over the summer, the gains made at the end of the school year were lost when comparing them to their untrained peers because none of the students were training during the summer months. Thus, interventions at each phase of development need to be continued if one is to have an age-related advantage. An absolute genetic ceiling exists for each age (e.g., the sixth-grade basketball player who is 6 foot 2 inches versus the 5-foot-2-inches teammate). Yet growth spurts occur for each athlete during their growth pattern over time.

While the primary purpose of this book is not to focus on the important phases of player development during childhood and early adolescence, it is important to understand that the basis of each athlete in a player development program is highly affected by what they have done in their youth. Therefore, understanding the basics of player development at young ages is paramount to understanding the context of any athlete as they enter post-adolescent age groups. The gain potentials of each age range are affected by prior interventions and genetic phenotypic expression as they approach their genetic ceilings for different variables.

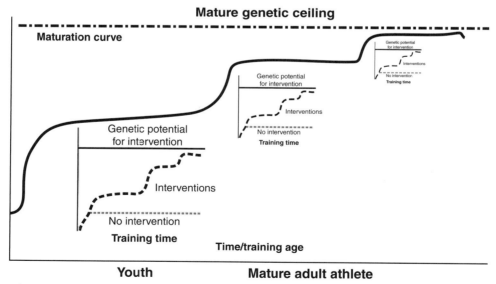

FIGURE 1.3 The athlete composite develops over the training age due to positive interventions by the player development team. The magnitude of gains in mutable characteristics is based on genetic composites at a given training age. As the athlete moves toward the genetic potential beyond the period of no training or intervention, even more attention is needed in the program's exercise prescriptions and auditing of stress to prevent unnecessary injury or overtraining due to newly developed higher capacities for physical performance. A lack of progress at one level of development as the athlete matures may in certain instances (e.g., motor skill performances) reduce the magnitude of gains in performance as the athlete ages.

Development of the Athlete from Youth to Adulthood

Athleticism is the ability to repeatedly perform movements that require a sufficient level of muscular strength, power, endurance, speed, agility, balance, coordination, and motor skill development (Lloyd et al. 2016). The athlete's development begins early in life (childhood and adolescence) and continues throughout adulthood. The National Strength and Conditioning Association (NSCA) defines *youth* as children up to age 11 for girls and 13 for boys and *adolescents* as ages 14 to 18 for boys and 12 to 18 for girls (Lloyd et al. 2016). Children should primarily participate in sports for fun and to experience different types of activities. Physical activity helps improve motor coordination and several health- and skill-related fitness components. The goal is to improve fitness and athleticism in children and adolescents and help them to carry these benefits and practices into adulthood. A positive relationship exists between physical activity in children and motor skill competency, so youth should be encouraged to be physically active even if they do not participate in competitive sports. Since opportunities for sport participation often decrease into adulthood, it is important that children and adolescents become involved in sports at an early age. Maintaining involvement in organized sports benefits youth in several significant ways—physiological, emotional, social, and psychological.

Athletic development stems from the nexus of physical education in school, physical activity outside of school, youth participation in organized sports, and strength and conditioning training. It is recommended that all youth accumulate at least 60 minutes of moderate to vigorous physical activity (MVPA) per day, consisting of aerobic, strength, and skill-related exercise (Faigenbaum et al. 2009; Faigenbaum, Lloyd, and Oliver 2020; Faigenbaum et al. 2020). However, youth participation in community and home physical activity is declining. Physical education classes have been removed in some areas or significantly reduced in intensity, frequency, and scope. Data from more than one million youth (ages 11 to 17) worldwide indicated that 80% were insufficiently active (Faigenbaum et al. 2020). As a result, the number of children who are "undertrained," obese, overweight, physically inactive, and demonstrate poor motor coordination, strength, and endurance (both aerobic and muscular) is increasing. The reduced level of muscular fitness (i.e., strength, power, and muscular endurance), resulting from a hypokinetic lifestyle has been termed *dynapenia* and poses several negative physical, social, and emotional consequences (Faigenbaum, Lloyd, and Oliver 2020; Faigenbaum et al. 2020). Approximately 90% of children with low motor function fail to meet MVPA recommendations, so it is clear that the road to optimal long-term athletic development begins with ensuring that youth participate in daily exercise.

A lack of exercise reduces neuromuscular function and fitness and poses several health risks, primarily if the hypokinetic lifestyle is maintained as an adult. The term *exercise deficit disorder* has been used to describe the association between low MVPA and health and fitness (Faigenbaum, Lloyd, and Oliver 2020; Faigenbaum et al. 2020). Low levels of physical activity may stem from various factors, including limited opportunities to participate in sports or outside activity, underuse, excessive levels of watching television and playing video games, excessive smartphone use, and limited physical education curricula in schools that do not focus on strength and conditioning activities. The lack of sufficient conditioning to play sports initially may put youth at greater risk of injury because they may be ill-prepared for the demands of the sport. Parents, teachers, and coaches need to recognize failing fitness levels and offer additional preparatory training for youth who are unfit to participate in a sport. Several athletic facilities with well-trained coaches and staff in pediatric exercise science have been established in the past 20 years. They offer programs that are instrumental in improving youth fitness and preparing youth for the demands of sports. Fundamental movement skills (e.g., stabilization, locomotion, and manipulation) are enhanced by muscular strength, power, and endurance levels. Physical conditioning and motor skill development are paramount to overall athleticism. Youth training should embark on many kinds of strength and conditioning activities. It should be noted that physical training does not negatively affect growth and development or increase the risk of injury (Lloyd et al. 2016).

Sport Specialization versus Sport Sampling

A key element to long-term athletic development in youth is the magnitude of exposure to different stimuli. Sports involve many motor skills and enhance motor learning, coordination, and various components of physical fitness. Exposure to different activities is augmented when a young athlete participates in multiple sports or begins developmentally appropriate strength and conditioning training to augment sport participation. *Sport specialization* is defined as intense year-round participation in a single sport to the exclusion of playing other sports. In contrast, *sport sampling* is defined as participating in multiple sports throughout the year under the supervision of qualified coaches. Specialization may subject youth athletes to higher volumes of repetitive training and practice that may provide the athlete with only a narrow spectrum of movement patterns compared to the wider range of movement patterns encountered when playing multiple sports. Jayanthi and colleagues (Jayanthi et al. 2015) developed a 3-point scale to specifically define and quantify the level of specialization—as low, moderate, or high—based on the following questions:

- Can you pick out a main sport in which you are involved (i.e., single-sport training)?
- Did you quit other sports to focus on the main sport?
- Do you train more than eight months a year for your primary sport?

Each question is worth 1 point, and the sum point total equates to the level of sport specialization; i.e., low (1 point), moderate (2 points), or high (3 points). This scale helps distinguish high specialization from participation in only one sport. For example, a youth athlete who plays one sport but does not focus on that sport during the off-season will have a different classification than one who participates in intense year-round practice and training for one sport. Issues arising from year-round sport specialization are more extensive than when a youth engages in only one sport but participates in other activities of interest or a strength and conditioning program throughout the year. A few studies using this scale have shown that 35% to 38%, 29% to 34%, and 28% to 36% of the thousands of youth athletes surveyed are classified as low, moderate, and highly specialized athletes, respectively (Bell et al. 2016; Jayanthi et al. 2015). The number of highly specialized athletes is greater among students who attend larger schools, which indicates that some youth athletes are forced to participate in only one sport because of the competition with more students vying for a fixed number of team positions or roster spots (Bell et al. 2016). Highly specialized athletes also start playing organized sports (their primary sport) at a younger age than less specialized athletes (Post et al. 2017).

The attraction for youth of focusing on one sport early in life has increased for several reasons. Given the perks and benefits accompanying elite athlete status, some youth athletes target only one sport, seeing it as the best way to maximize performance. For example, it is common for young athletes to see the fame and fortune surrounding elite college and professional athletes and shift their focus to one sport with the perception that it will be the best pathway to success. Pressure from coaches to specialize (they may prioritize team success at the expense of the athlete's best experience) and pressure from parents with hopes of college scholarships have led to some youth athletes specializing in one sport. In some cases, geographic location and the prohibitive cost of participating in some sports increase the likelihood that a youth athlete may focus only on one sport. Thus, deciding to participate in one or multiple sports depends on several social, economic, psychological, and geographic factors.

Although specialization may sound attractive on the surface, it does have several disadvantages. Specialization has been associated with increased injury risk across many sports (Jayanthi et al. 2015; Carder et al. 2020). Injury risks may be up to 37% higher in specialized youth athletes than in those who sample multiple sports (Carder et al. 2020). Both overuse and acute injuries to the lower and upper extremities are associated with higher levels of specialization. In addition, exceeding 16 hours per week of sports practice and competition increases injury risk regardless of whether the youth athlete is specializing (Myer et al. 2015; Post et al. 2017). Some have recommended that young athletes participate in sports for no more hours per week than their age. The concern over a high volume of practice and competition activity is to limit the risk of musculoskeletal injury. Many coaches are unaware of recommendations regarding the maximum number of months per year for one sport (it is recommended that youth athletes do not play one sport more than eight months per year), the hours per week for one sport, or the number of simultaneous leagues for an athlete to participate in to reduce injury (it is recommended that youth do not participate in multiple leagues of the same or different sports at the same time) (Post et al. 2020). It is thought that the chronic performance of a narrow range of motions, with insufficient rest and recovery and at the expense of other movements, may increase the risk of overuse and potential injury, in addition to making higher demands on competition. Sport sampling is associated with a decreased rate of sport dropout and burnout, injury risk, and depression as well as improved social and leadership skills (Myer et al. 2015; Carder et al. 2020).

Playing different sports exposes the athlete to different neuromuscular patterns and promotes greater long-term success and enjoyment. Studies show that sampling can augment motor skill development, muscular strength and endurance, and speed (Carder et al. 2020). It also enables the athlete to experience different movements, which may help in selecting the best sport for adulthood. For example, a potential high school American football player would benefit significantly from sampling in middle school or earlier. A sport such as wrestling elicits significant increases in muscular strength, coordination, speed, power, physical toughness, and muscular and aerobic endurance that could translate into better football performance down the road. Participating in track-and-field has a significant carryover to football, whether the athlete is involved in sprinting, jumping, or throwing events. Many sports have carryover effects between one another (e.g., for strength, power, mobility, balance, speed, quickness, agility, ability to change direction, and muscular and aerobic endurance). Sampling early for the youth athlete creates a well-rounded physical development that optimizes athletic performance when combined with a proper strength and conditioning program. This concept of *late specialization* may provide additional benefits that last into adulthood. Several major organizations, including the NSCA, the National Athletic Trainers' Association, and the American Academy of Pediatrics, recommend sport sampling for most sports (Jayanthi et al. 2019). As reviewed by Issurin (Issurin 2017), data from several studies examining elite or Olympic-caliber athletes have shown that a large number (58% to 94%) participated in two or three sports (for at least two to four years) before specializing in their respective sports.

Complicating the issue is that some sports rely on *early specialization*—that is, choosing a primary sport before age 12. For example, technical sports such as gymnastics, diving, figure skating, swimming, and dance require specialization before puberty, as optimal performance typically occurs in the teens to early 20s. Some organizations acknowledge these sports as exceptions to sport sampling recommendations. The key to young athletes benefiting from early specialization is to have a solid support system among family, coaches, medical staff, and friends and to use proper precautions when establishing a training and competitive program (Jayanthi et al. 2019). This could be accomplished, for example, by incorporating other conditioning activities and limiting some of the repetitive nature of the practiced movements, as well as by allowing athletes to take periodic time off (i.e., a few days per week or periodized weeks of altered activity) and to have a proper balance between training and extracurricular activities. An individualized, periodized resistance training program over the macrocycle of the athlete is vital to address the peripheral concerns of sport specialization and augment growth and development.

Models of Long-Term Athletic Development

The NSCA defines *long-term athletic development* as "the habitual development of 'athleticism' over time to improve health and fitness, enhance physical performance, reduce the relative risk of injury, and develop the confidence and competence of all youth" (Lloyd et al. 2016). Existing development models recommend that training focuses on acquiring rudimentary and fundamental motor skills and muscular strength (Lloyd et al. 2016). Participating in a single sport does not provide a sufficient stimulus to maximize athleticism. Muscular strength is related to several fitness components, such as speed and power. For example, research has shown that pre to post gains in motor skills resulting from resistance training in youth are ~50% greater than in adolescents (Behringer et al. 2011). Children are encouraged to be physically active through play and physical education at young ages. This builds fundamental motor skills and helps develop some foundational strength. Youth may participate in training programs at a young age. The recommendations include beginning training when the child is emotionally mature enough to follow instructions from their coach or a strength and conditioning professional and shows physical competence in balance and postural control, which is often around ages 6 to 7 (Lloyd et al. 2016). Youth participation in a well-rounded, multimodal strength and conditioning program (consisting of resistance training, balance, speed, agility, and power training) can decrease the risk of injury by up to 50%, presumably due to increased muscular strength, power, endurance, and improved movement biomechanics (Lloyd et al. 2016). For example, the risk for injury increases and peaks during the adolescent growth spurt as disproportionate bone growth rates precede adaptations to muscles and tendons (Faigenbaum et al. 2020). Increased body mass and height of the center of gravity, without accompanying increases in muscular strength and power, can result in excessive loading to the musculoskeletal system. A comprehensive strength and conditioning program can help safeguard athletes against periods of heightened injury risk. Studies have shown that children and adolescents can experience notable increases in muscular strength, power, endurance, speed, agility, and improved motor skills (Lloyd et al. 2016). Long-term athletic development entails a comprehensive, multimodal approach to achieving optimal fitness goals. This approach builds conditioning in excess of normal growth and maturation through a process termed *synergistic adaptation* (Faigenbaum et al. 2020). The following sidebar depicts the ten pillars of successful long-term athletic development (Lloyd et al. 2016).

Various models of youth athletic development have emerged over the years. Early athletic development models focused on young athletes participating in multiple sports up to age 13 and then specializing in one sport. However, models of sport training that only factor in strength and conditioning programs will not optimally develop a youth athlete or significantly reduce injury risk. In 2004,

Pillars of Long Term Athletic Development (LTAD)

- LTAD pathways should accommodate individualized growth and development
- Youth should engage in LTAD programs that promote physical fitness and psychosocial well-being
- Youth should be enccuraged to improve fitness from early childhood with a focus on motor skill and muscular strength development
- LTAD should encourage early sampling that promotes a broad range of motor skills
- Health and well-being should be a focus of LTAD programs
- Youth should participate in conditioning that reduces injury risk to increase participation in LTAD programs
- LTAD programs should provide youth with a range of modes to improve health- and skill-related fitness components
- Practitioners should use relevant monitoring and assessment tools as part of the LTAD strategy
- Practitioners should progress and individualize training programs for successful LTAD
- Qualified professionals and sound pedagogical approaches are critical to LTAD program success

Balyi and Hamilton proposed a long-term athletic development model that accounted for growth and development by using *peak height velocity* (age of maturity when the maximal growth rate in stature during adolescence takes place) to demonstrate training readiness. It consisted of 10 factors and 7 stages and provided a variety of pathways (e.g., elite and recreational) for participation, training, and competition (Balyi and Hamilton 2004). In 2012, Lloyd and Oliver proposed the *youth physical development model* (Lloyd and Oliver 2012). It emphasizes a development-based approach and provides more specificity than previous models. The model describes age, growth rate, maturation status, and type of training adaptation (e.g., neural or hormonal) relative to the development of the health- and skill-related fitness components. Strength, power, speed, and agility are the key components emphasized mostly during middle childhood, adolescence, and adulthood, whereas hypertrophy is targeted in adolescence and adulthood. Training structure progresses on a continuum from unstructured to highly structured, with maturation into adulthood.

The YPD model was developed to provide a more realistic and evidence-based training approach and was based on the contention that all fitness components are trainable at all stages of development. It is based on seven tenets: (1) fitness components are trainable at any age; (2) physical activity begins early in life; (3) muscular strength and motor development are prioritized throughout; (4) the focus shifts from fundamental movements to sport-specific performance; (5) training becomes more structured over time; (6) training prescription is individualized; and (7) youth specialists are needed for coaching (Faigenbaum et al. 2020).

The strength and conditioning element is focused on resistance, balance, power, speed, mobility, agility training, and hypertrophy (later in sequence). This multimodal approach is an example of *integrative neuromuscular training* (IMT). It is designed to address critical health- and skill-related fitness components in a comprehensive manner (Faigenbaum et al. 2020). The model emphasizes these fitness components—especially resistance training for maximal strength—beyond age 5. Muscular strength and motor skill development are critical priorities and serve as the basis for other components, such as speed, agility, and power. Mobility is defined as the integration of strength, power, and motor control to move the joints at a desired speed, in proper sequence, at a specific time, and in a specific direction for each movement (Faigenbaum et al. 2020). Despite its importance for health and fitness, mobility is not considered a training priority at any stage but is recognized as a key component that needs to be addressed. Muscular endurance and metabolic training should be training priorities addressed in physical education classes later in adolescence. An emphasis on hypertrophy training should increase for athletes after puberty.

A critical element in long-term youth athlete development is the increase of muscular strength via resistance training. Resistance training has a low risk of injury in youth who follow appropriate guidelines, such as qualified supervision from coaches and other personnel, appropriate program design and progression, and proper use of equipment. In addition, comprehensive youth training (i.e., resistance, balance, and plyometric training) decreases the likelihood of sport-related injuries for youth, possibly by 15% to 50% (Faigenbaum et al. 2009). Youth resistance training improves motor performance, such as jumping and sprinting ability, and can improve aerobic fitness when combined with aerobic training (Stricker et al. 2020). Much of the strength gains are attributed to neural mechanisms, especially in prepubescent youth, with hypertrophy playing a more significant role after puberty. Research shows that youth can increase muscular strength (approximately 30% on average over 8 to 20 weeks) beyond the increase associated with growth and maturation if training is of sufficient intensity, volume, and duration (Faigenbaum et al. 2009). Complex exercises, such as the Olympic lifts and their variations, may be used provided that qualified coaching is available and proper guidelines are followed. These exercises take considerable time to learn to perform correctly; recommended progressions should be followed. Plyometric training in youth is safe, provided that appropriate guidelines are followed. Plyometric exercises may be ranked on a continuum from low to high intensity. Beginning youth athletes benefit from low-intensity exercises because they do not have the augmented strength requirement for high-intensity exercises. Guidelines for youth resistance training have been published (Kraemer and Fleck 2004; Faigenbaum et al. 2009; Faigenbaum, Lloyd, and Oliver 2020; McHenry and Nitka 2022; Stricker et al. 2020). Recommendations were made for novice (limited experience), intermediate (3 to 12 months of consistent training), and advanced (at least one year of experience with substantial gains made) training statuses. Below is a summary of the key guidelines and recommendations for resistance and plyometric training:

- Qualified supervision and instruction are essential for exercise technique, program design, and ensuring safety protocols. Training programs should be enjoyable for youth.
- Workouts should begin with a 5-to-10-minute dynamic warm-up, followed by a specific warm-up and a cooldown to conclude the workout.
- Light weights or body mass should be used initially while learning proper technique—technique should always be emphasized. The Olympic lifts may be used and taught in an orderly progression with light weights or sticks to start with.
- Multiple- and single-joint exercises may be used that stress all major muscle groups and use dynamic (concentric or eccentric) and isometric muscle actions. Multiple-joint exercises are preferred for power development. The exercises may be bilateral or unilateral in performance. Large muscle group exercises can be performed before smaller body mass exercises, and multiple joint exercises should be performed before single-joint exercises. Exercises should be performed in a fully prescribed range of motion. Several pieces of resistance equipment or implements may be safely used by youth athletes.
- Performance of 1 to 3 sets of 6 to 15 repetitions for traditional resistance exercises and 3 to 6 repetitions for power exercises. The repetition number should match the loading and goals of the exercise. Intermediate and advanced training entails at least 2 to 3 sets per exercise or more.
- Loading should be light at first (less than 60% of the 1RM). The program can progress to heavier weights (60% to 80% of the 1RM for intermediate training and 70% to 85% of the 1RM for advanced training) depending on the exercise and its goals. Young athletes may be introduced to periodic heavy lifting provided that it is technique-driven and a strong foundation of muscular strength has been developed. For power training, 30% to 60% of the 1RM can be used to target the velocity component of power development. Heavier weights target the force component of the power equation (i.e., power = force × velocity).
- Youth may progress to more advanced training programs ~age 14 to 15 provided they have been training progressively and demonstrate proper technique.
- Loads may gradually be increased by 5% to 10% as strength improves.
- Youth recover faster than adults. Thus, short rest intervals (1 minute) may be used for several exercises but may progress to 2 to 3 minutes for intermediate and advanced resistance training for maximal strength with heavier loads.
- A controlled lifting velocity is recommended except for the Olympic lifts and power exercises for which high velocities are recommended.
- A frequency of 2 to 3 days per week is a good starting point for novice and intermediate training. Advanced training may entail 3 to 4 days per week.
- Training periodization is recommended where the acute program variables (i.e., volume, intensity, etc.) are systematically altered to accommodate training phases and goals.
- Training needs to be complemented with proper diet, hydration, sleep, and recovery.
- For plyometric training: Novices should perform 2 to 4 low-intensity exercises per

session, 8 to 10 repetitions per set, and 1 to 2 sets per exercise; intermediates should perform 4 to 6 low to moderate exercises per session, 4 to 8 repetitions per set, and 2 to 3 sets per exercise; and advanced athletes should perform 6 to 8 low- to high-intensity exercises per session, 4 to 6 repetitions per set, and 2 to 4 sets per exercise.

Strength and Conditioning and the High School Athlete

High school is a unique time for athletes. For some, it may mark the epitome of their athletic careers, while for others, it may serve as a building point for their collegiate careers and beyond. Regardless of athletic ability, the skills and performance gained through strength training and conditioning during high school should prepare the individual to improve physical literacy and fitness throughout life. Further, strength and conditioning during high school follows a similar pattern of progression; muscular strength, power, and hypertrophy are emphasized relative to the individual's training base. Speed and agility training form a substantial segment of the late off-season to preseason and in-season training. Technique is always emphasized, especially as the athlete progresses to more challenging exercises. In order that the acquisition of strength, power, and hypertrophy can be integrated with motor skill development, the proper periodization of training with sport participation and practice must be implemented. The NSCA has provided a framework for training objectives for high school athletes that fit within a long-term athletic development plan (McHenry and Nitka 2022). Recommendations include the following:

- First year: Optimize muscle activation, locomotive patterns, and balance, improve functional movement ability, develop a strength and stability base, and ensure proper technique for any activities related to strength and conditioning.
- Second year: Challenge fundamental locomotive movements, develop a high degree of strength and stability, and ensure excellent training techniques.
- Third year: Develop sport-specific strength and power, develop hypertrophy, optimize sport-related movement, and improve metabolic conditioning.
- Fourth year: Develop a high degree of sport-specific strength and power, and optimize sport-related movement and performance.

The College Strength Coach's Observations of the Quality of Youth Development

Implementing an appropriate long-term athletic development plan for youth benefits athletes when they play college sports. College strength and conditioning professionals must evaluate incoming first-year students on multiple levels. Depending on the sport, first-year students will be evaluated on several components, such as posture and mobility, flexibility, muscular strength and endurance, aerobic endurance, power, speed, agility, balance and coordination, ability to change direction, technique, and general knowledge of training, recovery, and nutrition. Strengths should be noted, but weaknesses must be identified and targeted as critical elements to address in the strength and conditioning program. The level of youth coaching will be reflected in the level of preparedness of the first-year college athlete. There is a cautionary tale, often now forgotten, in a study by Wade and colleagues at Bose State University (Wade, Pope, and Simonson 2014), who surveyed 57 collegiate NCAA Division I strength and conditioning coaches regarding major and minor issues seen in freshman athletes. They found that 33% of college first-year athletes had inadequate strength in the core and lower extremities, 37% lacked foundational technique in the Olympic lifts, and 19% to 23% lacked the flexibility or mobility and work capacity to complete higher-intensity workouts. In addition, 23% of the respondents believed first-year athletes lacked the mental toughness to engage in college sports training and had insufficient knowledge of proper nutrition and recovery. They recommended hiring certified high school coaches and strength and conditioning professionals who concentrate on teaching proper form, developing the posterior chain, increasing athlete work capacity, teaching appropriate nutrition and recovery, and increasing athletes' core strength and overall flexibility.

Strength and Conditioning In-Season: Motor Skill Adaptations

Motor skill performance will improve from playing sports and through the strength and conditioning program. What often may be misunderstood is how sport-specific motor performance skills adapt simultaneously to strength and conditioning. For example, a baseball player who begins a comprehensive strength and conditioning program at the beginning of high school will have developed baseball skills primarily from baseball participation, with complementary improvements from physical education classes, participation in other sports, and other outside physical activity. The baseball player then begins the off-season program and makes significant gains in muscular strength, power, speed, and endurance. When baseball season begins, this player has an improved 40-yard dash time, as well as improved strength and power measures, but also shows noted improvements in bat swing velocity, throwing velocity, and a few other baseball-specific performance tests. At this point, the improvements may be attributed to the off-season strength and conditioning program. However, when baseball season begins, the coach focuses almost completely on baseball activities and fails to prioritize the in-season strength and conditioning program, thinking that the improvements will carry over and be maintained throughout the season. Eight weeks into the season, the player may feel the loss of some of the added skills, despite practicing or playing almost every day each week. This scenario describes the potential for strength and conditioning *detraining* to negatively affect motor skill performance. Motor skill performance improvements are predicated on the athlete's conditioning level. The neural recruitment and coding strategies used in baseball may adapt to the athlete's conditioning level such that when the training stimulus has been removed or limited to the point that detraining occurs, there arises a possibility that baseball skills could be negatively affected at least for a specific period. This is especially true if the motor performance gains resulted from the strength and conditioning stimulus. The critical element for the high school and college coaches is to be aware of this and support the strength and conditioning professional to continue with an in-season strength and conditioning program to optimize sport performance over the season and limit any detraining effects.

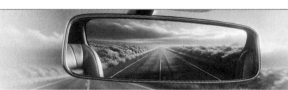

LOOKING IN THE REARVIEW MIRROR

- Understanding the mutable and largely nonmutable characteristics is an important part of helping youth play the most appropriate sports and be placed in the right positions. The development process must continue as athletes progress in their careers; otherwise, when the demands of the position change with increasing competition, the athlete composite may not succeed at the new levels of competition.
- Youth should be exposed to multiple sports (i.e., sport sampling) because the conditioning and motor skills gained from different sports contribute to overall athleticism and assist in development in a main sport in the future.
- Sport specialization should only occur for those sports that require peak performances at early ages. Youth should be exposed to quality PE programs, coaching, and potentially strength and conditioning facilities that feature youth training and adhere to the LTAD model.

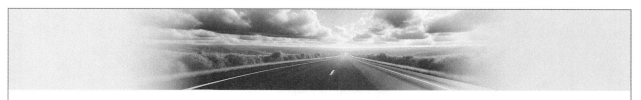

LOOKING AT THE ROAD AHEAD

After taking a careful look at the physiological systems and the factors that go into sport performance, we must start looking at the road ahead for the athlete composite. The optimal development of the athlete by the player development team arises from the different units, each having its own expertise and competence to contribute to the programs and interventions used. The developmental pathways from youth sports into adulthood in an athlete's career should be dedicated to promoting the athleticism and skill sets needed during the different windows of adaptation over time. Optimal individualized strength and conditioning programs are necessary to enhance the athlete's composite across an entire career. With the understanding of the mutable and largely nonmutable characteristics of the athlete composite, the next step is understanding how to match the athlete with the proper sport. In many sports, the position played on a team also affects success as a career moves forward. Thus, the road ahead involves many factors that need to be understood to properly place the athlete composite into a position where success in competition and self-esteem can be optimized.

Player Profiles, Sport Matching, and the Player Development Team

Matching the athlete with the sport is vital to player development. The choice of a sport is relevant even when, as a young athlete, the development of athleticism is promoted with multiple sports. With the motor skill development needed for different sports (e.g., golf, tennis, and baseball), few successfully take on a new sport in their 20s unless their athlete composite plays into the sport demands (e.g., crew, bobsled, and track events).

An *athlete composite* is the total sum of largely nonmutable and mutable characteristics. It is what the athlete brings to competition at any time and is dynamic due to environmental and situational context at the time of competition. The many factors that affect performance potential noted in chapter 1 (see figure 1.2) are also dynamic, with acute modulation of the composite in many ways. An athlete may have all the strategies or capabilities to compete at a given level, but environmental (e.g., acclimatization) or psychological factors (e.g., performance pressure or new venue) may be present that reduce the optimization of that athlete's composite for that point in time. Thus, preparation is ongoing for both the development of the athlete composite but also the readiness of the composite for competition at a specific time. Thus, the athlete composite is a dynamic entity constantly modulated by multiple positive and negative influences from everyday life.

In a study conducted by Patton et al. in 1990, the focus was on the relationship between an athlete's physiological and biomechanical strategies and their performance variable; specifically, lower body power output using the Supercycle (Knuttgen et al. 1982; Knuttgen, Patton, and Vogel 1982). The study found that the average maximal power was 771 +/- 149 W, ranging from 527 to 1125 W. Interestingly, the results indicated that there were no significant correlations between the percentage of type II fibers, relative area of type II fibers, or fat-free thigh volume, and maximal power or endurance times at any percentage of maximal power. However, weak but significant relationships were observed for fat-free mass, which showed a positive correlation with both maximal power ($r = 0.57$) and a negative correlation with endurance time at 73% of maximal power ($r = -0.47$). Overall, the findings suggest that maximal power appears to be more dependent on factors related to an individual's body size rather than specific muscle-fiber characteristics. However, the relatively low correlations for many of the relationships imply that athletes may employ diverse combinations of these factors or utilize other strategies to generate high power during sports performance. Ultimately, the point is that each athlete brings their own set of strategies to the sport, and this athlete composite and its adaptability will dictate success or failure in a task.

Every aspect of the athlete composite has mutable and largely nonmutable traits. These traits coalesce synergistically or antagonistically to aid or diminish the capacity to perform a task. In early human civilization, tribes with the greatest adaptability and resilience to a threat or stress had the greatest chance of survival. During the nomadic period, towns, cities, and countries stood the greatest chance of defending their land by calling on the sum of their resources to fight off threats of food shortages, famine, and being conquered. As each century progressed, the specialization and individualization of needs became increasingly

The Physiological Athlete Composite

The concept of a *physiological athlete composite* has gained significant attention in athletics as a reliable indicator of an athlete's potential for success. This measure considers an individual's physical attributes, such as strength and speed, as well as their mental and emotional capabilities, including their motivation, focus, and ability to work effectively with a team. Research has shown that athletes with a stronger physiological athlete composite are more likely to perform well at higher levels of competition and to be able to adapt to new demands of the game (figure 2.1). Relying solely on an athlete's past individual achievements and statistics, particularly in team sports, is an insufficient predictor of future performance. This is because production at any level results from a complex combination of factors, and simply looking at awards and stats does not provide a complete picture. Coaches need to consider the broader context and evaluate an athlete's potential by considering the physiological athlete composite and the player's willingness to work hard, learn, and grow. It is essential to consider the resources and support available to athletes as they progress to higher levels of competition. Participating in a sport at a high level requires a significant commitment and can be a demanding full-time job. A strong support system (i.e., the player development team), including performance staff and coaches dedicated to helping athletes commit to the work, is crucial. By considering these factors, coaches and strength and conditioning professionals can make well-informed decisions about which athletes are most likely to succeed and thrive, given the standards and expectations of the team at that level of competition and the support services they will have access to.

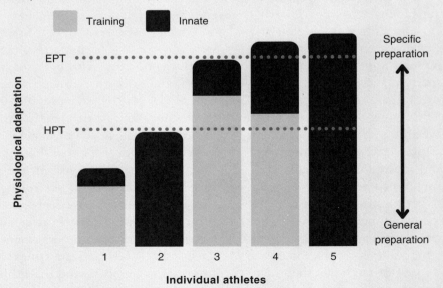

FIGURE 2.1 Physiological adaptation is plotted as a function over time in six individual athletes. High-performance and elite threshold performances are noted. This figure demonstrates that each athlete possesses a specific contribution of innate versus training attributes that take them to their highest level of performance. Note that few athletes reach elite performance capacity. The physiological athlete composite considers both physical training and innate attributes.

Adapted from R. Tucker and M. Collins, "What Makes Champions? A Review of the Relative Contribution of Genes and Training to Sporting Success," *British Journal of Sports Medicine* 46 (2012): 555-561.

focused. Formal education even went as far as to create dedicated learning tracks for liberal arts, technical engineering, and medicine. These formalized training programs were designed to take selected individuals with an intrinsic interest in a subject area and transfer knowledge and expertise to them in order to advance the field and improve the body of human knowledge. It has been the application of this knowledge to solve problems and enhance health and human performance that has framed the basis of applied sciences including exercise and sports sciences.

This same identification, selection, and development process occurs in athletics. As a sport gains popularity and economic significance, the prerequisite traits become statistically scarcer. Too often, coaches and others argue that a successful athlete was not the tallest or fastest in order to refute the underlying reality that some prerequisite nonmutable traits are required to be a viable candidate for on-field production or success at the highest level in a sport. To make matters more complicated, having these traits only allows one to compete. This is why, time and time again, genetic testing for athletic success is still not thought to be possible (Guth and Roth 2013). As noted in this book, many factors contribute to the athletic composite and its readiness for success in competition at a given time point. While largely nonmutable characteristics must be there for an athlete to compete, multiple factors affect development and readiness for competitive success. Whether one possesses ACE I/I, the genotype for endurance, or the ACTN3 R/R genotype for power, or the ACT-3 warrior gene, focus and intentionality also play vital roles in player success to maximize genetic potential.

Dr. Baker relates a cautionary tale about the mix of science and its dangers to overstate or interpret beyond what is appropriate: "At a time when epigenetic science is being taken up enthusiastically by Indigenous groups, and when we are reassessing the kinds of science that are necessary or desirable, the warrior genes controversy forms an instructive warning regarding the power of fiction to shape scientific realities and about some of the dangers of reductive genetic thinking. Scientists and writers alike must remain vigilant about where their narratives might take us, and with the age of post genomics comes a heightened responsibility to develop more sophisticated ways of analyzing and interpreting scientific 'knowledge'" (Baker 2020).

Additionally, depending on the sport and the position, an individual with exceptional drive and desire to compete may be genetically gifted and just in the wrong position in a sport to achieve success. During my (Tom Newman) time at Yale University, we analyzed our positional profiles and assessed that there was an individual who, while never playing meaningful minutes as a linebacker, could be an exceptional tight end. In collaboration with the head coach, an unexpected decision was made to move the player in his senior season. Just as the data forecast, the individual won several regional awards and signed a deal with a professional American football team. This entire journey was made possible by the practical analysis of the positional profile and alignment with the coaching staff to put every player in the best position for a chance of success. Ultimately, success will be determined by the individual walking through the doorway opened by the data, a concept conveyed by the following quote by an unknown author: "Athleticism gets you a seat at the table; your effort and commitment to excellence will determine success."

The athlete composite is a set of strategies the athlete brings to the competition at a given time. For example, the athletes on the starting line for the 100-meter Olympic gold medal race will have an athlete composite that allows them to perform at the level that puts them in the race. The athlete would have largely nonmutable characteristics, including body size, muscle length, fiber type, limb lengths, tendon origins, and insertions. They should have optimally trained the mutable characteristics of strength, power, and speed as elite athletes, yet any deficiencies in training could be detrimental in such a competition. Other factors may influence the athlete's composite, such as the psychological environment of the race, how favored the athlete is by the media, the amount of press coverage, social media hype, environmental heat and track conditions, and any medical issues, such as foot blisters or a prior strained muscle from preliminary heats. As competition looms, the athlete composite's mutable characteristics are developed for a sport both acutely and chronically. Therefore, mutable characteristics can positively or negatively influence the athlete's composite. It is then the nonmutable characteristics that act as

How to Build Your Composite

Athlete development magic lies in successfully enhancing one or several facets of an individual's composite. This chapter delineates human traits into two categories: mutable and nonmutable attributes. The often-misunderstood aspect is the synergistic or antagonistic interplay between these traits. Moreover, while some attributes have high potential for growth, the timing and sequence of adaptation can be even more crucial than any single trait. Many coaches grapple with determining training priorities. Over the past decades, the performance industry has been inundated with misinformation and misunderstood science. With digital platforms amplifying the spread of information, many now disseminate content for personal gain. Alarmingly, young coaches often gauge expertise by social media following rather than knowledge.

Coaches can counter this by recognizing that biology and physics are truth-bound. Regardless of the noise, athlete development's core remains anchored in tangible results.

Getting Started

Before devising any plan, staff must dissect the unique elements of their sport. Assess the team's current state, compare players against upcoming opponents, and determine the coaching staff's commitment to implementing suggestions. Properly crafting an athlete composite can guide future recruitment and can be fortified with an all-encompassing training strategy.

Recruiting

Dr. Chris Eskridge's cohort methodology is invaluable for profile creation. This method, first employed for the Epley Advantage Performance Index at the University of Nebraska, analyzes athletic traits to determine impactful field tests. At Yale, this approach pinpointed vital nonmutable traits for numerous sports. Traits were categorized by position and prioritized for recruitment. This was replicated for mutable attributes, producing a comprehensive training and recruiting guide. To choose your nonmutable traits:

Step 1

- Document current nonmutable traits (e.g., height and wingspan).
- Collect all data relevant to athletic development (e.g., players' upbringing environment or support system). Don't limit yourself to "weight room" metrics.
- Gather as many metrics as possible in a spreadsheet, each column representing a unique metric.

Common mistakes among coaches include averaging these values or calculating standard deviations and Z-scores. Such methods, though research-suitable, may mislead in practical settings by favoring physically gifted athletes over top on-field performers. The composite's objective is recognizing the basic standards required for an athlete to excel in their sport, not just identifying the most athletic.

Step 2

Categorize into cohort groups:

    3: Athlete recognized at a national or professional level

    2: Athlete recognized at league or conference level

    1: Athlete participated above the team's 50% participation mark (minutes/games)

    0: Athlete played below the 50% mark or was injured

Step 3

Initially, some coaches were wary of this approach. However, when they noticed younger players getting more playing time, they embraced the methodology. This wasn't because senior athletes underperformed; they were simply outrecruited. By pinpointing both mutable and nonmutable traits of top performers, coaches can focus on recruiting those with abundant favorable nonmutable traits and give them the performance team traits that if properly developed can make an immediate impact. While no trait stands alone in importance, a collection of beneficial traits can dramatically affect the win-loss column. If executed correctly, each recruiting year should bring in athletes with superior physical attributes. Within three years, by elevating the team's athletic baseline, your program should be on an upward trajectory.

the basic framework for the initial match of the athlete with a sport for optimal performance. As will be shown in this chapter, analyzing the sport is necessary when matching the athlete composite with the sport.

Program Alignment

Alignment must start with the athlete understanding the program and then continue to the multiple elements involved in the developmental process. It also extends to the family and friends; everyone should be brought into unison on the program goals and objectives. The need for alignment among the different units in the player development team is important; otherwise, there can be major disruptors to the quality of care and service delivery to the individual athlete. Conflicts between professionals on the team are disruptors, and evidence-based solutions need to be in place for unit-to-unit disagreements, especially regarding individual care of the athlete. Many mistakes are made from tunnel vision and a lack of understanding of, as they say, "the whole playing field." At worst, this can lead to malpractice and, at best, to subpar decisions for an athlete, limiting the athlete composite acutely or chronically.

Organization of the Team

Organizational alignment can be structured in "org charts." To be effective, leaders must keep in mind the demands for leadership, cooperation, and understanding of the core values of the player development program (see chapter 1, figure 1.1). Competency in each of the expertise and practice areas is of paramount importance. Expertise has to be genuine and not a function of social media or posturing. Hiring in each area is a potential minefield for developing a truly effective and competitive group of professionals. Professionals in each area need to know what they know and, more importantly, what they do not know, and also be willing to learn and contribute from their experience and perspective. Leaders in the different expertise areas or units need to promote communication and respect. The top priority should be to use effective interactions to communicate and provide the best care and management of the individual athlete.

Communication and Interactions

The success of the player development program depends on the communication and alignment of the different program elements. A lack of communication can tear apart any cohesion of the program and limit the positive impact for the individual athlete. The player development team, from the athlete to the different units involved, must be on the same page for it to work. Communication is the key to the rapid flow of information and effective decisions from local professionals making day-to-day changes to workouts, recovery, and nutrition, as well as systemic or whole-group decisions that address program principles, values, and innovations and technology that affect all units. For a player development program to work, all professionals must have a communication system, a decision-making process, and respect for each area's expertise. Additionally, implementation pathways have to be determined. Failure to achieve alignment on common goals and objectives for each sport and athlete in the program makes such a program impossible.

Coordination of the different programs and implementing the technology and knowledge base at the practical level (the athlete's training, eating, studying, practicing, and recovering) is a challenge for any player development team. How much of the science reaches the athlete in the programs designed by the player development team is key to success. Improving the timeliness of the program interventions is a significant factor in the program's organization and success. Due to the rapid changes in all aspects of the athlete's daily demands, quick answers are needed along with implementation strategies to address the needs, objectives, and goals of each athlete's program. What used to be called "total conditioning" might now also be understood as "total programming."

Total programming involves the player development team meeting each week to set the stage for what is happening. It also requires unit meetings and meetings with consultants from other units and outside resources. While this appears cumbersome, meetings are necessary—if not in person, then by video call (Zoom or Teams meetings). Involvement with the sport coach and coaching staff also has to be part of this process so that buy-in is achieved. Each unit has to be aware of the expertise around them and understand that there is immediate access to other player development team members. The decision-making process has a hierarchical role. Day-to-day decisions begin with grassroots professionals but draw, when appropriate, on the input of expertise from other areas.

For example, the strength and conditioning professional should be well aware of the sport nutrition unit and the programs they have in place. They may want to consult with them on the efficacy of a new approach for weight loss (e.g., a ketogenic diet) for one group of athletes in a weight-class sport. If the sport nutrition unit has no expertise in this area of practice, they can default to a larger group, using an evidence-based practice approach to determine how that group's expertise can be used or if it can be used for the question at hand. Failure of the nutrition unit to admit limitations in their professional understanding, in this case, would be an example of posturing or not doing their due diligence on a question for the athletes. Many such examples could be given on a host of different player development unit interactions (or lack thereof).

While mistakes are made, it is the ones that could have been prevented with due diligence that negatively affect the individual athlete composite and the efficacy of the player development program. Remember, these interactions can be complicated by issues related to self-esteem, power, and control in the organization. Still, the expertise of, for example, the nutrition unit should be respected if evidence-based practices are used to come to an initial decision. The strength and conditioning professional should respect the approach decided upon. However, it does not end there; the impact of the decisions is evaluated with monitoring and testing to determine if the expected responses and adaptations have been achieved. If they have not, the evidence-based process is repeated to find answers and another solution for an effective dietary approach. With groups of athletes, searching for answers to questions may come down to an individual athlete who is not responding to the general nutritional practice being implemented. Thus, searching for answers can range from a team to an individual athlete. Determining the effectiveness of the intervention requires testing, monitoring, and continual tracking of data to understand the progress toward the target goals.

Decision-Making Process on Questions in Player Development

Using a team approach to evidence-based practices has proven essential for answering questions with team members' perspectives on research, practice, and insights (Amonette, English, and Kraemer 2016). Getting the needed perspective on the question is crucial because it might lead to the correct answer. Still, problems might then exist in its implementation for the team (e.g., massage might be the answer for stress reduction). To implement the perspective for the whole team, we may need more staffing and expertise in this area. Keeping the initial answer in mind while finding an effective alternative may be necessary until the "best" solution can be implemented. As an example, related to equipment, the player development team may not have a DEXA machine to do body composition, but an evidence-based practice may find that underwater weighing, a Bod Pod, or even effective skinfold measurements can be used while the program transitions to more direct measurement systems. But the key point is that any program should be implemented at the highest level of efficacy for its use. Its limitations and error factors should be known in order to understand the context of the decisions made regarding it (e.g., skinfold body fat measures can have a 4% to 5% error factor when properly measured, so evaluations with this body composition technique must consider this).

This can be done within a unit of the player development team (e.g., sport performance) for a specific question. Conversely, for a more extensive global question, members of each unit can be involved along with the coaches to address and give their perspectives. For example, if the coach opposes having an in-season strength and conditioning program, the athletic trainer might explain the role of conditioning in injury prevention, and the strength and conditioning professional can share their expertise on the benefits of in-season training. Each professional and the entire group can use this process locally when combined expertise is needed to decide on questions arising from a particular sport or issue with an athlete.

The key is getting multiple perspectives, assessing knowledge, and making decisions based on the best available knowledge. Decisions are not static but dynamic because science progresses with time on various topics. Many decisions must have a structural background for their approach in a particular area of player development, such as using a periodization model in strength and conditioning programs. Questions may then drill down on the type of model and training cycle, but a structure must be set. Each unit's professionals must have freedom to work within their lanes as they know best, but competence and best practices must be at the core of each professional in a unit. When questions arise, the player development team can examine evidence-based practices with this procedure. Some questions may be local but may need to consult with another unit to gain perspective on the approach. Hence, there must be support and consistency throughout the player development team. Here is where major issues and conflict can arise, but it is the efficacy and facts that need to be considered before the judgments of professionals with specific expertise are involved.

The basic steps of this evidence-based practice are as follows:

- Step 1: Develop a question that includes a population, novel intervention, comparison, outcome, and time variable. Examples include the following:
  - *Local Unit Questions:* What periodization model should we use for women's lacrosse?
  - *Global Player Development Team Question:* What types of recovery technologies should we invest in? What kinds of software programs do we need for our player development team?
- Step 2: Search the peer-reviewed research literature, using databases such as PubMed or Google Scholar for supporting peer-reviewed evidence to answer the question.
- Step 3: Evaluate the evidence for its design, quality, and bias with a ranking based on its merit and relevance.
- Step 4: Incorporate or do not incorporate the evidence into practice. By evaluating the strength of the research evidence in conjunction with their own practical experience, the player development team or unit professional determines if the intervention warrants incorporation into an athlete's programming.
- Step 5: Confirm the evidence for the individual athlete. With a systematic testing routine already in place, the sport scientist and analytic team members can monitor the effectiveness of the new intervention and provide information to the player development team. Decisions can then be made to continue or discontinue accordingly.
- Step 6: Reevaluate the evidence. The evidence-based approach implies the need to reassess the literature regularly. With thousands of papers published each month, the answer to a question may change over time based on emerging research. The sport scientists can then call for meetings of units or the whole team to examine the new data and reevaluate the current approach being used.

The Player Development Team Model

Historically, success with such player development programs has been observed in Olympic training centers around the world since the 1950s. This type of Olympic model has been adopted by different organizations and has been called the *high-performance management model* in sports (Smith and Smolianov 2016). Many countries use this model for club and professional sports player development. However, while this was known in the early 1980s in collegiate athletics, such multidisciplinary models, due to the silo effects of the different disciplines in athletics and academics, did not evolve. In athletics, the evolution arose from the strength and conditioning professionals as well as athletic training units within sports medicine beginning in the 1970s (Shurley, Todd, and Todd 2019).

In 1989, Penn State developed a Center for Sports Medicine that included multiple units, including nutrition, research, academics, team physicians, and orthopedic surgeons, to work comprehensively with the athletic teams and Dr.

Kraemer, one of the first sport scientists hired by athletics in such a program. This extended sports medicine model was one of the early evolutions of a type of player development model in which sports medicine was extended beyond clinical interfaces. This first attempt incorporated sport science, research, and nutrition units inside a sports medicine model, interfacing directly with athletics to develop work with teams, coaches, and athletes in different sports. This type of Olympic training center model has slowly grown in university settings as more funding has become available (see chapter 8 on models). As the demands of addressing the athlete composite for competition have increased, interdisciplinary interfacing has become a critical factor. As with the development of strength and conditioning in the late 1970s, larger schools have more aggressively started to put such multidisciplinary programs together.

Units in the Player Development Team

As sport science and sport analytics evolved, it became apparent that the athletic composite was far more complex than historically addressed. As noted in chapter 1, figure 1.1, various areas need expertise contributing to the player development team. While each institution or organization establishes the configuration and reporting lines, the professionals in a player development team are essential. The amount of time each professional spends with the athlete is also a key factor, owing to the sport's governing body rules and regulations as well as the administrative structures.

Strength and Conditioning, Sport Performance, Sport Science, and Sport Analytics

The professionals in these areas of expertise spend the most time with the athletes at the grassroots level and implement many training, testing, and monitoring metrics needed in a player development program. These titles are often earned through certifications and degrees, along with experiential backgrounds, slightly differentiating each title. These titles have evolved from the strength and conditioning field and have not yet been entirely determined in the player development model.

The strength and conditioning coach position arose in the 1950s with the National Strength and Conditioning Association (NSCA) solidifying the profession in 1978 and offering the first certification in strength and conditioning (i.e., the Certified Strength and Conditioning Specialist, CSCS) in 1985. Thus, a strength and conditioning professional has a well-defined task analysis and is defined as a physical performance professional who uses exercise prescription—resistance training for maximal strength, aerobic conditioning, and other methods—to improve the performance of competitive athletes or athletic teams.

Arising from this designation was the sport performance professional, generally defined as a professional who specializes in physical, mental, and emotional fitness training designed to improve an athlete's ability to perform a specific sport. It includes resistance training, aerobic training, corrective exercise, and mindset training. This expanded the expertise of the strength and conditioning professional. Thus, the two professionals are often indistinguishable, and can even be the same person, but other domains of expertise were added to the strength and conditioning specialist. Certifications specifically for a sport performance professional do not yet exist but are typically tied into various movement specialties or sport science disciplines and strength and conditioning certifications.

The sport science professional again grew out of the strength and conditioning field with testing and monitoring technologies, most notably global positioning systems (GPS) and heart rate monitoring. Certifications again arose for this title from different organizations, including the NSCA, which offers the Certified Performance and Sport Scientist (CPSS) credential. Similarly, degrees for each of these professionals range from baccalaureate degrees in exercise and sport science to master's degrees in the same areas. Doctoral degrees, which typically are related to undertaking and directing experimental studies in an area of expertise, also exist in this genre of sport science. Thus, the practice, expanse, and duties can vary depending on individual backgrounds. Not all those with a PhD or EdD are research-specific. They can be a generalist and not an investigator. Their research expertise can be evaluated by their Google Scholar

H scores. Often this unit can benefit from interfacing with academic departments and experts in various areas of sport and exercise science that are based in different types of expertise (e.g., thermal regulation, hydration, neuromuscular function, endocrinology, biomechanics, cardiovascular, and environmental). A PhD does not mean high-level expertise in all areas but should indicate training in research and a global understanding of exercise and sport science. Another PhD from faculty in another department may, for example, provide resources from nutrition, psychology, sociology, and engineering.

In general, the sport analytic professional is a phenomenon reflected in the popular 2010 movie *Money Ball*. This profession is defined as someone working in a field that applies data analysis techniques to analyze various components of the sports industry, such as player performance, business performance, recruitment, and more. The sport analytic professional has been famous in both collegiate and professional sports. This professional works in television audience appeal and gambling businesses to add more dimensions to the viewer's experience with sport competitions. With expertise from engineering, business, and statistics, this professional can be involved with database development, big data, algorithms, machine learning, and other characteristic profiles.

Many say these professionals have become too expansive and overextended in their role on the field (e.g., telling baseball managers when to pull players and pitchers from the field, or field alignments taking out the coaching element). In sports, analytic professionals can benefit player development by testing, monitoring, and accounting for the mutable and largely nonmutable characteristics that are so crucial to the goals and objectives of training cycles and long-term projections. This professional can also set the stage for recruiting metrics for each position in a sport.

Interestingly, these different professions are often combined in one evolved strength and conditioning specialist who has developed additional skill sets for professional survival and improved pay. In more extensive programs, these sports professionals are broken into distinct elements of practices, which is a more ideal structure for a sport performance model.

Sport Nutrition

Sport nutrition has become essential to the player development program. Typically, a registered dietitian or RD is the standard for this professional in this unit. However, an RD is not necessarily an expert in sport nutrition, which has a more varied use of dietary approaches and supplements compared to the clinical field of the typical RD. The university training for the RD with a sport nutrition specialty contributes to the expertise level. Thus, sport nutrition internships, fellowships, genuine certificates, and experience working with various athletes are essential. With the plethora of certificate programs, care is needed to determine who is truly a sport nutritionist. The educational background and experience define the level of expertise for professionals in this unit.

Sports Medicine

This area is one of the more highly defined units. Certified athletic trainers (ATCs) by the National Athletic Trainers Association (NATA) and many states' licenses define this professional expertise in dealing with athletic injuries. The doctor of physical therapy (DPT) degree is also a well-established degree but with specialties in different areas of expertise, which should be noted as some degrees focus more on neuromuscular therapy and are better related in their training to sports. Physicians with varying specialties, from team physicians to orthopedic surgeons, have had residencies or fellowships pertaining to sports medicine. Specialist physician referrals for eating disorders to psychiatrists have also been at the forefront of medical interfaces with athletes in different sports.

Sport Psychology and Sport Sociology

A sport psychologist is typically defined as someone who investigates how participating in sports can improve health and well-being. They help athletes use psychology to improve athletic performance and mental wellness. The professionals in the sport psychology area of expertise typically have master's or doctorate degrees in sport psychology and experience working with athletes. Sport psychology—in the competition venue, in performance preparation, and as a provider of coping mechanisms for dealing with and treating anxiety and depression—has become vital to the player development program. Appropriately trained and licensed clinical psychologists are also crucial for treating depression, which has come to the forefront over the past several years and can result in suicide when left untreated. This has become an essential element needed for monitoring and treatment referrals. Imagery, precompetition preparations, and recovery aspects are just a few interfaces between athletes and sport psychology. Degrees based in psychology, clinical licenses, certifications, and experience all indicate the level of expertise of professionals in this unit.

With the plethora of social media, press, and microscopic analysis of athletes' personal and social lives, the sport sociologist has become an essential professional in this unit. Sport sociology has generally been defined as a discipline of sociology that studies sports as a social phenomenon. Sport sociologists critically examine the functions, impacts, and roles of sports on different societies. In a player development program, this professional works with coaches and athletes to help develop the team culture and interface with outside elements like family, entertainment, and social media. Degrees, licenses, certifications, and experience working with athletes define the expertise of professionals in this area.

The Need for Individualization of Programs for Player Development Success

Various capabilities are associated with these professionals and certifications in the total player development team. Extensive task analyses for the job have delineated the profession. The number of professionals in each unit is reflected by college or university resources and the number of athletes and teams served by the program.

Individualization of program implementation is a significant challenge for this type of program, no matter how organized the level of expertise is in the player development program. Thus, the major challenge is the need for well implemented individualization of programs, which is crucial for optimizing player development, as the singularity of the term implies. This aspect of the program has become almost mandatory for today's athletes because there are individual variations among responses to workouts, recovery metrics, and progressions addressing daily needs and needs across the different training cycles.

A critical member in today's sports player development team has a PhD, experience in experimental research and testing, and experience with athletes. Such members can be found among faculty in a department trained in exercise and sport sciences as well as statistical and laboratory research. Their expertise in laboratory equipment and testing modalities over many years of training is helpful to a player development team. Even more critical is their competence and ability in interpreting data with context for other members of the player development team, along with coaches and athletes. Thus, a player development team must have the advanced expertise of a doctoral-trained investigator to help understand the validity and reliability of testing as well as the context and meaning of data from instruments. We will cover testing modalities more in chapter 3. Such understanding is vital because not every instrument (e.g., force plates, isokinetic dynamometers, strain gauges, and GPS units) is identical in its type and data output. Testing using a random force plate may not measure power in watts like other studies or national standards have done. If not correctly calibrated and if testing is not performed appropriately, the data will be invalid. Additionally, interpretation is essential. We learned this long ago with isokinetic dynamometers, where the peak torque value on one brand of dynamometer did not equal the peak torque if tested on another brand. Understanding the validity and reliability of a testing modality is essential; any measure is only a starting point or one point on the progression toward an achievable goal. Discounting an athlete based on one metric is foolish if a developmental program has not been created from a strength and conditioning perspective.

Sport Coaching

The head sport coach and assistants play a vital role in the player development team. Their background, interest, and buy-in to the program are essential. Their involvement should be mandated by the athletic administration, and they must share the values for optimizing the athlete's well-being and potential; otherwise, optimal player development programs cannot be established or implemented for the sport. It is well known that sport coaches can represent a significant disruptor to the player development program, even at the level of strength and conditioning, if programs are not coordinated (Moore and Fry 2007). Thus, communication and evidence-based practices must be respected, or else disruptions can occur (e.g., a coach does not want an in-season resistance training program, or a coach brings in dozens of donuts to a team trying to change body composition and reduce fat, or a coach has their own ideas on training and implements them in conflict with the advice of their strength and conditioning professionals, or a coach does not want to participate in evidence-based decision-making). The sport coach needs to play an essential role in their programs, understand what is going on, and overtly support the program with their athletes. Thus far, historically, participation in a complete player development team is not common in most sports organizations. This role has not been very well established, nor are practices taught that go beyond an authoritarian position and viewpoint.

Academic Advising and Community

Another ancillary group that can be an essential part of the player development team is the interface with the university academicians and the larger communities related to player development. Thus, in some cases, the needed area of expertise can come from faculty members with athletic backgrounds and research expertise that can specifically contribute to the program. From research collaborations to academic programs feeding the player development programs with student volunteers and interns, this relationship can provide what we call in the military "force multipliers," from physiology to nutrition to engineering. The university's community, the city, its associated businesses, and citizen groups can also help with financial support to interface with charities and volunteer activities.

Level of Competition

It is essential to understand the level of competition for which the player development program is attempting to prepare the athlete composite. Each sport will have largely nonmutable characteristics that will define the general requirements for a sport and a position. Remembering chapter 1, the levels of adaptation that can be achieved with the mutable characteristics can only go so far in taking the athlete composite to the next level. Thus, the starting point of that athlete composite must have the potential to reach the level of competition the athlete will be competing in. Therefore, the first steps are evaluating the mutable and nonmutable characteristics and setting up the criteria for what is needed in a particular sport or position.

Initially, it's crucial to evaluate the mutable and nonmutable characteristics, establishing criteria based on the needs of a specific sport or position. In every sport, there are always "unicorns" – exceptional talents who defy conventional metrics and norms. These players are rare, and while their unique skills might shine brighter in team sports, it's not because they need to hide their weaknesses. Rather, it's that their extraordinary abilities can significantly contribute to overall team performance, thereby making their rarity even more impactful.

Each sport needs to set its criteria for mutable characteristics as target training goals and objectives. Additionally, for recruiting, the threshold for the largely nonmutable characteristics needs to be developed for each sport. Figure 2.2 shows a spider graph that can show athletes and coaches where the values for testing measurements are positioned. There is a distinct need to have honest and ethical conversations with athletes, as well as their parents (when appropriate), to help place them in the proper sport and position. This is vital in recruiting and when the player development team works with the athlete.

The Epley Athletic Performance Index

The Epley Athletic Performance Index (EAPI) is a valuable metric to get a feel for an athlete's athleticism. While developed for American football, it has been amazingly informative for other sports. Figure 2.3a depicts some average ranges from untrained to elite athletes. This figure shows that a top Division I athlete has dramatically higher scores than an average Division III athlete. Elite athletes may score 1,700 or more. Figure 2.3b shows that the population of elite athletes dwindles to very few, underscoring why recruiting and elite competitions have a minimal number of

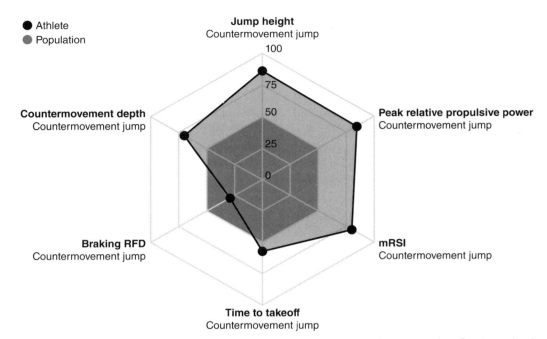

FIGURE 2.2 Data from force plate testing for the sport can be compared to the testing data for the individual athlete to see where deficiencies exist. These deficiencies would need to be addressed in a training program. In this case, the athlete had only one deficiency in these parameters: the braking rate of force development.
Courtesy of HAWKIN Dynamics.

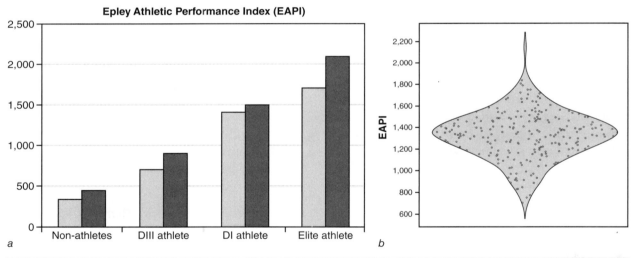

Color	Proficiency	Relative strength			Performance				
		Back squat	Bench press	Power clean	EAPI	Vert	Pro	10	Percentile
Blue	5	2	1.5	1.5	1,528.6	33.5	4.07	1.69	90
Green	4	1.75	1.3	1.3	1,456.2	31.75	4.14	1.73	80
Orange	3	1.5	1.2	1.2	1,337	29.75	4.24	1.78	60
Yellow	2	1.25	1	1	1,224.6	28	4.36	1.83	40
Red	1	1.25	1	1	1,086	25.5	4.56	1.91	20

c

FIGURE 2.3 (a) The different levels of the index can indicate the level of inherent athletic potential for the athlete. The gray bars represent a range of scores per population. The color code represents the percentile rank. (b) Distribution of athletes from the top 0 to ultra-elite at the bottom of the parametric distribution. (c) Sample profile of men with performance testing standards and index measures.

athletes that achieve the level of the athlete composite needed to participate at the highest level of a sport. Figure 2.3c shows a sample profile with performance standards and the EAPI. The ability to improve only 100 points each year indicates that competing at that next level could be difficult at best if the performance index is too low in a sport.

Talent Identification Role in Player Development Programs

As noted in chapter 1, youth development of physical capabilities concerns different physical, motor, and strength capabilities. The concept of talent identification and specialization has been extensively studied and written about for quite some time. Many moving parts affect the identification of young talent and their potential for given sports, with maturation and fundamental movement skills being paramount and on different time scales for other young athletes (Vaeyens et al. 2008). In this book, the athlete's development at any age is the goal of a player development program. Talent identification is separate from the process, except for the use of recruiting metrics and the placement of athletes in the right team positions, especially at the high school and collegiate levels. Many times, an athlete who is a slow developer with a later maturation timeline is only discovered later on. Maturation in all of its dimensions is very important and is often discussed in the talent identification literature. In many collegiate player development programs, the redshirt junior or senior makes the difference in team success, if given the time for developing their physical capabilities.

Anthropometry, Talent Identification, and Sport Performance

Sport performance results from a composite of numerous variables identified throughout this book. Complicating matters is that some sports are composed of different positions, each bringing a unique blend of skills and somatotypes to the table. For example, a cornerback in American football possesses a specific athletic profile that allows that individual to excel at that position. However, that same athlete may struggle or not be able to play another position within the same sport (e.g., defensive or offensive tackle). Thus, each position within a sport requires a specific profile that will lead to athletic success. In addition, each component of the sport may require its own specific profile. For example, there may be better profiles for displaying high levels of agility in other aspects of the game than a biomechanical profile that favors a large service velocity in tennis. Thus, the complete athlete will display the best profile components and excel in each to optimize sport performance. The profile consists of several mutable and largely nonmutable characteristics. Player development consists of training the mutable components while maximizing the largely nonmutable components through practice, technique enhancement, and training.

Some examples of largely nonmutable characteristics include selected body composition and anthropometric variables such as height, body segment, limb lengths and proportions, and wingspan. Body composition and anthropometric assessments are standard practices for coaches and athletes and gain valuable information about percent body fat, fat distribution, lean body mass, segment and limb lengths, proportions, and girths and circumferences. Body composition tests may help evaluate training, diet, or athletic performance or reduce the risk factors associated with musculoskeletal injury. *Body composition* describes the relative proportions of fat, bone, and muscle mass in the human body. *Anthropometry* describes the measurement of the human body in terms of dimensions such as height, weight or body mass, circumferences, girths, and skinfolds. Although genetics contributes to all of these from a moderate to a great extent, some characteristics are predominantly genetic, meaning there is little possibility of changing them, regardless of athletic or training status.

These largely nonmutable characteristics form a composite for proper self-selection of athletes into sports where they are best suited. It has long been recognized that sports are dominated by elite athletes with specific somatotypes and skeletal dimensions. Interest in analyzing the physiques of elite athletes dates back to the 1920s, although it took another 30 years before early studies of physique differentiation were published (Stewart 2011). This element of physique specialization is a critical part of the recruiting process for athletes. One often hears a motto like "you can't coach height." To a large extent, this is true (although athletes have to be coached on how to use their height and skeletal dimensions properly), which is why an athlete's frame yields vital information about the potential to excel in a specific position or sport. Thus, the anthropometric assessment of athletes provides critical information on their potential for success in sports and different sport positions.

An athlete's body size influences maximal strength and power production. Generally speaking, the larger the body size, the larger the absolute strength and power potential, and the more likely to carry additional body mass, which could be advantageous for some strength and inertial sports. For example, the size of NFL linemen has increased greatly (Kraemer et al. 2005). The increased size provides an advantage to these athletes. We have documented the body mass and lean body mass values of some of the strongest men in the world. The average body mass of these athletes was approximately 152.9 kilograms (± 19.3 kg), and lean body mass was 118 kilograms (± 11.7 kg), showing that elite strongmen are among the largest male athletes capable of carrying large amounts of tissue mass (Kraemer et al. 2020). Although skeletal size relates to specific sport performance characteristics, lean muscle mass positively relates to strength and power production. Relative strength and power measures are critical to some sports, especially those that involve weight classes or sports where athletes compete against gravity (e.g., long jump, high jump, gymnastics, and pole vault). Larger athletes may have a higher absolute segment of their body mass in the form of bone mass. The greater skeletal dimensions have a significant impact on the biomechanics of performance. Depending on the sporting movement, the larger athlete may display greater segment mass and leverage to the point where performance is maximized at the expense of relative energy or reliance on neuromuscular mechanisms to optimize strength, power, and speed. Figure 2.4 depicts the average sizes of various male athletes.

While body composition describes the relative proportions of fat, bone, and muscle mass in the human body, analysis of how these relate to the physique type (i.e., shape and composition) is called *somatotyping*. Somatotyping involves categorizing athletes into variations of physique types using anthropometric and photoscopic measures. The basic physique types include (1) *endomorph* (round physique, high fat), (2) *mesomorph* (muscular), and (3) *ectomorph* (lean body build). Ten anthropometric measures are taken to calculate the anthropo-

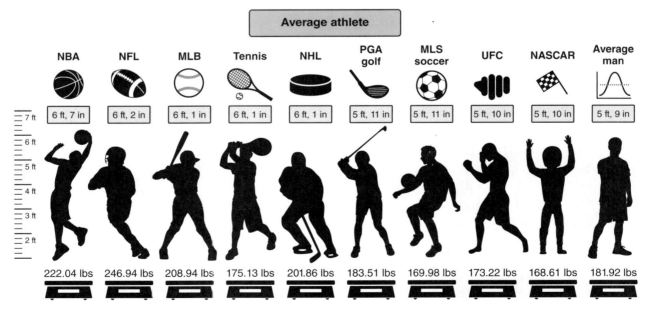

FIGURE 2.4 Average sizes of various male athletes.

Adapted by permission from "Male Body Image and the Average Athlete," PsychGuides.com, accessed June 21, 2023, www.psychguides.com/interact/male-body-image-and-the-average-athlete/.

metric somatotype for endomorphy, mesomorphy, and ectomorphy: stature, body mass, four skinfolds (triceps, subscapular, suprailiac, medial calf), two breadths (biepicondylar humerus and femur), and two limb girths (arm flexed and tensed, calf) (Carter and Heath 1990). Ratings are given for each somatotype and then plotted. Athletes are then placed into one of 13 categories, including *balanced mesomorph, mesomorph-endomorph, mesomorphic endomorph*, and *endomorphic mesomorph*. Rankings of 0.5 to 2.5 are considered low, 3 to 5 is moderate, 5.5 to 7.0 is high, and greater than 7 is very high.

A blend of somatotype categories is seen among athletes. Mesomorphy is positively related to muscular strength, whereas the magnitude of ectomorphy negatively relates to strength measures (Ryan-Stewart, Faulkner, and Jobson 2018). Strength and power athletes, in general, will demonstrate significant degrees of mesomorphy. A large degree of mesomorphy is seen in athletes such as bodybuilders, powerlifters, Olympic weightlifters, strongman competitors, American football, rugby, track-and-field throwers, wrestlers, and gymnasts (Stewart 2011). In weightlifters, high levels of mesomorphy are seen with rising endomorphy and mesomorphy, and decreasing ectomorphy is seen with increasing weight classes (Orvanova 1990). Mesomorphy is seen at moderate to high levels in athletes requiring speed, such as track-and-field sprinters and jumpers, American football players (i.e., running backs, wide receivers, defensive backs), basketball players, MMA fighters, martial arts fighters, boxers, and baseball and softball players. The interaction of mesomorphy with moderate to high ectomorphy is more commonly seen in these athletes who are lean and compete in light to middleweight classes or compete against gravity. Also, this combination may be seen in some hybrid sports where both aerobic and muscular endurance are important fitness components for success. The interaction of mesomorphy with moderate to high endomorphy is more commonly seen in heavy to super heavyweight classes for MMA fighters, boxers, and wrestlers and in inertial sports and positions such as offensive and defensive linemen in American football and sumo wrestling. Aerobic endurance athletes display high levels of ectomorphy with lower levels of mesomorphy and endomorphy (Stewart 2011). Specifically, team handball players display high levels of mesomorphy (5.35 to 6.0) with lower levels of ectomorphy and endomorphy (1.99 to 2.3) (Lijewski et al. 2021). Professional male soccer players display moderate levels of mesomorphy (4.9 to 5.2) and lower levels of endomorphy (1.9 to 2.0) and ectomorphy (2.7) (Campa et al. 2020). Elite male volleyball players display low levels of mesomorphy (2.2 to 2.5) and moderate levels of endomorphy (2.9 to 3.2) and ectomorphy (2.8 to 3.1) (Giannopoulos et al. 2017). Greco-Roman wrestlers have shown high levels of mesomorphy (6.3 to 6.8) with low levels of ectomorphy (1.1 to 1.3) and endomorphy (1.7 to 2.2) (Sterkowicz-Przybycien, Sterkowicz, and Zarow 2011). Given the 13 categories of somatotypes, significant variation may be seen within a sport because athletic success is predicated upon the integration of somatotypes with other anthropometric and physiological variables.

Bodily Proportions

An athlete's stature plays an important role in performance. Longer limbs, torso, and relative ratios alter moment arm lengths, which may pose an advantage or disadvantage depending on the task. For example, long arms and brachial index create a larger resistance arm and require the athlete to displace the barbell farther and perform more work for an exercise such as the bench press. Thus, it is difficult for a very tall athlete to achieve elite-level bench press performance. However, longer arms could assist an exercise such as the deadlift because they help place the trunk and legs in a more biomechanically favored position during the triple extension of the ankle, knee, and hip joints. In addition, longer limbs may yield greater velocity. This is advantageous for basketball, volleyball, and pitching in baseball. In biomechanics, the tangential linear velocity of an object at its point of release is a product of the limb's angular velocity and the radius's length. The angular velocity is a composite of the strength, power, mobility, and speed capacity of the athlete's limbs, trunk, and lower extremities (e.g., a function of the interaction of the athlete's physiology and biomechanics). The radius length depends on limb length and the athlete's technique during the throw, strike, kick, and release. Thus, maximal velocity is a function of the optimal interaction between the body's angular velocity capacity and radius length. A taller athlete (with longer limbs) who can generate high angular velocity has an advantage in some sports, which proves highly attractive to coaches and recruiters. In addition, longer limb lengths contribute to greater stride length and foot contact time, reduced energy expenditure in running, and greater stroke length, frequency, and efficiency in swimming. Limb length is a largely nonmutable genetic attribute that is not coached but increases the likelihood of success in some sports.

Another critical extension of limb length considerations is the contribution of individual segment proportions, which affect the ratios of segments to other segments or to height. Proportions contribute, in part, to the success an individual will have in athletics. For example, segment proportions affect performance in several ways, including altering the moment of inertia about the rotation of the hip, spine, or shoulder axes. In biomechanics, the moment of inertia is the product of the segment's mass and the square of the radius of gyration, which is a measure of mass distribution. Smaller moments of inertia facilitate rotation, while larger moments of inertia have the opposite effect. The moment of inertia is affected by technique as well as the sizes and proportions of the limbs. Although an athlete may have long limbs, the relative mass distribution and proportional segment lengths play key roles in the performance. For example, a larger crural index is thought to reduce the moment of inertia and facilitate faster leg motion. Bodily proportions are stable in adulthood; thus, an athlete can modify technique or train specifically to accommodate or compensate for genetic structural attributes. Relative proportion is an area of interest to coaches. Comprehensive anthropometric evaluation can be used to rank athletes by how they compare to other athletes. It may also be used to place athletes in appropriate sports or individual positions within a sport. Some commonly used ratios include the following (see chapter 3 for measurement directions):

- Tibia length to femur length (crural index)
- Forearm length to upper arm length (brachial index)
- Trunk to upper or lower extremity
- Lower limb to trunk
- Leg length to sitting height (skelic index)
- Seated height to stature
- Biacromial breadth to biiliocristal breadth (androgyny index)
- Arm span to height (relative arm span)
- Sitting height to height (cormic index)
- Lower or upper limb to height
- Hand length to height (relative hand length)
- Second digit to fourth digit

Relationships between selected anthropometric variables and performance measures have been shown in several studies. Some studies have looked at pooled data; others have found significant relationships demonstrated in men or women but not the other. In some cases, anthropometrics had minor effects on measures such as vertical jump (Davis et al. 2006). Some studies (but not all) have demonstrated the following relationships:

- Vertical jump height and lower limb length
- Vertical jump height and toe length
- Vertical jump height and heel length
- Vertical jump height and foot length in men
- Shorter heel length, longer forefoot bones, and shorter lower legs in some sprinters
- Sprint speed and relative height and length of calcaneus
- Relatively longer forefoot bones and shorter Achilles tendon moment arms to improve running economy in aerobic endurance runners
- Smaller digit size (the ratio of the second digit to fourth digit, which is a general marker of prenatal exposure to testosterone) in men, negatively related to grip strength, sprint performance, aggression, power, and various measures of sport performance in, for example, tennis, wrestling, surfing ability, and rugby (Kim and Kim 2016)
- Hand length, breadth, finger length, finger span, and grip strength
- Ratio of arm span to height and basketball and MMA performance (Monson 2018)
- Propulsive forces in swimming and arm span and height (Moura et al. 2014)

- Swimming speed and arm span and biacromial breadth
- Handball performance and upper limb length
- Hand size and receiving performance in American football
- Elite handball performance and length of hands, arms, forearms, and lower limbs, as well as arm span and height (Lijewski et al. 2021)

Determining Sport Demands

Player development is a multifaceted concept. It entails optimizing the player composite by proper talent identification and placing athletes in the right sports and positions, but it also involves optimizing the mutable and largely nonmutable characteristics through training, practice, and competition. The strength and conditioning program must match the demands of the sport and the position within the sport. Thus, the player

Body Proportions: What to Look for in Different Athletes

- Tennis: Long limbs are an advantage with high-velocity shots; shorter limbs may be advantageous for some measures of agility.
- Swimmers: Large stature. Sprinters have a higher brachial index, arm span, ratio of foot to lower leg, and lower leg and foot length compared to middle-distance and distance swimmers. Freestyle and backstroke swimmers have longer limbs, and butterfly swimmers tend to have longer trunks.
- Gymnasts: Shorter statures with a low crural index and ratio of lower limb to trunk.
- Weightlifters, powerlifters: Long trunks, low crural index, low ratio of lower limb to trunk, low brachial index, and high ratio of sitting height to stature. Exercise specificity is seen where a large relative arm span may help for the deadlift but not for the bench press.
- Sprinters: Low ratio of lower limb to trunk with an average-to-high crural index compared to middle-distance runners.
- High jumpers and triple jumpers: A high ratio of lower limb to trunk and a high crural index.
- Discus and javelin throwers: Longer arms with normal trunk lengths.
- Cyclists: High crural index that increases mechanical advantage during pedaling.
- Baseball, American football: Variable based on the diversity of different positions. Tall statures, limbs, wingspan, and hand size help for several positions, including pitchers in baseball and linemen, tight ends, wide receivers, and quarterbacks in American football. Other positions in both sports may benefit from high stature. Moderate stature may work for running backs for lower center of gravity (COG). Hand size is important for a running back. Middle infielders and center fielders in baseball have moderate stature for added agility requirements of the position. High crural index for speed positions.
- Basketball, volleyball: Tall stature and long upper and lower limbs, large hands and fingers, large arm span and ratio of arm span to height, and a high crural index.
- Wrestlers and judo athletes: Low ratio of lower limb to trunk and a low crural index to assist in maintaining a low COG.
- Boxers, striking athletes (depending on style): Large arm span and ratio of arm span to height create a potential reach advantage.
- Handball players: Tall stature and greater arm span, upper and lower limb length, arm length, hand length, biacromial and biiliocristal breadths, and lower brachial index.
- Bodybuilders: Higher androgyny index and ratio of torso length to height.

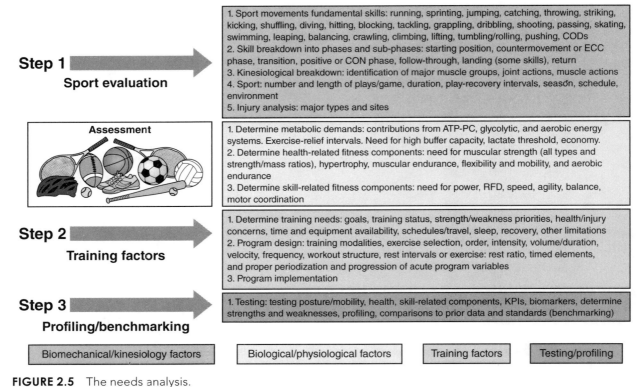

FIGURE 2.5 The needs analysis.
COD = change of direction; CON = concentric; ECC = eccentric; RFD = rate of force development; KPIs = key performance indicators

development team must perform a biological, biomechanical, nutritional, and psychological breakdown of the sport. The sport's specific needs must be addressed through practice and the strength and conditioning program. This is accomplished by performing a *needs analysis*. A needs analysis consists of answering questions based on goals and desired outcomes of training, assessments, access to equipment, health, and the demands of the sport. It helps establish training priorities and guide sport- and training-related decisions regarding the athlete. An overview of the needs analysis process is presented in figure 2.5.

The Needs Analysis

The needs analysis must address the demands of the sport as well as the health- and skill-related fitness components that are critical to the sport and the athlete's composite. The technical training of an athlete can only take them so far. It takes a well-planned, individualized strength and conditioning program targeting the health- and skill-related fitness components to maximize athletic performance. Several descriptive studies comparing different competition levels of athletes have shown that the higher the competition level, the better the fitness testing scores. For example, Garstecki and colleagues compared Division I and II collegiate American football players (Garstecki, Latin, and Cuppett 2004). They showed that Division I players had higher levels of 1RM maximal strength (by 9% to 12%), vertical jump (by 12.5%), and sprint speed (by 3%) (Garstecki, Latin, and Cuppett 2004). Fry and Kraemer (1991) showed similar results where Division I players were 5.3% to 6.4% and 8.1% to 11% stronger, able to jump 4.8% and 7.4% higher, and 1% and 1.6% faster than their Division II and III counterparts (Fry and Kraemer 1991). Thus, several health- and skill-related fitness components serve as discriminant factors separating competition levels in athletes. Optimal player development must target these mutable components from youth through adulthood.

The needs analysis involves a breakdown of the sport but also poses questions that the strength and conditioning program should address (Kraemer et al. 2012; Ratamess 2022; Scroggs and Simonson

2021). Figure 2.5 depicts a sequence of conducting and implementing the needs analysis. Part of breaking down the movements is identifying the fitness components contributing to each. Sample needs analyses are presented in figure 2.6 for a college men's American football player and a college women's volleyball player. The needs analysis consists of three basic steps: (1) sport evaluation, (2) training factors, and (3) profiling and benchmarking.

Sample Needs Analysis: College Men's American Football Player—Tight End

Player Profile
- Height = 6'5"
- Weight = 260 lbs
- Age = 21 yrs
- Football exp = 8 yrs
- Training exp = 6 yrs (advanced status)
- 40 yd dash = 4.76 sec
- Vertical jump = 32 in
- 1RM bench press = 245 lbs
- 1RM squat = 365 lbs

- Sport/Position Need: Sprinting, route running, blocking, pushing, receiving, running after catch, tackling (on turnovers or special teams), jumping, hand fighting, diving, rolling
- Major Muscle Groups: All muscle groups emphasized—special attention for lower-body strength for speed and power, core and upper-body strength for blocking, breaking tackles and yards after contact, neck and grip strength
- Muscle/Joint Actions: All major actions, focus on strength for all muscle actions—may target additional training for eccentric and isometric strength
- Common Injury Sites: Shoulder, knee, ankle, foot, lower back, head (concussion)

- Metabolic Demands: Predominately ATP-PC, glycolysis, good buffer capacity
- Fitness Demands: High muscular strength, hypertrophy, high intensity endurance, power and jumping ability, linear speed, acceleration, deceleration, mobility, reaction time, balance, coordination, agility moves (i.e., side shuffling, side sprint, hops), cutting (side-step, cross-over, split-step) and change of direction ability; good flexibility and aerobic base; moderate-to-low percent body fat

- Goals: Muscular strength, hypertrophy, speed, power, endurance, agility, reduce body fat
- Limitations: None, no injuries, well-equipped facility for training
- Testing Results: Scored well on most tests, needs to increase strength
- Training Needs: Integrated periodized strength and conditioning program consisting of resistance training (structured around Olympic lifts, basic strength exercises, ballistics, implements, sport-specific and assistance exercises), plyometrics, speed, and agility; off-season strength focus

a

(continued)

FIGURE 2.6 Sample needs analysis for *(a)* a college men's American football player (tight end).

Sample Needs Analysis: College Women's Volleyball Player—Outside Hitter

Player Profile

Height = 6'0"
Weight = 145 lbs
Age = 20 yrs
Volleyball exp = 7 yrs
Training exp = 4 yrs (advanced status)
Vertical jump = 17 in
Approach jump = 9 ft
Block jump = 9 ft
1RM bench press = 115 lbs
1RM squat = 205 lbs

- Sport/Position Need: Passing (bumping), setting, spiking, blocking, digging, serving, jumping, diving
- Major Muscle Groups: All muscle groups emphasized—special attention for lower-body strength and power, core and upper-body strength and power for blocking, spiking
- Muscle/Joint Actions: All major actions, focus on strength for all muscle actions—may target additional training for eccentric strength for better landing kinetics
- Common Injury Sites: Shoulder, knee, ankle, lower back, fingers

- Metabolic Demands: Predominately ATP-PC, glycolysis, good buffer capacity
- Fitness Demands: Muscular strength, high intensity endurance, power and jumping ability, quickness, mobility, reaction time, balance, coordination, agility, cutting/pivoting, flexibility; good aerobic base; low percent body fat

- Goals: Muscular strength, power and jumping ability, endurance, agility, reduce body fat
- Limitations: None, past knee injury, well-equipped facility for training
- Testing Results: Scored well on most tests, needs to increase strength, power, vertical jump

- Training Needs: Integrated periodized strength and conditioning program consisting of resistance training (structured around Olympic lifts, basic strength exercises, ballistics [e.g., jump squat], sport-specific and assistance exercises, injury prevention), plyometrics, agility; off-season strength and power focus

b

FIGURE 2.6 *(continued)* Sample needs analysis for *(b)* a college women's volleyball player (outside hitter).

Sport Evaluation

Sport evaluation involves an examination of each sport or position by identifying the biomechanical and kinesiological demands and the metabolic, biological, and physiological demands that target critical health- and skill-related fitness components.

Each position within each sport brings a unique blend of fitness qualities and motor skill applications to its optimal performance. Breaking down a sport begins with identifying the critical movements fundamental to play. Figure 2.6*a* and *b* depict some common fundamental movements paramount to many sports. For example, in baseball and softball, some of the major sport actions include throwing, pitching, catching (from multiple positions), hitting, bunting, base running, defensive play (e.g., a plethora of positions depending on where the ball is hit), sliding, diving, sprinting, jumping, squatting (for catchers), and integrated motions involving multiple components (i.e., charging a ball, catching, adjusting position, crow hop, and throw). The defensive play could involve movements such as linear sprints, side shuffles, backpedaling, cutting, change-of-direction and agility movements, hops, jumps (bilateral and unilateral), lunging, reaching, bending, and combination movements that allow the athlete to get in position properly, catch the ball, and throw. Identifying the basic movements allows the player development team to develop appropriate training measures to target improvements.

In many sports, specific analysis of each phase or sub-phase may be necessary; that is, breaking down a global locomotor skill into its units can identify weaknesses or areas that need targeting for improvement. Each phase and subphase serves as a target for training and allows the athletes to pinpoint specific elements of the movement to improve the skill's performance. For example, a powerlifter training to maximize their 1RM bench press must target each phase. Briefly, this entails targeting the negative phase, the pause, and the positive phase (max velocity, sticking region, and area of max strength) with specific training methods (e.g., heavy negatives, paused repetitions, partial repetitions, lockouts, and speed repetitions). Skill enhancement begins globally with general practice but proceeds to more specific training in each phase to maximize performance. This can only be accomplished once the phases and subphases are analyzed.

The next step is to analyze the underlying kinesiological elements. The kinesiological evaluations include identifying the major muscle groups involved in each skill and their roles (i.e., agonist, antagonist, stabilizer, and neutralizer), the major joint actions (i.e., flexion, extension, adduction, abduction, internal and external rotation, protraction and retraction, tilt, pronation, supination, combination movements), and the major muscle actions (i.e., concentric [CON], eccentric [ECC], and isometric [ISOM]). Although each skill involves most or even all of the muscles and actions, exercises are prescribed in training that stress each muscle group and the movements against a resistance that may enhance the strength, power, and speed of performance. For example, some athletes require higher levels of ECC and ISOM strength. These qualities may be targeted specifically with a variety of exercises. Exercise performance also entails powerful repetition velocities to mimic the neural drive needed to maximize motor unit recruitment, which is essential to transferring the training effects to movements specific to the field, court, pool, track, or gym.

The sport must also be analyzed for its temporal components. The nature of the sport helps determine the metabolic needs and potential interval nature that can be targeted through conditioning. The duration of the competition or game, number of quarters or halves, length of each game, number of plays per game, whether the sport involves continual motion (e.g., aerobic endurance sports), competitions per day (for tournaments or doubleheaders in baseball and softball), and play-recovery intervals need to be considered when developing the strength and conditioning program. For example, a college American football game consists of four 15-minute quarters with a 20-minute halftime; an offensive series averages 4.6 plays per series with approximately 14.4 series per game; each play averages 5.5 seconds (range of 1.9 to 12.9 seconds) with approximately 32.7 seconds in between plays (Kraemer and Gotshalk 2000; Hoffman 2008). These values may vary depending on the level of competition and the type of offensive strategies employed. Still, they provide a good framework for the coaching staff and strength and conditioning team to design interval programs to address the metabolic needs of the American football player. Other macrovariables such as season length (off-, pre-, and in-season periods, including potential for postseason play), competition schedule, and time of year (with environmental challenges) must be considered.

The last segment of the sport evaluation is the injury analysis. Analysis of the sport through research or one's team data enables the staff to identify the major sites and types of injuries seen in the sport. The mechanisms leading to the injury may be identified so that the strength and conditioning program can target susceptible areas and prehabilitate the athlete to avoid injuries in the long run. For example, female athletes are far more likely than their male counterparts to sustain a tear of the anterior cruciate ligament (ACL). Special attention can be given to strengthening the kinetic chain to prevent ACL injuries in female athletes. Concussions are concerns for collision athletes, combat athletes, soccer players, and catchers in baseball and softball. Including neck strengthening exercises in the program can reduce concussion risk significantly. Hamstring strains are common in athletes who sprint, accelerate, decelerate, and change directions at high velocities. Including an exercise such as the reverse hamstring curl (i.e., Russian or Nordic leg curl) in a training program has also been noted to reduce hamstring injuries. This is a short list of potential benefits accompanying the targeting of susceptible areas, and specific training recommendations are discussed in later chapters. Routine evaluation of team injuries enables the staff to ascertain the efficacy of the prehabilitation segment of the strength and conditioning program.

Metabolic, Biological, and Physiological Demands The needs analysis should also address the sport's metabolic, biological, and physiological demands. This involves targeting the critical health- and skill-related fitness components through the strength and conditioning program. The acute physiological responses and subsequent chronic adaptations to training enable improvements in the fitness components.

The metabolic demands of the sport refer to the contributions of energy systems to the activities. The major energy source in the human body is adenosine triphosphate (ATP), which is limited and must be replenished by three major energy systems: the *ATP-PC, glycolysis,* and *aerobic systems*. The first two systems are *anaerobic* (without oxygen) and help athletes sustain high-intensity exercise and sport performance. The *aerobic* (with oxygen) system is constant but provides long-term energy yield, especially for prolonged aerobic endurance exercise. All energy systems are engaged at all times, regardless of the activity. However, one may predominate at a specific moment based on the intensity, volume or duration, and recovery intervals of the sport or exercise. Table 2.1 depicts the metabolic demands of various sports that a coach may use for conducting a needs analysis of the sport to determine which energy systems need to be targeted or emphasized in training. Training programs can be designed to target each system by manipulating the intensity, volume or duration, and rest intervals used. An athlete whose sport requires the majority of energy from the ATP-PC system should target this system specifically with high-intensity, short bouts of explosive exercise. Metabolic specificity is critical to athletes' off-season, preseason, and in-season training. Interval training allows the athlete to train at higher intensities for periods using prescribed rest intervals. The athletes can dedicate more time to high intensities than continuous training, which may limit the intensity and depend on fatigue. Exercise-to-rest ratios of 1:10 indicate that athletes rest 10 times longer than the exercise interval. An explosive bout lasting approximately 8 seconds requires the athlete to rest for approximately 80 seconds. The exercise-to-rest ratio can target energy systems such that 1:12 to 1:20 ratios target ATP-PC, 1:3 to 1:5 ratios target glycolysis, 1:3 to 1:4 ratios target glycolysis and aerobic oxidation, and 1:1 to 1:3 ratios target the aerobic system.

Energy systems, primarily glycolysis, produce acids (H^+) that cause fatigue in human skeletal muscle. Another critical consideration of training (especially programs targeting glycolysis) is to improve *buffer capacity*, which refers to the body's ability to buffer or neutralize acids (and resist changes in pH), thereby delaying fatigue and improving aerobic endurance performance. Several substances in the blood and skeletal muscle (e.g., chemical buffers) and the lungs and kidneys (e.g., physiological buffers) help to buffer acids and maintain pH. Through training, these components are enhanced and allow the athlete to maintain performance at higher levels of acidosis. This is a critical component of preseason and in-season training. High-intensity interval training, also called *metabolic training*, targets the glycolysis

TABLE 2.1 Metabolic Demands of Sports

Sport	ATP-PC system	Anaerobic glycolysis	Aerobic metabolism
Baseball	High	Low	—
Basketball	High	Moderate to high	—
Boxing	High	High	Moderate
Diving	High	Low	—
Fencing	High	Moderate	—
Field events	High	—	—
Field hockey	High	Moderate	—
Football (American)	High	Moderate	Low
Gymnastics	High	Moderate	—
Golf	High	—	—
Ice hockey	High	Moderate	Moderate
Lacrosse	High	Moderate	Moderate
Marathon	Low	Low	High
Mixed martial arts	High	High	Moderate
Powerlifting	High	Low	Low
Skiing:			
Cross-country	Low	Low	High
Downhill	High	High	Moderate
Soccer	High	Moderate	Moderate
Strength competitions	High	Moderate to high	Low
Swimming:			
Short distance	High	Moderate	—
Long distance	—	Moderate	High
Tennis	High	Moderate	—
Track (athletics):			
Short distance	High	Moderate	—
Long distance	—	Moderate	High
Ultraendurance events	Low	Low	High
Volleyball	High	Moderate	—
Wrestling	High	High	Moderate
Weightlifting	High	Low	Low

Note: All types of metabolism are involved to some extent in all activities.

Reprinted by permission from N.A. Ratamess, "Adaptations to Anaerobic Training Programs," in *Essentials of Strength Training and Conditioning*, 3rd ed., edited by T.R. Baechle and R.W. Earle (Champaign, IL: Human Kinetics, 2008).

energy system, exposing athletes to high levels of acidosis and thereby promoting an environment conducive to adaptation. Athletes in sports that rely on glycolysis to a significant extent must focus on increasing buffering capacity. The needs analysis must reflect this during preseason or precompetition training phases.

Health-Related Fitness Components

The critical health-related fitness components include muscular strength, muscular endurance, aerobic endurance, flexibility, and body composition.

Muscular Strength Muscular strength is the maximum amount of force one can generate during a specific movement pattern at a specified contraction velocity. Acute muscular strength varies depending on the muscle action (ECC > ISOM > CON), range of motion, and contraction velocity; thus, strength variations can be measured. Critical physiological and biomechanical variables that contribute to muscular strength include the following:

- Neural drive and motor unit recruitment, firing rate, and temporal firing
- Muscle fiber type (fast-twitch > slow-twitch)
- Muscle fiber number, arrangement, and size
- Metabolics (i.e., substrate storage, such as ATP-PC, glycogen, and enzyme activity)
- Connective tissue support
- Anabolic hormone concentrations (testosterone, growth hormone superfamily, IGF-1, insulin) and signaling properties
- Muscle length and tendon insertion location (leverage)
- Stretch-shortening cycle potency

Based on the factors mentioned earlier that affect acute strength expression and the force–velocity relationship, where maximal force output depends on the movement velocity, different strength measures may be assessed and identified. Figure 2.7a depicts the concentric force–velocity and power–velocity relationships, and figure 2.7b represents the force–velocity curve for all muscle actions showing that strength is greater at a faster ECC velocity, and max ISOM force (depending on ROM) crosses the y-axis at 0 m/s velocity. At the low end of the velocity spectrum, maximal absolute dynamic strength is seen. This is assessed by the one repetition-maximum (1RM) for an exercise, defined as the maximal amount of weight lifted in one all-out effort and the limit of the physical capacity of an individual for a specific exercise. When maximal strength is expressed relative to body mass or lean body mass (the mass of nonfat tissue like muscle, bone, and water), it is defined as *relative muscular strength*. Relative muscular strength (or the *strength-to-mass ratio*) is critical for many athletes who compete in weight classes or against gravity because the higher the ratio, the more advantageous it is for that athlete. A high

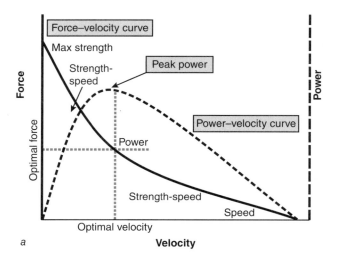

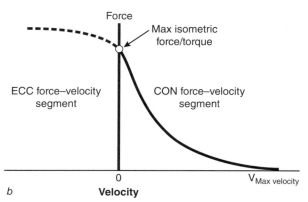

FIGURE 2.7 (a) The concentric force–velocity and power–velocity relationships. The segments of the force curve (max strength, strength-speed, power, speed-strength, and speed) are also labeled. (b) The eccentric (ECC) and concentric (CON) force–velocity (V) relationship.

strength-to-mass ratio enables high levels of force production without the addition of substantial mass gains where strength gains exceed increases in body mass. Relative strength measures have been used to compare lifting performances among athletes of different sizes and for benchmarking. For example, we have found that a 1RM back squat of at least 1.8 to 2.0 times body weight for female and male athletes respectively is a good threshold applicable to maximizing power and speed performance in athletes. Thus, both absolute and relative measures of maximal strength can be helpful to assessment tools and key performance indicators (KPIs) that can be tracked over time and used for their transfer effects to other sport-specific movements.

Maximal Isometric Force Maximal isometric force (strength) is ROM-specific. It can be determined in many ways and has high applications to athletes requiring significant levels of ISOM strength. For example, measures of grip strength, hip and back strength, and barbell exercises such as max ISOM mid-thigh pull, squat, and deadlift on a force plate can provide meaningful data to the player development team. Figure 2.7 shows that the CON force is reduced as movement velocity increases. This has formed the basis for the popular *velocity-based resistance training* methodology discussed later in this book. Shifting to the right, we see the *strength-speed* zone. This zone is where moderately heavy loading (80% to 90% of the 1RM) can be moved as fast as possible. The term *explosive strength* has also been used to describe the maximal velocity of movement with higher loading. Next, we see the *peak power* zone (30% to 80% of the 1RM), where the optimal interaction of force and velocity is seen. *Speed strength* is seen next (30% to 60% of the 1RM), where force and loading are reduced but the movement velocity is significantly faster. Lastly, we see the *speed zone* (less than 30% of the 1RM), where maximal velocity or speed of contraction is seen but substantially less force is produced as a result. Here we see the zone where body weight plyometrics, speed, and agility training take place. In addition, when velocity is controlled (e.g., isokinetic), strength output will differ. *Isokinetic strength testing* has been very popular for many years and is used as an assessment tool primarily in research and rehabilitation settings. However, some isokinetic devices (especially those that enable multiple-joint exercises) have become popular and have been used by some in training and assessment. Lastly, the term *functional strength* has been used. Functional strength describes the athlete's ability to display high levels of strength during sport-specific movements. Although practice and competition assist with functional strength development, the strength and conditioning program may target this specifically with loaded motion. For example, wearable resistance can help with speed (and related motion) development, weighted vests can be used to load many different locomotor movements, and implements have become popular for training muscular strength at many loading vectors or angles.

All types of muscular strength have significant implications for athletes. As mentioned in chapter 1, a key element of the long-term youth development athletic model is the focus on increasing muscular strength. Maximal muscular strength is a discriminant factor separating several groups of athletes at different competition levels. A case can be made that increasing strength is paramount for every athlete. This becomes obvious for sports requiring high levels of strength, such as powerlifting, American football, track-and-field throwing events, and wrestling and combat sports. However, muscular strength contributes to speed and power development, and the additional strength helps athletes in sports such as baseball and softball, soccer, volleyball, basketball, lacrosse, field hockey, and track-and-field sprint and jump events. For the aerobic endurance athlete, increased muscular strength helps increase exercise (e.g., running, cycling, swimming, and skiing) economy. Research has shown that the "big three" for the aerobic endurance competitor are $\dot{V}O_2$max, lactate threshold, and exercise economy. Although several factors contribute to the exercise economy, muscular strength is one of them and a major reason aerobic endurance athletes resistance train to increase their strength-to-mass ratio. A stronger athlete may epitomize the sport and take athletic performance to new heights. Thus, strength enhancement via resistance training should be a key priority of the needs analysis for all athletes.

Muscular Endurance Muscular endurance is the ability to sustain performance over time and to resist fatigue at multiple levels. The intensity (or difficulty of exercise) of the activity plays a substantial role. *Submaximal muscular endurance* is characterized by the ability to sustain low-intensity muscular activity for an extended period (e.g., the repetitive motion of an aerobic endurance athlete). *High-intensity endurance* or *strength endurance* is the ability to maintain high-intensity muscular activity over time. For example, it entails the ability to run repeated sprints (*repeated sprint ability*) with similar times or perform a specific number of repetitions for a resistance exercise over a number of sets despite a rest interval in between sets. Both types of muscular endurance are critical to many sports involving aerobic endurance (e.g., cross country running, skiing, and cycling) or intermittent bouts of explosive activity followed by lower-intensity activity (e.g., basketball and soccer). Some degree of endurance is also required for predominate ATP-PC athletes, particularly repeated high-intensity endurance. For example, a lifter will have three attempts to achieve a 1RM for two to three exercises (in weightlifting and powerlifting). A baseball player may have several intense intermittent bouts of activity spaced over a period lasting a few hours (except pitchers and catchers). Thus, the athlete must have adequate aerobic endurance to recover between extensive rest intervals but perform at a maximal level once the sport demands require it. Endurance testing is multidimensional and can form a key element in profiling. Muscular endurance may be tested using body weight tests over time (e.g., push-up, pull-up, and sit-up), repetitions to failure with standard loading, and sustained maximal duration trials that are especially useful for assessing core or trunk stability and muscular endurance (e.g., plank and side plank tests, Biering-Sorensen test, etc.). Other tests assessing other components (i.e., repeated jump tests and repeated sprints) may also have a muscular endurance component. Overall, increasing muscular endurance is critical to optimizing sport performance and often is targeted later in the periodization cycle as the season or competition approaches.

Aerobic Endurance Aerobic endurance is the ability to perform prolonged exercise at moderate to high exercise intensities. Aerobic endurance is highly related to the functioning of the lungs, heart, and circulatory system, as well as to the capacity of skeletal muscle to extract oxygen and thereby sustain performance. The key measure of aerobic endurance, or *aerobic capacity*, is maximal oxygen uptake or $\dot{V}O_2$max. $\dot{V}O_2$max is the product of systemic factors (cardiac output; i.e., heart rate × stroke volume) and peripheral factors (arterial-venous O_2 difference), also known as the *Fick equation*, and it depends on many factors, including sex, age, mode of activity, and body size. A high or moderately high $\dot{V}O_2$max is critical for success in aerobic endurance athletes, and a good aerobic base can also enhance recovery from anaerobic exercise. For example, aerobic endurance athletes have the highest measured relative $\dot{V}O_2$max values (60 to 85 ml/kg/min and beyond), whereas hybrid athletes such as soccer players, basketball players, and wrestlers (50 to 65 ml/kg/min) as well as ATP-PC athletes such as baseball players and powerlifters (40 to 55 ml/kg/min) tend to have lower values with values higher in male than in female athletes. Since 20% to 50% of the variance in $\dot{V}O_2$max values is explained by genetics, training will have a profound effect on the athlete as increases of 10% to 30% may be seen during the first six months of training (Ratamess 2022). Aerobic training is the best way to increase $\dot{V}O_2$max and is paramount for aerobic endurance athletes.

Flexibility Flexibility is the ability of a joint to move freely through its ROM. *Static flexibility* refers to ROM at a joint or joints during active or passive movement where the final position is held. *Dynamic flexibility* refers to the ROM during movement and includes ballistic flexibility during fast movements. Enhanced joint flexibility can reduce the risk for certain types of injury (but not all), improve muscle balance and function, increase performance, improve mobility and posture, and reduce the incidence of low back pain. The best ways to increase flexibility are to perform exercises in a full ROM (especially those requiring high levels of joint ROM) and engage in a proper flexibility or stretching program (e.g., with myofascial release, static and dynamic stretching, proprioceptive neuromuscular facilitation [PNF] stretching, and yoga), preferably at the end of an aerobic or anaerobic workout when the muscles are thoroughly warmed up or as a part of a flexibility, mobility, and corrective exercise workout. Athletes such as gymnasts and dancers require very high levels of flexibility (figure 2.8). Other

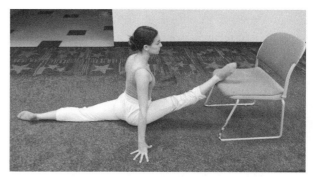

FIGURE 2.8 Flexibility is highly variable from athlete to athlete.

Photo courtesy of Jenna Ingui and Dr. Nick Ratamess.

athletes need sufficient flexibility to perform various skills within a sport. For example, flexibility in the shoulders, spine, and hips is required for the proper performance of an overhead squat or snatch as well as for wrestling, and good hip flexibility is required for hurdling in track-and-field. Thus, the needs analysis should determine which areas of the body require flexibility so that the strength and conditioning program can target these areas.

Body Composition *Body composition* refers to the proportion of fat and fat-free mass throughout the body. Fat-free mass (or lean body mass) consists of bone, muscle, water, and other nonfat tissues. For most athletes, desired body composition involves minimizing the fat component while maintaining or increasing the lean body mass component. We previously described the anthropometric elements of sport performance. Here, we focus primarily on lean tissue mass and percent body fat. The most effective way to enhance body composition is to eat correctly and train regularly. Resistance training, as well as other forms of anaerobic training, is effective for improving body composition because it increases lean body mass (muscle and bone components) while reducing fat. *Hypertrophy* is another desired component for some athletes who need high levels of strength or size in their respective sport or position. Aerobic training plays a significant role in reducing fat mass and a lesser role in enhancing lean tissue mass. Body composition plays a crucial role in those sports where weight classes are used (e.g., wrestling and weightlifting), where athletes have to overcome their body mass for success (e.g., high jump, gymnastics, and aerobic endurance sports), or where athletic competition is based on physique development (e.g., bodybuilding).

Skill-Related Fitness Components

The critical skill-related fitness components include power, balance, reaction time, speed, and agility.

Power *Power* is the rate of performing work. Because power is the product of force and velocity, there is a strength component to power development (strength at low-to-high velocities of movement). Figure 2.7a depicts the relationship between power, force, and velocity. The curve is parabolic, as peak power is produced at the optimal interaction of force and velocity. Light-to-moderate loading performed as fast as possible for many exercises leads to maximal power expression. The optimal expression of muscle power relies on the correct exercise technique. Although the terms *power* and *strength* are sometimes used interchangeably, this must be corrected. Power has a time component; thus, if two athletes display similar strength, the one who expresses strength at a higher rate (higher velocity or shorter period of time) will have a distinct advantage during the performance of strength and power sports. In addition, power has been described in terms of strength. For example, terms such as *speed strength* and *acceleration strength* have been used to define force development across a spectrum of velocities. *Starting strength* describes power production during the initial segment of the movement. The *rate of force development* represents the time needed to reach a threshold level of force or the amount of energy produced per second. The velocity component of the power equation indicates that high contraction velocities (or at least the intent to contract at maximal velocities even against a heavy resistance) of muscle contraction are imperative. Therefore, power development is multidimensional, involving the enhancement of both force and velocity components. Muscle power may be enhanced via resistance training, speed, agility, and plyometric training and through sport-specific practice and conditioning. Power measures are crucial in testing, profiling, and benchmarking athletes. For example, vertical and broad jumps are commonly used as power measures and, ultimately, stretch-shortening cycle capacity. When coupled with force plates, jumps may be used to ascertain critical KPIs over time. For example, dual force plates allow for bilateral and unilateral components for examining potential asymmetries. Jump data can be used to determine key metrics such as *reactive strength*, *reactive strength index-modified*, *ECC utilization ratio*, and *prestretch augmentation percent* (discussed later in this book). The use of linear position transducer technology enables power assessment during the ballistic jump squat (and other exercises). Upper-body power may be assessed on a force plate using the plyo push-up, ballistic bench press (bench throw), or medicine ball–throwing tests. In addition, power tests have been instrumental in determining workout types within a flexible nonlinear periodization training model.

Balance *Balance* is the ability of an individual to maintain equilibrium. Specifically, *static balance* requires the athlete to remain upright and stable during a static position, whereas *dynamic balance* requires the body to remain stable during active motion. It requires control over the athlete's center of gravity, line of gravity, and base support and allows the athlete to maintain proper body position during complex motor skill performance. The needs analysis should determine the types and magnitudes of balance needed. Balance can be enhanced by strength and power training, plyometrics, flexibility, sprint and agility training, specific balance training (with unstable equipment, unilateral exercises, exercises with small base supports, and combination exercises), and sport-specific practice. *Gross motor coordination* refers to the ability of an individual to perform a motor skill with good technique, rhythm, and accuracy. Critical elements of coordination include balance, spatial awareness, timing, and motor learning. Likewise, coordination can be improved by similar training methods. Sport-specific practice is crucial because repetitive exposure to different motor patterns is essential to improving motor coordination.

Reaction Time *Reaction time* is responding rapidly to a stimulus; that is, it involves the ability of the brain and nervous system to identify the stimulus and form a corrective strategy in response. Part of reaction time is rapid visual processing. Reaction time is critical to sport performance. The quicker an athlete reacts to a stimulus, the more likely success will be obtained. Some athletic skills require response times of less than half a second (e.g., hitting a 95-mph [153 kph] fastball in baseball). The ability to react quickly is necessary and can be used to separate athletes of a different caliber. Complicating matters is that reaction time can be impaired by fatigue but improved with pre-exercise energy supplements (Hoffman et al. 2009; Hoffman et al. 2010). The reaction time may be enhanced by explosive exercise (e.g., power, sprint, agility, and quickness training) and sport-specific practice. We have seen advances in technology address reaction time testing and training, including equipment that requires the athlete to respond to a stimulus (at different levels and temporal patterns), such as lights or sound (e.g., light-emission training systems and stroboscopic visual training); dynamic visual training; and virtual reality training and gaming that place athletes in simulated real-life situations. Complete player development entails athletes taking advantage of new technology to maximize performance. *Stroboscopic visual training* was designed to provide a training tool to improve an athlete's visual, perceptual, and cognitive skills and athletic performance. It is based on visual interruption via strobing lights to improve visual-motor control by forcing athletes to rely less on their vision and make better use of the limited visual information available (Appelbaum et al. 2011). Reaction lights and similar devices can be used for many drills and incorporated with strength and conditioning exercises and sport-specific movements. For example, reaction lights can enhance hand speed and reaction ability in boxing, MMA, and other striking sports. Varying the locations, timing, pattern, and several lights can create a stimulus capable of improving performance. Lights may be used to create a specific cadence for exercise (e.g., tapping the light at the end of a reaching drill or strength and conditioning exercise such as a sit-up). In addition, incorporating lights into a workout circuit creates a scenario where the athlete must display good reaction time during a fatigued state, which is common in real-life sport performance. Several elite athletes from many sports have included visual and reaction light training in their strength and conditioning programs and found it vital.

Speed *Speed* is the capacity of an athlete to move as rapidly as possible and is an essential component of the sport. For example, linear running speed is composed of three phases: (1) acceleration, (2) maximum speed, and (3) deceleration (if the sprint is at least 60 yards or meters). The *acceleration* phase is characterized by an increase in speed and relies on strength, power, and reaction time. The *maximum speed* phase is characterized by the individual's attainment of their fastest speed and how long they can maintain it (e.g., speed endurance). The *deceleration* phase results from fatigue and is characterized by the individual involuntarily decreasing speed after maximum speed has been attained. Speed may be enhanced by a combination of methods, including nonassisted and assisted sprint training, strength and power training, plyometrics, technique training, and sport-specific practice. Routine assessment of speed is critical to athlete profiling and benchmarking.

Agility *Agility* is the ability of an athlete to change direction rapidly without a significant loss of speed, balance, or bodily control. Being agile requires power, strength, balance, coordination, quickness, speed, visual scanning, perception and anticipation, and neuromuscular control. Agility is a critical component of any sport that requires rapid changes of direction, decelerations, and accelerations. Agility training is multimodal and composed of predetermined drills (*closed drills*) and drills that force the athlete to anticipate, adjust, and react explosively (*open drills*). Developing change-of-direction ability (control of the body during cutting, pivoting, and directional changes), agility movement technique (e.g., backpedaling and side shuffling) from different body positions, mobility, acceleration, deceleration, and linear speed is critical to agility training. Likewise, agility can be enhanced by plyometrics, multidirectional agility and reactive drills, strength and power training, balance training, and sport-specific practice. The needs analysis must determine the level and types of agility needed for the sport, and specific training may be added to the strength and conditioning program.

Training Factors

The second major component of the needs analysis is determining the training factors. The information gained will give the player development team pertinent information regarding the following questions that need to be answered:

- *What is the training status of the athlete?* This includes years of sport participation plus years spent with each training modality implemented. Training status is determined not only by years of experience but also by the associated technique and gains made by the athlete.

- *What are the athlete's training goals?* Improved performance, muscular strength, hypertrophy, muscular endurance, aerobic endurance, flexibility, mobility, body composition, injury prevention, health, balance, speed, agility, power, reaction time, coordination, and sport-specific KPIs (e.g., punching power, throwing and kicking velocity, and tennis serve velocity) are common goals. More detailed goals may be associated with each one of these major goals.

- *Are there health and injury concerns that may limit the exercise or intensity?* An injury or health concern may limit some exercises and training intensity until sufficient recovery has ensued. Exercises can be selected to work around an injury.

- *What type of facility will the athlete be training at?* Equipment availability is paramount to exercise selection. Although effective programs can be developed with minimal equipment, knowledge of what is available allows one to select appropriate exercises and variations. In addition, it is good for the athlete to train with teammates in a well-equipped team facility with trained staff supervision.

- *What is the training frequency, and are there any time constraints that may affect workout duration?* The total number of training sessions per week needs to be derived initially because this will affect all other training variables, such as exercise selection, volume, and intensity. Some athletes may be scheduled at specific blocks of time. If this block of time is 1.5 hours, then the program must be developed within that time frame. The exercises selected, the number of exercises and total sets performed, and rest intervals between sets and exercises will be affected.

- *What areas require special attention?* All major muscle groups need to be trained, but some may require prioritization based on strengths and weaknesses or on the demands of the sport. It is important to maintain muscle balance, especially among those muscles with agonist–antagonist relationships, primary stabilizer roles for large muscle mass exercises, and small muscles that are often weaker than larger muscle groups. The sport injury analysis yields results that can be used to emphasize areas susceptible to injury (e.g., stressing the core and hips to reduce knee injuries in female athletes, or strengthening the neck to reduce concussions in American football players).

- *What is the team training and competition schedule?* The yearly macrocycle must be determined around the needs of the sport. Determining the off-season, preseason, and in-season periods, as well as subsequent activities, is paramount to designing the training program and optimizing recovery for team-sport athletes. This planning considers practice, competition, and travel schedules. For single-competition sports, preparatory and competition periods must be determined and applied to the number of competitions in one year. College student-athletes have the rigors of academic study to fit into their schedules, so training must consider the extracurricular load and stressors on the athlete. The players' position and playing status need to be acknowledged. For example, some positions in sports have special requirements that need to be addressed through training. Also, starter versus nonstarter status is important. Nonstarters may require more attention and training time in-season to stay in shape, whereas starters dominate playing time and are exposed to higher activity levels.

- *What are the environmental concerns and limitations?* The locations of the athlete's training, both indoors and outdoors, need to be established. Information related to the weather conditions (e.g., heat, humidity, precipitation, cold, and wind), outdoor surfaces (e.g., track surface, grass, sand, and concrete), inclinations and declinations (e.g., for hill or speed training), and altitude need to be determined because these can influence the training program implementation.

The information above sets the table for designing the program. The player development team must consider all this information while preparing the training plan. Program design begins with selecting and organizing the targeted training modalities. For each modality, the acute program variables must be addressed. These include the exercise selection, order, intensity, volume and duration, training velocity, frequency, workout structure, set structure, rest intervals or the ratio of exercise to rest, and timed elements (for circuits, intervals, and time trials). The system of monitoring and use of technology must be determined. For example, programs may be given to athletes and tracked with iPads and tracking software. For resistance training, sets, repetitions, and loads can be monitored. Linear position transducers may be used to measure bar velocity and power. Heart rate and kinematic data (e.g., displacement, peak velocity, and velocity) may be tracked with GPS or LPS—global and local positioning systems—to monitor player load (see chapter 3). The training must be designed using an appropriate periodization plan. The specifics of training program design and monitoring are discussed later in this book. Ultimately, the training program will be implemented and supervised by staff that is certified and proficient in strength and conditioning.

Profiling and Benchmarking

The needs analysis provides the initial information needed for program design and the profiling and benchmarking of athletes. *Profiling* involves creating a composite of an athlete based on KPIs that can be monitored over time and used to compare norms, standards, or previous data from the athlete (i.e., *benchmarking*). For example, the initial screening of the athlete, testing results, determination of strengths and weaknesses, and goals determined by the needs analysis form the initial profile of the athlete. Upon implementation of the strength and conditioning program, workouts and performance of KPIs are monitored over time and used to determine progress. Profiling and benchmarking can be used for short- and long-term training, from an individual workout to specific use for the entire macrocycle. Benchmarking assists the player development team in identifying areas that need more training attention, and it is essential that staff benchmark accurately, by comparing, for example, athletes to norms from athletic samples that are similar in age and maturation, competition level, weight class, and sport position.

The KPIs used in sports can be extensive, especially as the sport data analytics field and evaluation technology evolve. Because KPIs include measurable values to indicate the efficacy of how specific training and sport objectives are being met, they are tracked over time, help form the athlete composite or profile, and are compared for benchmarking over desired periods of time. KPIs should be valid, reliable (i.e., trained staff should use standardized procedures and equipment), and consistently measured to provide an accurate means of benchmarking and gauging athlete performance changes over time. Considering that KPIs are benchmarked, they should be realistic and based on the appropriate outcome. The player development team must identify critical KPIs used in their programs to quantify the success of their strength and conditioning and athletic development programs. KPI determination is a dynamic process that changes as goals, strategies, and knowledge change. Given that KPIs envelop the complete player development process, they should match the philosophy of the coaching staff and the strength and conditioning or sport science team.

KPIs are used to evaluate the needs analysis implementation. Given that the needs analysis consists of sport evaluation, biological and physiological demands, biomechanical and kinesiological factors, and training program design and implementation, KPIs may vary depending on the segment of the needs analysis. For example, sport-specific data may be obtained and used as KPIs. Sport-specific KPIs may be *skill-based* or *strategy-based*. Skill-based KPIs can be used as an assessment of technique analysis. Video analysis is a large component of athlete monitoring. In some sports, all competitions may have some element recorded for further analysis. Expert observations by coaching staff are essential to providing a valid means of technical evaluation. Coaches may compare the performance video to a reference standard or desired method of performance and form their evaluation. Video analysis may be compared over time as a form of benchmarking to evaluate progress. This will allow the coaching staff to identify errors, maximize performance, and reduce injury risk. Thus, skill-based KPIs rely in part on subjective information. Although high-tech 3D motion analysis may be used to determine specific joint angles, displacements and ROM, linear and angular velocities, and accelerations, motor skill performance is still interpreted by the coaching staff. Skill-based KPIs can be determined throughout the year for athletes involved in single-competition sports or aesthetic sports. In team sports, skill-based KPIs are more commonly used in preseason and in-season periods because some athletes may focus on the strength and conditioning program rather than the sport itself during the off-season.

Strategy-based KPIs refer to quantifiable attributes relevant to the player and team success, especially for team-sport athletes and athletes for whom performance data are available (e.g., weight lifted in lifting sports, race times, etc.). These metrics are commonly seen in sports as a form of tracking performance. For example, Major League Baseball uses a plethora of metrics to gauge performance. Some examples include batting average, home runs, runs batted in, stolen bases, strikeouts, walks, on-base percentage, slugging percentage, OPS (on-base percentage plus slugging), and many other advanced batting performance metrics such as launch angle, ball exit velocity, hard-hit rate, batting average on balls in play, wins above replacement (WAR), expected batting average, and many more used to monitor hitting performance. KPIs for all aspects of the game exist and are used in-season to analyze performance. Individual and team statistics are also used, and since the rise in popularity of *sport data analytics* (see below), many teams have employed an analytics team to monitor KPIs and evaluate performance. This information is used primarily to evaluate talent for recruiting, for professional sport contracts, and for management and coaching of the sport. In professional sports, the data analytics department is part of the player development team. Other sports have similar extensive KPIs. Thus, strategy-based KPIs are those determined at several points throughout a competitive season as part of the evaluation of sport performance (see figure 2.9).

Physiologically-based KPIs represent data obtained from testing and monitoring internal and external load. As previously discussed, several health- and skill-related fitness components exist, and there are several ways to test each component and sub-component (see chapter 3 for testing). Some examples include 1RM strength testing, vertical jump, 40-yard (37 m) dash, percent body fat, and $\dot{V}O_2$max. The player development team must develop a realistic testing schedule consistent with regular training and practice. Testing-based KPIs have been commonly used in athletes for many

Key Performance Indicators (KPIs)

Internal (KPIs)

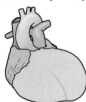

- Heart rate (resting, exercise) and TRIMP
- Heart rate variability
- Blood lactate
- Blood biochemistry (hormones, damage markers, immune cells, etc.)
- Body composition
- Sleep
- Mood state
- Effort perception (RPE, session RPE)

External (KPIs)

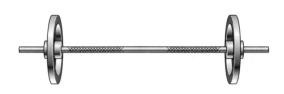

- Weight lifted/repetitions performed
- Repetition velocity and power
- Ground reaction force measures and jump height
- Distance covered
- Time, speed, and acceleration parameters
- Foot contacts and throws
- GPS/LPS data
- Sport-specific measures

FIGURE 2.9 Sample KPIs.

years. The second element of physiologically-based KPIs is data derived from the daily monitoring of athletes. Monitoring involves collecting data from athletes regularly to quantify the extent of *internal* (e.g., physiological and psychological) and *external* (e.g., workout performance output) loads. Some examples of internal load include heart rate (resting and during exercise), heart rate variability, blood pressure, ratings of perceived exertion, blood biomarkers (lactate, hormones, damage markers, etc.), and sleep quality. Some examples of external load include weight lifted, repetitions performed, repetition velocity and power, ground reaction force measures, distance covered, time parameters, foot contacts, throws, and GPS and LPS data.

Managing internal and external load and the extraordinary amount of data that can be generated with modern technology is essential for the player development team, especially for the sport scientist who may collect, analyze, and present the results to the rest of the strength and conditioning team and coaching staff. Matching load to player performance is critical to optimizing training, performance, recovery, and reducing injuries. It is important to note that the monitoring of KPIs may exist at different intervals. For example, sport-specific KPIs are determined primarily during or close to the season or competition. Training-related KPIs are determined mostly year-round, coincide with athletic testing and monitoring, and may be determined in-season as part of the maintenance training program. Thus, it is important to note that KPI determination via testing should not disrupt regular training. Extra testing is unnecessary to derive more data points for comparison. Instead, testing and KPI determination should fall within the athlete's regular training and competition macrocycle.

Impact of Athlete to Sport to Position Matching

Matching an athlete to a sport becomes easier as the athlete's age increases. As discussed in this book, participation in multiple sports and a properly designed and supervised strength and conditioning program can benefit the athlete in the early phases of a sports career. As the competitive levels increase, the optimal placement and position in a sport is vital as the demands of competition challenge the athlete composite. A host of examples exist of mismatches made due to proximal needs in

Sport Data Analytics

Sport data analytics (SDA) is the study of how player attributes and performance data affect outcomes and team success for team-sport athletes. Strengths and weaknesses can be determined (similarly to performing a needs analysis) and targeted through training and practice. The SDA market size is now billions of dollars and growing rapidly. In combination with the rise of technology, machine learning, and artificial intelligence, SDA has created a lucrative field in which teams can assess many components of the sport. Colleges and universities offer majors and certification programs in some facets of SDA. Data are readily available and serve to help athletes perform better. For example, during a Major League Baseball game a player may be in the dugout watching their previous at-bat on an iPad or getting digital scouting reports on the new pitcher who just entered the game. Combined with the increasing availability of data from video, wearable sensors, and other monitoring systems, the SDA team has played an increasingly important role in the player development team. Coaches constantly receive data from the SDA team and use it to influence coaching strategy. SDA is commonly used for numerous aspects of sports, including team strategy, player evaluations and recruiting, professional player contracts, the strength and conditioning program, and injury prevention. Coaches use SDA for scouting and game strategy, while front offices use it to prioritize player development.

SDA should serve as a complementary guide to coaching and should refrain from dominating every coaching decision made regarding the team. In some sports, there are disagreements between the traditional coaching staff and the SDA departments. Sometimes, the SDA is viewed as the deciding factor for coaching decisions. The coaching staff needs to balance the SDA with the current game scenario to make the best possible decisions for the team. For example, in baseball, a "hot" pitcher may be taken out of a game (after yielding no runs and a few hits) because of a certain theoretical pitch count, but the next pitcher who comes in then gives up several runs. After the game, the coach may ask why the first pitcher was taken out. "The SDA says his performance decreases at this pitch count level." In this scenario, although the coach noticed no signs of fatigue, the SDA was used anyway and produced a poor decision because the current environment was not taken into account. The old expression "That's why you play the game" means that matchups on paper do not determine the game's outcome. SDA and scouting reports can be used to influence decision-making, but many things determine the final outcomes, some of which are not in the SDA reports or in any foreseeable circumstances. Predictability in sports should be approached with suspicion. Even multiple SDA reports do not always provide accuracy. If they did, coaches would never lose and anyone could be a millionaire from sports betting and fantasy sports. The expression could be amended in the following way: "Games are not played on paper or on a computer." If computer decisions based on SDA were the sole factor for coaching, we probably would no longer need coaches. The human factors should not be removed from coaching. Instead, coaching should complement science. Historically, the "it factor" or the mark of a great coach has been the ability to make the right decisions at the right time.

a particular sport in a school, club, or community where the number of possible participants is low. Thus, the athlete who would never be a starting center on the high school basketball team at 5 foot 10 inches (178 cm) in a large school may play the position at a small school. The transition to other positions at the next level is likelier in basketball than in other sports. But if that athlete then competes in that position against the 6-foot 8-inch (203 cm) center, the results would be consequential due to the mismatch of largely nonmutable characteristics. Therefore, mismatches can have both acute and chronic effects on the athlete's competitive potential and development.

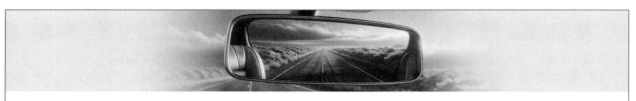

LOOKING IN THE REARVIEW MIRROR

It is crucial to understand the athlete composite and match the athlete with the sport by analyzing and being aware of the importance of talent identification, anthropometrics, and sport performance. The player development team should be built up to include coaching staff, athletic trainers, physical therapists, physicians, strength and conditioning staff, sport scientists and analysts, sport nutritionists, sport psychologists and sociologists, and academic advisers. An effective needs analysis involves breaking down the kinesiological, metabolic, physiological, and biomechanical elements of the sport and relating it to practice, the strength and conditioning program, and the profiling and benchmarking of the cthlete.

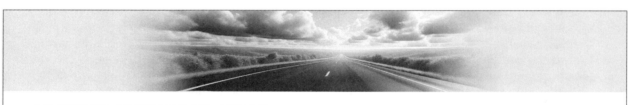

LOOKING AT THE ROAD AHEAD

Testing is needed to accurately understand the athlete's composite and to use it to monitor the effectiveness of training programs. Accurate testing is often sacrificed for the notion that approximation is good enough, but in reality, it is not good enough for decisions that affect the athlete's player development. Therefore, it is crucial for the player development team to understand the available tests, what those tests reflect, and the standardization protocols for each testing profile. The road ahead involves intense study of the area of testing and its role in player development.

Testing and Assessments in Player Development

Assessments and testing in a player development program are only effective if they have purpose and intentionality to respond to the data. The assessment domains help characterize the athlete composite to better understand who that athlete is. As presented in chapter 2, testing data are essential for optimally placing an athlete in a sport or a position in a team sport and can also help establish the sport's recruiting needs and position profiles. The athlete composite's testing and assessment database should be developed with secure repositories and historical archives for later study. Data collection, monitoring, and evaluation are time-intensive efforts if the player development team is to be effective in optimizing the athlete composite. Player safety and care in any testing assessment are the necessary top priorities. Sports medicine unit members should be ready to address any injury situation with emergency procedures.

A fundamental concept, referred to as the *three Cs*, must be addressed by the player development team. The three Cs represent the primary drivers of an individual player development team member to contribute to the group dynamic's success or failure. It is imperative to honestly assess each stakeholder's ability, commitment to the cause, and roles within the team.

- *Credentials:* Formal education, degrees, certifications, special skills, and mentorship experience. High-level performers have each of these types of credentials.

- *Competence:* Beyond credentials, the ability to evaluate and solve problems, implement the science, and understand one's own limitations while working to develop professionally each day is key to competence in a specific professional field. Competent professionals understand the necessary principles of their area of expertise, keep up with continuing educational opportunities, and have the ability to apply theoretical understanding and execute skills at an industry-leading level.

- *Commitment:* Commitment is almost always situational and has a shelf life. Highly competent people with credentials must also put in the effort to push through adversity and hardships. They must be committed to giving the individual athlete the best product of their professional skill sets and be competitive enough to desire to be the best in the industry in their roles on player development teams.

In every group setting, individuals are expected to combine their roles and produce a sum that is more significant than its parts—however, a failure at any level of the three Cs results in underperformance and interpersonal friction. Elite professionals will become frustrated and leave the group if underperformers are promoted not by their output but by selective tribalism. Great organizations must prioritize recruiting, rewarding, and retaining

> ### The Three Cs to Athlete Development:
> ### Winning Championships Through Group Dynamics
>
> During the creation of this book, we developed a new framework for understanding group dynamics, which we call the 'Three Cs.' This framework posits that the success or failure of any group is contingent upon three critical elements. For a team to function effectively, it is vital that these elements are cultivated and maintained among all stakeholders:
>
> - **Credentials:** This encompasses the formal education and mentorship experiences that individuals bring to the table. Such background ensures that the foundational knowledge necessary for the group's objectives is present.
> - **Competence:** More than just academic understanding, competence is about effectively applying skills and delivering at a level that sets industry standards. It's the practical execution that transforms theory into results.
> - **Commitment:** Unlike the relatively static nature of credentials and competence, commitment is dynamic and can fluctuate with the context. It refers to the willingness to persevere through challenges and is not indefinite—it has a lifespan that requires renewal through motivation and engagement.
>
> In group settings, each member is expected to contribute in a way that the collective outcome surpasses the sum of individual efforts. However, shortcomings in any one of the Three Cs can lead to underperformance and interpersonal conflict. Elite professionals may become disenchanted when contributions are overshadowed by internal politics or "selective tribalism"—a situation where decisions are influenced more by group loyalty than by merit. This can lead to their departure from the group.
>
> For organizations striving for excellence, it is vital to prioritize the recruitment and ongoing support of top-tier talent. An objective assessment of the Three Cs should be a continuous process, offering a robust foundation for leadership and team development. By recognizing and nurturing these core qualities, organizations position themselves to foster a culture of high performance and commitment.

top performers on player development teams by providing internal and external evaluations of the three Cs. The level of expectations related to the three Cs provides an excellent foundation for any evaluation and composite of the team leadership structure.

Once in the program, the player development team must set goals for each athlete. After examining the goals, the interventions need to be designed and determined for the start of the individual athlete's training cycle. Monitoring the progress of the many programs through different training and competition cycles becomes the primary demand for the player development team. Workouts, practices, and game demands must be monitored and evaluated (French and Torres Ronda 2022). It is a time-demanding but crucial task for the strength and conditioning professional to work daily with the data. Assessments and monitoring of workout performance and recovery, as well as determining the prescriptions for the next workout, influence how effectively the interventions achieve the athlete's goals and will be covered in more detail in chapter 5.

Setting the Standards for Testing and Assessments

The player development team members must be committed to developing a valid testing and assessment program and then responding to the data. Therefore, player development program professionals must hold to the program's core values and standards. This means that the evidence-based practice paradigm must be used in decision-making and in guiding choices. When the player development team administers a test, it must meet the highest standards of safety, efficacy, and responsibility for implementing precise testing methods and data analysis.

Testing protocols must be determined for each sport, and procedures must be carefully scrutinized. The multitude of tests available to a program can be daunting and requires an evidence-based process. Testing should be of laboratory quality, whether in maximal strength testing or survey assessments. Accuracy of record-keeping and proper techniques is vital for all testing protocols and exercise sessions (French and Torres Ronda 2022). The data generated from testing and workouts will be used for making important decisions. The seriousness of such a process must be understood by each member of the player development team.

It is essential that all testing follows the standards and guidelines set forth by science and the industry (e.g., the American College of Sports Medicine, the National Strength and Conditioning Association, and the National Athletic Trainers Association) so that tests of physical performance or biomarkers of physiological systems are valid (Liguori 2021; Miller 2012; NSCA 2017). Field and laboratory testing protocols have also been extensively examined in books on this topic (Fukuda 2019; Janot and Beltz 2023; French and Torres Ronda 2022). Protocols should be listed in specific steps and practiced by the player development team members involved with testing.

Certified professionals, experienced and trained in administering the tests within their scope of practice, are responsible for supervising and teaching assistants who are helping in any testing sessions. Testing and assessment data will be collected for daily use and evaluation by some units, such as strength and conditioning and athletic training, with other data coming from other player development units at different points in a training or competitive cycle (e.g., nutritional intake, formal testing protocols, psychological mood states, sleep profiles, and sports medicine physicals). In this case, a unified database is essential for each athlete in a sport. As the saying goes, "everything affects everything," so there can be no blind spots in the data availability from a computer database when working daily with an individual athlete.

In many cases, a university faculty adviser working in sport science and human performance can assist a player development program, especially when trained scientists are outside the organized player development team or when funding and costs demand alternative organizational structures. Another benefit of coordinating with faculty adviser units could be getting the data collected approved by the local ethics or institutional review board. Such data can then be used in formal research papers. Informed consent is a crucial factor in getting approval for the use of data in research. Using data from research with human subjects in scientific publications must have the permission of an ethics board or an institutional review board.

Additionally, medical data must adhere to local government laws and regulations in the United States and comply with the Health Insurance Portability and Accountability Act of 1996 (HIPAA), a federal law to prevent sensitive health information from being disclosed without the patient's consent or knowledge. All data should be collected with the athlete's knowledge and with the same level of care and precision as if it will be used for research purposes. All the data in a player development program needs to be stored, handled, and secured as medical data for an athlete. Finally, such a database development process takes funding, thought, optimal use of available software technology, education, and a systematic approach by the player development team. It is the foundation for visually and analytically "bringing to life" the player development program for the different professionals within the team as well as to the athlete, sport coaches, and athletic administration.

The athlete needs to understand the purpose of each test and how to perform it. It is also essential that athletes practice the tests several times before they are tested. This can be difficult in some cases, but testing done without adequate practice on a different day can lead to very low reliability in the actual score, in which case the true capability may be dramatically lower than what is shown in the test. Additionally, it is essential to discuss with athletes why tests are vital to their development. The risks involved with the test can also be discussed in this process.

With any physical performance test, it is well known that there is always some risk. However, the player development team member needs to discuss how the risks of the test will be limited or reduced if the athlete pays attention and works with the testing team to prepare for the actual test. Enough time should be allotted for each athlete to personally interact with a player development team member involved in the testing to ask questions, practice the tests, and feel comfortable with each test's proper techniques and demands. With trained professionals performing the tests, several steps can be taken to reduce or limit potential risks for any tests being performed. The steps include the following:

- Athletes medically cleared
- Testers certified in CPR and first aid
- Emergency procedures documented and practiced
- Emergency equipment, such as an automated external defibrillator (AED), checked and available at the testing site, steps documented, and procedures practiced
- Athletes have practiced the tests
- Performance technique is standardized (i.e., range of motion, grip and foot spacing, and rest intervals)
- The appropriate number of qualified testing assistants are present to conduct the test
- Proper hydration is available
- Proper nutritional intake and timing are standardized before testing
- Appropriate testing equipment is available, with safety checks, calibrations, and backups performed
- Proper testing surfaces are available
- Environmental conditions are safe
- Proper player-standardized footwear is available
- Proper general and specific warm-ups (e.g., dynamic stretching, rolling, and light aerobic exercise) performed
- Proper cooldown exercises (e.g., static stretching and foam rollers) performed

Preparing for the Testing Sessions

The first question that must be addressed is whether the athlete is ready for the test. This can be an issue with the youngest athletes in youth programs (Barker and Armstrong 2011; McHenry and Nitka 2022). Is their prior training background conducive to their performance on the test? The next question is whether the test is appropriate for the sport. Often, the significant problem with testing profiles is that the actual athlete composite is not reflected in the testing profile. Sport specificity can be extreme if each element of the athlete's composite is not assessed (e.g., maximal strength, anaerobic capacity, and aerobic endurance). Each test will fall into a different domain for profiling the athlete's composite. Still, the rationale for each test must be carefully determined by the evidence-based practice process (Amonette, English, and Kraemer 2016). One must also consider testing demands, logistics, and the point during the year when each test will be administered. This can be challenging with large teams.

Is the athlete ready for the test, and is it the appropriate time for the test? More conditioning preparation is necessary if the athlete is coming off a long rest cycle or vacation or has just recovered from injury. Under such conditions, care is required to make sure the athlete is ready physically. In the worst-case scenarios, rhabdomyolysis or death have occurred with extreme exercise protocols used for testing, conditioning, or even punishment after coming off a break (Casa et al. 2012; Parsons et al. 2020). Practicing tests several times on days before testing is necessary to become properly familiar with them. Workouts provide an optimal opportunity to assess different aspects of performance. Thus, workout quality, exercise technique, and proper intentionality in recording and logging data are of significant importance and will be covered more extensively in chapter 5.

Testing Protocols

All player development team members must have a basic understanding of exercise physiology and research. This is vital for having an optimal context for many aspects of player development (Armstrong and Kraemer 2016; Kraemer, Fleck, and Deschenes 2021). When one starts to evaluate this part of the domain of the player development program, the team must have access to the online software (e.g., PubMed, SPORTDiscus, and Google Scholar) related to scientific literature searches. Additionally, basic statistical and graphing software (e.g., SPSS and Excel) are needed by members who are trained and qualified to use it for different types of analysis and for player monitoring and accounting, which will be discussed in greater detail in chapter 5.

While determining the validity of a test and equipment is typically beyond the scope of many player development teams, every team should measure the various reliabilities needed to make a test stable and consistent in its results. A host of different management schemes are possible when working with testing and workout data, and these have been extensively discussed elsewhere (French and Torres Ronda 2022). A critical issue for testing arises from the buildup of errors in the results used to monitor progress and make decisions on programming. In this lies the importance of certain validities the player development team needs to be able to evaluate. These are at the heart of the efficacy of data for use.

Testing Validity

Here is where a player development team with different kinds of expertise can greatly help understand the types of validity in testing. This is a crucial area of study and work for the team because errors in test choice and measurement destroy the effectiveness of evaluating, monitoring, and assessing the actual player composite. It is, as we say, where the rubber hits the road for serious thought and evaluation. Research has many types of validity (e.g., construct, face, content, criterion-referenced). For further reading, one should refer to an edited book by Armstrong and Kraemer on all aspects of the research process (Armstrong and Kraemer 2016).

In this chapter, we are interested in understanding *validity*. This means we are interested in how well the test gives data closely related to the well-established criterion or "gold standard" measure. How well can this variable be correlated to the gold standard by using simple regression analysis, or what is the statistical "r" for its relationship? The closer it is to the gold standard measure, the closer it is to a perfect $r = 1.0$ or 100%. When one sees a criterion r value for a measure with the gold standard, one squares the value to see how much it is related to it, which is called shared variance. Thus, an "R-value" of 0.89 between a chosen test and the gold standard (squared) means that the selected test has a similarity or closeness of 79.21%. It is often stated that a test should be over 70% to be considered high enough for use. Validity between the gold standard and a given test can vary among the different tests. In this chapter, we present tests from the gold standard for a given variable (e.g., body composition, speed, and maximal strength) and then continue with the other tests to measure the same variable but moving away from the use of gold-standard technology. Many call this *direct measurement* (i.e., using the gold standard) versus *indirect measurement* (i.e., using other tests). As we will see, tests can be reliable but not valid. Tests must be validated; otherwise, a lack of a high relationship could be seen if the methods and use of the test technologies are not performed at the highest level. This may happen, for example, if calibrations are not used or if strict testing techniques are not employed (e.g., one needs to touch the line in a pro agility test, and not just reach for it, if it is to be considered a good test). Inaccurate or wrong data has serious implications if used in player development assessments or in decisions on intervention programs.

The player development team can use scientific literature to find out if a test is valid. If the instrumentation has not yet been evaluated, then depending on the resources one may be able to perform a validation test with a scientific group, potentially one from the university or institute adviser unit. Suppose no data exist as to the test or instrumentation validity. In that case, it is questionable to use it because doubts remain about what it reflects regarding the variable of interest. Thus, the first few questions for the evidence-based practice process are as follows:

- What is the valid test needed for this specific variable of interest?
- How is the equipment or instrumentation we have to measure a variable related to the gold standard for this test?

The farther away the test is from the gold standard of its validity, the lower the measure's sensitivity will be for reflecting the variable that one wants to evaluate. This adds error factors to the testing profile and can limit comparisons to other normative data used in profiling a player or team. Additionally, one's own data and the data reported in the literature must originate from the same test and equipment if valid comparisons are to be made. Other relevant contextual factors like sex, time of day, age, training level, etc. must also be shared for comparisons to be valid. As discussed later in the chapter, the choice of tests should reflect the evaluation of the largely nonmutable and mutable variables in an athlete composite (Haff and Triplett 2016).

Reliability of the Test

There are many different reliabilities for the player development team to assess and evaluate. Many factors affect the *reliability* of a test. The basic concept is that if we give a test and then repeat it, it should produce the same or nearly identical result under the same conditions. The results are related to the sensitivity of the instrument used (e.g., stopwatch timing versus electronic timing), conditions (e.g., hot versus cold or time of day), and other factors. Typically, we determine variance in the results by using a simple regression, or the Pearson-product-moment correlation coefficient, or a simple r statistic (a calculator may be found at the following website: www.socscistatistics.com/tests/pearson/). This value should be close to $r = 1.0$, which would mean that there is no variance in the test results. The player development team must determine the reliability of each test on its own and not rely on the literature (Haff and Triplett 2016). Additionally, while the test may be reliable, if more than one tester performs the test and the scores are close to identical, this is called *inter-rater reliability*. If we track the test day to day or week to week and the scores are maintained, this is called *test–retest reliability*.

Inter-Rater Reliability

This is the reliability when one uses different testers performing the same test. It should be an r value of close to $r = 1.0$ to reduce the variance in the measures. Variance between different testing sources make tests hard to interpret, which is why we always attempt to have the same group of testers perform a test in research. While this is often not feasible, the inter-rater reliability should be high, meaning all testers must be highly trained and practiced in doing the test.

The player development team needs everyone involved with a testing group to practice, whether they are a whole unit measuring vertical jumps or an individual testing a flexibility measure. Suppose different test units or individuals will be testing athletes (e.g., three units measuring pro agility). In that case, for a test group of athletes being tested by all the units, the r must be determined for the inter-rater reliability using a simple r calculation. Ideally, the regression r should be ≥ 0.95, allowing only a 5% error between units or testers for the same test variable. If r is lower, error factors enter the testing process and lower sensitivity. The player development team must determine the inter-rater reliability for each test.

Test–Retest Reliability

While all of the different reliabilities are very important, if the test–retest reliability is not known, monitoring progress and making decisions is almost impossible (Armstrong and Kraemer 2016). In other words, this reliability indicates whether giving the test on one day and then giving it again a couple of days later using the same technologies, testing methods, testers, and environment (e.g., temperature or audience encouragement) results in a very similar or identical value. If no intervention or environmental changes occur over this period, we should get nearly identical values on the two test days. This is called the *interclass correlation*, or ICCR, typically noted as a capital R to differentiate from a simple r, which uses a different equation to calculate the R-value. One then calculates an ICCR R-value between the two time points. This is always done to show the stability of a variable so that any changes observed in subsequent tests can be attributed to interventions rather than unreliable testing methods. We want the R-value from one day or even week to the next to be about $R = 0.9$ or ideally 0.95 or higher when there have been no interventions. The key here is to reduce all errors daily and weekly in our testing values. If we have an ICCR of 0.85 and our intervention shows only a 3% or 5% increase, it is an improvement but unfortunately not above our test–retest reliability error, which is 15%. Thus, when gains become small, sensitivity and errors in testing reliabilities become a limiting factor in interpreting an intervention's effects. Test results must be interpreted with error factors in mind when making decisions.

Impact of Additive Errors in Testing and Training Protocols

Considering all of the sources of error discussed in the above sections, it is easy to see how they become additive and make subtle changes in an intervention almost impossible to detect. 10% here, 10% there, and then another 5%, and one has built up a 25% accumulation of error that can mask an intervention effect as the athlete moves up toward their genetic potential. At this point one can only look at the largest changes from an intervention, typically occurring in the early phases of a training program or a training cycle with a supercompensation effect. Athletes who are not yet highly trained have large windows of adaptation for a given variable. To understand when an athlete is peaking or if an intervention is having any effect, one must reduce errors at every stage of a testing and training program so that the data are accurate and sensitive. Thus, understanding these and other statistical analyses and approaches in testing and data management is vital (Brown, Kaiser, and Allison 2018; Armstrong and Kraemer 2016). A player development team should have a member with the credentials, competence, and commitment to work in this area (French and Torres Ronda 2022). This may require a university or faculty adviser that can help address these issues. Extensive write-ups on this topic in sport science are available (French and Torres Ronda 2022; Fukuda 2019; Miller 2012).

Importance of the Accuracy of Values Derived from Testing and Training

Electronic timing is the gold standard in determining a task's speed (i.e., how long it takes to get from point A to point B). The values derived from electronic timing will have absolute validity for that particular variable if all of the electronics are calibrated and working. Some electronic timing devices used in sports like swimming can measure in microseconds so that time differences can be attributed to factors besides the accuracy of the device in a race or test for speed. As these data are produced by trained personnel conducting and supervising tests, one can use them to determine the effects of an external variable, such as training intervention, time of day, jet lag, or environment. One can see why it is essential that the variable measured is valid and that its reliability has been made solid by taking the human error in gaining the measurement out of the equation. Any error should be attributable only to environmental or external factors other than human error.

In comparison, skinfolds are not the gold standard for determining body composition because there is a variance in comparison to the accepted gold standard of dual-energy X-ray absorptiometry (DEXA), which means there will be an inherent error related to criterion validity. Errors made by individuals who are not highly proficient in the skinfold's technique can then add to this error. More errors can result from multiple people taking skinfolds. The daily and week-to-week variance in the skinfold procedure can add even more error. One will then have many errors getting in the way of deciding whether an intervention altered the variable. Even high-tech determinations, such as magnetic resonance imaging of muscle for changes in volume and hypertrophy, can be in error if measurements are not appropriately taken with enough slices or views of the muscle. Such an error can be beyond the gains made in a resistance training program.

It has to be clear that while team reports and assessments of positions are important for profiling a standard athlete composite, we are primarily concerned with determining the individual's profile and, more importantly, whether progress is being made in the athlete's development. Validity and reliability errors must therefore be kept to a minimum, and testing has to be obsessive about reducing errors in the values determined. The context of the values can then be known relative to a testing environment used with proper procedures and techniques, and the values can be used to make decisions.

Testing Organization

All testing conditions must be replicated for each test battery (Haff and Triplett 2016). This is vital if the impact of different interventions is monitored over the athlete's training cycles. Typically, indoor testing offers the most reliable conditions, but the conditions of the test must still be documented (e.g., temperature, humidity, clothing, footwear, surface, and audience) (Fukuda 2019). Each factor can affect the results, as we have discussed on the topic of reliability, and can move the needle artificially either because of error or from an actual response to the intervention's adaptation toward set goals over a training cycle.

Testing sessions are a logistical challenge and have to be developed with multiple factors addressed, including the following:

- Number of athletes to be tested
- Whether instructions are given before the test
- Equipment readiness
- Time of day
- Time to complete each test
- Order of the testing sequence
- Recording technology to be used
- Number of testers
- Activities in the 48 hours prior to the test
- Nutritional intakes, hydration, and sleep level before testing
- Audience (e.g., no audience, athletes, coaches, or administrators) and its role and instruction

Order of Testing

The testing order is a vital and often last concern when organizing a day or days of testing. Fatigue from one test can be carried over to the next and dramatically affect performance. Fatigue arises from both psychological and physical sources; therefore, the order of the tests and the number of tests used in a given session are important. Unfortunately, the testing window is set by sport coaches who want to get it over with, which can again affect the actual value of a test. Furthermore, the testing order should begin with the least stressful test, and the tests should be spread out over multiple days. The NSCA ranks fatigue testing as follows (Haff and Triplett 2016):

1. Nonfatiguing tests (e.g., height, body mass, flexibility, skinfolds, girth measurements, and vertical jump)
2. Agility tests (e.g., *t*-test, pro agility test)
3. Maximum power and strength tests (e.g., 1RM power clean, 1RM squat)
4. Sprint tests (e.g., 40-yard, 100-meter)
5. Local muscular endurance tests (e.g., push-up, sit-up)
6. Fatiguing anaerobic capacity tests (e.g., repeat sprints, 300-yard [274 m] shuttle)
7. Aerobic capacity tests ($\dot{V}O_2$max, 1.5 mile [2.4 km] run, or Yo-Yo intermittent recovery)

It is ideal to only have one very fatiguing test (five to seven) on a given test day and surround it with other tests, but it all depends on the sensitivity needed to gain a peak score. What is the priority for a testing measure? To meet logistical demands, testing is often done at the beginning of a planned workout session, thus allowing one to focus on the test at hand. However, prior exercise, sleep, and nutrition for the preceding 24 to 48 hours must be carefully documented because these factors also affect reliability.

Taking the best effort score when multiple trials are given is essential to not penalizing the athlete for less than maximal efforts. This statistical approach was determined appropriate for multitrial tests (e.g., three attempts at a vertical jump), and is used in the NHANES testing grip strength protocol from Bethesda, MD, the NIH statistical group, and in our (WJK) studies of strength in the U.S. population (Perna et al. 2016).

Number of Testers

As noted in the chapter's reliability section, one must train testers who have experience administering the test battery (Haff and Triplett 2016). Furthermore, one must ensure there are enough testers for each test to make accurate records and measurements (French and Torres Ronda 2022). Additionally, one needs testers that determine whether the test is good and whether the athlete has followed the exact directions to perform the test (e.g., touched the line or cone).

Audience Effects

Athletic and military testing scenarios have shown that the audience effect can play a significant role in testing. Whether during strength testing with a bench press or an endurance Yo-Yo test, cheering and encouragement by peers can make a big difference in the results (Rhea et al. 2003; Leitzelar et al. 2016). Therefore, every attempt should be made to standardize the testing situation each time a test battery is administered.

Audience effects can be very intimidating as well and add stress to the situation when head sport coaches or senior-level athletes are present when younger athletes are being tested. Jokes and criticism, rather than encouragement, can have a negative effect on the testing environment and should not be allowed. An audience's usual effect is to raise the arousal levels of athletes and improve their performance, but for some competitors the audience can be a source of considerable stress and can cause anxiety (Epting et al. 2011). It has been reported that gender may play a role in sport performance (Heinrich et al. 2021), so the gender of testers and athletes should be carefully considered. Who the testers are and their relationship to the athletes being tested must be considered as important environmental factors. The expertise of the sport psychology or sociological unit in the player development team can address these aspects of the testing environment. The player development team must carefully orchestrate who is present for test days and what exactly their roles will be with regard to the type and amount of encouragement.

Equipment Used

All testing equipment must be chosen and evaluated for its safety and validity for use by the player development team. As noted before, the testing equipment used will be related to the gold standard and be valid for use and comparisons to other normative data (French and Torres Ronda 2022; Fukuda 2019; Haff and Triplett 2016).

As one puts together a testing program, the cost of the benefit of any equipment is a concern. Weight room equipment can be helpful because of its dual purpose in various tests (e.g., strength testing or plyo ball throws). Investing in other instruments (e.g., skinfold calipers, jump mats, and electronic timing devices) gives dimension to the testing program and addresses variables that are needed for a better understanding of the athlete composite. Remember that one has a testing program to visualize the athlete composite. Safety is the primary concern for any testing protocol and for equipment used in a testing program or weight room (French and Torres Ronda 2022; Fukuda 2019; Liguori 2021; Myer et al. 2009).

Equipment needs to be piloted before it is used to test athletes in the program. All testers must practice with the equipment and be trained in its proper use. If feasible, identical backup equipment should be ready in case a malfunction occurs (e.g., an electronic gate in speed testing goes down, a skin caliper breaks, a stopwatch breaks, or replacement batteries are needed).

All equipment needs to be checked for safe structure and function, including resistance training equipment (e.g., benches, pulleys, boxes, collars, and bands) and testing equipment (NSCA 2017; McHenry and Nitka 2022). Prevention of injuries in testing or in the weight room is a priority; the player development team is directly responsible for athletes' safety and well-being (McHenry and Nitka 2022; Haff and Triplett 2016; Liguori 2021).

Instrument Calibrations

Equipment must be calibrated according to the requirements and procedures outlined in the manufacturers or company's guidelines. Calibrations should be done before each day's testing, or even before each test if this is recommended by the guidelines from the equipment manufacturer (Fukuda 2019).

Surfaces for Tests

The surfaces used should allow for appropriate movements in all directions without slippage or sticking when they interact with footwear (Newton et al. 2002). Often, surfaces will be relevant to sports with grass, artificial turf, or other composites. When comparing test data to normative data, the same surface must be used (e.g., NFL or NBA combines). Testing sport surfaces has become a significant issue in sport performance over the years (Fleming and Young 2006) because of differences between, for example, grass and typical track surfaces (Brechue, Mayhew, and Piper 2005).

Clothing and Footwear

Clothing and footwear should be the same each time testing is conducted. Decisions about what footwear is appropriate for a given surface affect performance (Gains et al. 2010). Clothing should not restrict the movements performed during a test. Clothing should be thermal-neutral and not affect heat dissipation or retention in a neutral environment.

The sport dictates what equipment is used in various field-testing scenarios (e.g., ice hockey, downhill skiing, and swimming). Equipment should be chosen for its relevance to the thermal safety demands of the external environment (e.g., for downhill skiing, biathlons, or road races). Field testing should use the equipment type and configuration appropriate to the sport. American football equipment, for example, can impair speed, and surface type in a 40-yard (37 m) sprint can affect performance (Brechue, Mayhew, and Piper 2005).

Environmental Conditions

The environmental conditions must be the same each time a test battery is administered. The average room temperature is typically around 20 °C or 68 °F, with humidity between 30% and 60%. This is an excellent ambient temperature to aim for, but it is crucial to remember that different rooms will need to be heated to specific temperatures. Safety is the key to any testing environment. Heat and humidity stressors are the most critical aspect of safety and preventing sudden death (Casa et al. 2012; Hosokawa et al. 2021; American College of Sports et al. 2007). Athletes need to be acclimatized to the environmental conditions they are being tested in for safe and optimal results. For crucial environmental physiology and exercise background, please study the source cited here (Kraemer, Fleck, and Deschenes 2021).

Time of Day

The time of day at which testing takes place is also a crucial decision that needs to be made and replicated for any longitudinal test battery that is being used to evaluate the progress made in an athlete composite. Speed and power are higher later in the day (Zarrouk et al. 2012). Testing in the early hours of the morning (e.g., 6 a.m.) may not be optimal due to the impact of the sleep hormone melatonin, which is higher in the early morning. To compensate for the melatonin, the adrenal glands produce more epinephrine (a.k.a. adrenaline) to offset its negative effects on power (Kraemer et al. 2014), but this can cause adrenal stress if it happens repeatedly and is not accommodated by a change in the sleep pattern. When using workouts to re-evaluate changes over the training cycles, the same workout time and the previous day's activities (e.g., academics, sleep, nutrition, and exercise training) must be standardized. Ideally, a rest day should come before a test day.

Choice of Tests for the Player Composite

To build a historical player composite, there is a need to test for the athlete's largely nonmutable and mutable characteristics. The choice of tests for the player or athlete composite is based on the concepts related to validity and reliability managed by the performance development team. Continuing the process is an issue of availability. With the rapid technological advances being made, the instrumentation and methods chosen to test for a specific variable must be completely understood and strictly followed. Again, being just "good enough" does not cut it in the world of testing and assessments. The performance development team must research whatever is the topic at hand. For example, not all hand grip dynamometers are identical, nor are the protocols used interchangeably. Testing grip strength is different for a standing position than for a seated position, just as straight arm testing is different than bent arm testing. When comparing norms, one must use the right testing protocol (e.g., NHANES grip strength norms or Canadian norms). The major mistakes made in testing are related to some of the following issues:

- The athlete not knowing how to perform the test or not having the opportunity to practice it on a different day to become comfortable

- Athlete safety and readiness to test not being individually determined
- Not understanding the previously discussed factors related to the testing organization
- Disregarding the importance of validity and reliability in testing protocols
- The use of testers who have not been trained and screened for competence
- Improper ordering of multiple tests on a given day
- Lack of needed reliability data using the chosen order of testing
- Not understanding the strengths and weaknesses of technology chosen for evaluating a specific variable
- Not understanding that even some advanced technologies cannot validly or reliably measure everything despite being the gold standard for some variables (e.g., differences in what certain DEXAs can measure for body composition)
- Not understanding the software used in an instrument to determine outcome variables
- Not knowing how to correctly measure standing reach for a vertical jump test, proper skinfold technique with different levels of subcutaneous fat, proper hand or foot touching required in agility tests, and other basic concepts

The point here is that details matter in testing protocols!

Development of the Player Composite

Periodic athlete testing is essential to portraying the athlete's composite fingerprint. The athlete composite is predicated on the mutable and largely nonmutable characteristics that make up the athlete's phenotype and work together to form critical components of successful performance. Although training targets mutable characteristics, testing can assess the program quality and monitor the athlete's composite over time. In general, testing can be used to do the following:

- *Identify athletic strengths and weaknesses:* Training programs may then be designed to target and correct weaknesses and produce a balanced athletic development.
- *Evaluate progress:* Testing is critical to evaluating progress in the athletes' training programs. Testing can assess each major health- or skill-related fitness component. In addition, sport-specific tests may be used to represent sport performance accurately. For example, different technologies have been developed to measure punching and striking force and power. Sport-specific test technology for the martial artist or striking athlete (e.g., MMA, boxer, and kickboxer) provides meaningful data directly related to the sport. Thus, fitness and sport-specific tests should assess and monitor the athlete.
- *Identify training loads:* The results of assessments may serve as the basis for intensity prescription for anaerobic (e.g., % of the 1RM) and aerobic training (% $\dot{V}O_2$max or $\dot{V}O_2$R). In addition, pre-workout testing can determine the type of workout performed that day within a flexible, nonlinear, periodized program design.
- *Assess athletic talent identification:* Testing results can help the coach correctly identify athletes participating in certain sports. This may be particularly true for younger athletes. Testing can be used as a form of athletic identification for specific sports and can significantly assist with recruiting.
- *Motivate athletes to train harder:* Coaches and athletes may establish goals, and testing enables evaluation and comparison to other athletes, hopefully providing a level of motivation "to be the best."

Testing Athletes

The testing of athletes can generally fall into three categories of tests: (1) those that target some facet of the *health-related fitness components*, (2) those targeting *skill-related fitness components*, and (3) *sport-specific tests* that simultaneously test multiple fitness components concerning how the sport is played. As previously mentioned, coaches must pick the tests that are most critical to their athlete's performance and select metrics most valuable to their training goals. Ideally, tests representing the gold standard of the measure will be selected—that is, the test should be the most reliable and valid measurement of that specific component (e.g., direct measurement versus prediction from regression analysis). This entails proper selection of equipment, testing methods, and testing staff. Only reliable data can be used to assess and monitor athletes over time. Testing staff must be competent and agree about proper testing procedures, especially when large groups of athletes are being tested simultaneously. Ideally, a single coach or training staff member should supervise and conduct the testing of an athlete. For example, if body fat percent is tested six times over the course of the macrocycle and three different coaches perform the skinfold tests during this time on one athlete (inter-rater reliability), the data will vary not only due to changes resulting from training and diet but from other testing techniques as well. Each testing day should also be as identical as possible to previous testing days regarding environment, clothing, and equipment. Calibration of testing techniques for the testing staff is necessary when members of the athlete development team are testing groups of athletes over time.

Testing Health-Related Fitness Components

Testing of health-related fitness components is part of the testing battery for athletes. These include body composition and anthropometry, muscular strength and local muscular endurance, aerobic endurance, and flexibility and posture.

Body Composition and Anthropometry

In chapter 2, we defined body composition and anthropometry as part of mutable and largely nonmutable characteristics affecting sport performance and talent identification. Here we will discuss the assessment of each of these concepts. Body composition and anthropometric assessments are standard practices for coaches and athletes. Valuable information regarding percent body fat, fat distribution, lean body mass (LBM), limb and segment lengths and ratios, somatotypes, and circumferences are gained through body composition assessment. Body composition tests may help evaluate training, diet, and athletic performance, or reduce injury risk factors. All fitness components depend on body composition and anthropometry to some extent. For example, an increase in LBM through hypertrophy contributes to increased strength and power and may contribute to speed and agility depending on how much mass is gained (these components are related to relative strength increases). Reduced body fat can help enhance muscle and aerobic endurance, speed, mobility, and agility development. Thus, body composition assessment and improvement significantly increase athletic performance, especially in aerobic endurance athletes and athletes who require high strength-to-mass ratios.

Height and Body Weight (or Mass) Standing height is assessed with a *stadiometer* (a vertical ruler mounted on a wall with a wide horizontal headboard). Height can vary slightly throughout the day, with higher values in the morning. When measuring height, the athlete must remove shoes, stand as straight as possible with heels together, take a deep breath and hold it, and stand with head level. Body weight (expressed in pounds or N) or mass (expressed in kilograms) is best measured on a calibrated physician's scale with a beam and movable weights. Clothing is a major issue and should be standardized (shoes removed, minimal clothing, and items removed from pockets). Body weight changes at various times of the day due to food and beverage consumption, urination, defecation, and dehydration or water loss. A standard time early in the morning is recommended. *Body mass index (BMI)* is used in health settings to assess body mass relative to height. It has little practical value in athletes because it does not factor in LBM (muscle mass), commonly seen in athletes, as a significant contributor to body mass. It is calculated with the following formula:

$$\text{BMI (kg/m}^2) = \text{body mass (kg)} / \text{height squared (m}^2)$$

Seated Height, Lengths, and Breadths In chapter 2, we discussed several lengths, breadths, and ratios related to various fitness components. These largely nonmutable characteristics do not serve as part of the regular testing battery because they do not typically change; however, they are routinely assessed when recruiting athletes. These anthropometric measures provide a segment of the picture of the athlete's composite and contribute to the biomechanical profile of the athlete. They include tape measures, *anthropometers* (for measuring the vertical heights between specific anatomical landmarks on the athlete and the floor or sitting surface), *segmometers* (for measuring segment length), and *sliding calipers* (for measuring breadths) (Norton 2018). Likewise, skilled practitioners must use precision when using specific landmarks. At each location, two or three measurements should be taken (on the right side of the body) to the nearest 0.1 centimeter, with the average value being used for analysis, when measuring the following:

- *Seated height:* The athlete is seated on a box in an erect position with head straight and looking forward. The measurement is taken from the box to the head's vertex while the athlete takes a deep breath. This is used as a measure of trunk height.
- *Arm (wing) span:* The athlete stands with back to the wall, feet together, and heels, buttocks, and upper back touching the wall while arms are outstretched laterally. The measurement (linear distance) is taken from the tips of each hand's middle finger from left to right as the athlete holds a deep breath.
- *Upper arm length:* The athlete stands erect with the palms slightly off the thighs. Using a caliper, the measurement is taken from the acromial (top of the most lateral part of the acromion process of the shoulder) to the radiale (proximal lateral border of the head of the radius).
- *Forearm length:* The athlete stands erect with the palms slightly off the thighs. The measurement is taken from the radiale to the stylion (the distal point on the lateral radius) using a caliper.
- *Hand length:* The measurement is taken as the distance from the crease of the hand to the fingertip of the middle finger while the fingers are outstretched. The hand may also be traced on paper for subsequent measurement.
- *Thigh length:* The athlete stands upright in a relaxed position, with evenly distributed weight and arms folded across the chest. The measurement is taken from the superior part of the greater trochanter to the superior part of the lateral border of the head of the tibia.
- *Lower leg (tibia) length:* The athlete is seated with the right ankle crossed over the left knee. The measurement is taken from the most superior part of the medial border of the head of the tibia to the inferior part of the distal tip of the medial malleolus.
- *Leg length:* This may be derived by subtracting the seated height from the standing height. It can be measured in different ways, so standardization is critical. Example methods include measuring the locale of the greater trochanter of the hip to the floor and measuring from the ASIS to the medial (or lateral) malleolus of the ankle.
- *Arm length:* The measurement is the distance from the tip of shoulder (acromion) to the tip of the middle finger of one arm.
- *Biacromial breadth:* The athlete stands in a relaxed position with arms hanging at the sides. The measurement is taken from the lateral points, from the right to the left acromion processes, using a caliper.
- *Biiliocristal breadth:* The athlete assumes a relaxed standing position with arms folded across the chest. The measurement is taken from the most lateral points on the iliac crests using a caliper.
- *Biepicondylar breadth of right humerus:* The athlete assumes a position with the shoulder and elbow flexed to 90°. Using a caliper, the width between the medial and lateral epicondyles of the humerus is measured.
- *Biepicondylar breadth of right femur:* The athlete assumes a seated position with knee flexed to 90°. Using a caliper, the width between the medial and lateral epicondyles of the femur is measured.

- *Foot length:* While the athlete is standing, the measurement is taken from the most posterior part of the heel to the tip of the longest toe.

Girth Measurements Girth measurements provide useful information regarding changes in muscle size and body composition. The advantages of taking circumference measurements are that they are easy, inexpensive, do not require specialized equipment (other than a tape measure), and are quick to administer. The tape measure is applied tautly in a horizontal plane, and the circumference is read to the nearest half of a centimeter while minimal clothing is worn. Duplicate measures are obtained at each site, and the average is used. If readings differ by more than 5 to 10 mm, an additional measurement may be taken. Critical is the correct placement of the tape measure at each site for the following measurements:

- *Chest:* around the chest at the level of the fourth ribs after the athlete abducts the arms back to the starting position at the end of respiration;
- *Shoulder:* horizontally at the maximum circumference of the shoulders while the athlete is standing relaxed;
- *Abdominal:* over the abdomen at the level of the greatest circumference (near the umbilicus) while the athlete is standing relaxed;
- *Right thigh:* horizontally over the thigh below the gluteal level at the largest circumference (upper thigh) while the athlete is standing;
- *Right calf:* horizontally over the largest circumference of the calf midway between the knee and ankle while the athlete stands relaxed;
- *Waist:* around the smallest waist area, approximately 1 inch (2.5 cm) above the navel;
- *Hip:* around the largest area of the buttocks (with minimal clothing);
- *Right upper arm:* horizontally over the midpoint of the upper arm between the shoulder and elbow while the athlete is standing, relaxed, and the elbow is extended; and
- *Right forearm:* horizontally over the proximal area of the forearm where the circumference is the largest while the athlete is standing relaxed.

Dual-Energy X-Ray Absorptiometry *Dual-energy X-ray absorptiometry* (DXA) is based on the exponential attenuation of X-rays at two energies as they pass through the body. The DXA is considered the gold standard of body composition. In many cases, it requires a trained or certified professional to operate the instrument based on local government and university requirements. Following system calibration and removal of metallic objects, the athlete lies motionless and is secured with Velcro straps on the lower legs and feet on a scanning bed. The athlete is scanned rectilinearly from head to toe for a duration of 5 to 25 minutes, depending on the type of scan. A DXA scan generates pertinent information regarding the mass (in grams) of fat, lean tissue, and bone mineral content and density (g/cm^2) for the total body and specific regions like the head, trunk, and limbs. DXA has many advantages: it is easy to administer, the software provides a great deal of information for the user (including regional measures), regional measurement of LBM is attractive for assessing hypertrophy, it uses low-level radiation, and it is safe, fast, and accurate. For women, pregnancy tests will need to be given prior to a DXA scan; however, in some cases, because of its emission of low-level radiation, a physician's prescription or a licensed or certified technician may be required to perform DXA scans depending on local legal requirements. For high reliability of measurements, it is strongly recommended that DXA scans be performed on the same machine and software for repeated measures.

Underwater Weighing Underwater weighing was for a long time the gold standard for body composition analysis, when performed correctly by trained practitioners, but its popularity has waned with the advent of DXA technology. It requires no technique certifications, but highly trained technicians are needed for optimal testing. It is based on Archimedes' principle for determining body density: A body immersed in water encounters a buoyant force that results in weight loss equal to the weight of the water displaced during immersion.

Subtracting the athlete's body weight in water from the body weight on land provides the weight of the displaced water. Body fat contributes to buoyancy because the density of fat (0.9007 g/cm^3) is less than water (1 g/cm^3), whereas lean tissue mass (1.100 g/cm^3) exceeds the density of water. Lean tissue density varies based on ethnicity and maturation. Body density is calculated and then converted to percent body fat using an equation such as the Siri or Brozek equations. Population-specific equations have been developed to convert body density data into percent body fat more accurately. A tank made of stainless steel, fiberglass, ceramic tile, Plexiglas, or a swimming pool (the temperature of the water should be between 91.4 and 96.8 °F [33 to 37 °C]) that is at least 4 × 4 × 5 feet (1.2 × 1.2 × 1.5 m) is needed, along with a seat suspended from a scale or force transducer for weighing. *Residual volume* (the amount of air left in the lungs following full expiration) must be determined via spirometry. Water density, the amount of trapped gas in the GI system (a predicted constant of 100 milliliters is used), dry body weight, and body weight in the water need to be known.

The procedures for underwater weighing include the following:

- Athletes wear minimal clothing (i.e., a tight-fitting bathing suit). All jewelry should be removed, and the athlete should have urinated and defecated.
- Athletes should be 2 to 12 hours postabsorptive and have avoided foods that increase gas in the GI tract. Menstruation may pose a problem for females due to associated water gain; they should not be tested within 7 days of menstruation.
- The athlete is weighed on land to determine the dry weight, enters the tank, removes potential trapped air, and is seated on the chair to be weighed (the athlete fully expires as much air as possible before leaning forward to be weighed).
- The athlete is weighed 5 to 10 times while submerged underwater for 5 to 10 seconds. The highest or average of the three highest weights is used (the weight of the chair and belt are considered in the calculation).

- Residual lung volume can be measured directly via spirometry (which increases accuracy) in some systems or estimated based on height and age using the following formulas:

  Males: RV (L) = [0.019 × ht (cm)] + [0.0155 × age (yr)] - 2.24

  Females: RV (L) = [0.032 × ht (cm)] + [0.009 × age (yr)] - 3.90

- Body density is calculated using the following equation:

  BD = Mass in air (g)

  ([Mass in air (g) - mass in water (g)] / density of water) - (RV in mL - GI gas (100 mL)

- Body fat can be calculated using the Siri, Brozek, or population-specific equations.

Skinfold Assessment *Skinfold assessments* are one of the most popular and practical methods to estimate percent body fat. Skinfold assessment can be relatively accurate, provided a trained coach measures with high-quality calipers. Although not considered a gold standard for body composition (since it involves estimation), its practicality makes it far more likely to be used with athletes, given the high cost and restrictions of some other body composition equipment. Skinfold analysis is based on the principle that the amount of *subcutaneous fat* (fat immediately below the skin) is directly proportional to total body fat. Regression analysis estimates total percent body fat (with ±3% to 5% accuracy). Body fat varies with gender, age, race or ethnicity, training status, and other factors, so numerous regression equations have been developed to predict body density and percent fat from skinfold measurements. Skinfold assessment for athletes is most accurate when the prediction equations closely match the population. The number of sites ranges from three to seven. Prediction equations estimate body density, and body density calculation is used to estimate percent body fat. *Body density* is described as the ratio of body mass to body volume.

The number of sites and the equation are first selected. Depending on population and gender, common sites include abdominal, triceps, biceps, pectoral, mid-axillary, subscapular, medial calf, suprailiac, and thigh. A fold of skin is firmly grasped between the thumb and index finger of the left hand (about 8 centimeters apart) while the athlete is relaxed. The jaws of the caliper are placed over the skinfold 1 centimeter (0.2 in) below the fingers of the tester, released, and the measurement is taken within 2 to 3 seconds. All measurements are taken on the right side of the body two to three times for consistency to the nearest 0.5 mm. It is important to rotate through all the sites first instead of taking two or three measurements sequentially from the same site. Each site is averaged and summed for several tests to estimate body density and percent body fat via a regression equation or prediction table. Percent body fat can be calculated once body density has been determined. Most often, the Siri or Brozek equations are used, although other population-specific equations have been developed.

Air Displacement Plethysmography (ADP) Body volume can be measured by air displacement. The Bod Pod (a commercial ADP system) uses a dual-chamber plethysmograph that measures body volume via changes in air pressure within the closed two-compartment chamber. It includes an electronic weighing scale, computer, and software system. The volume of air displaced is equal to body volume. It is calculated indirectly by subtracting the volume of air remaining in the chamber when the athlete is inside from the volume of air in the chamber when it is empty. Reliability is good, but sources of error include variations in testing conditions, the athlete not being fasted, air that is not accounted for in the lungs or trapped within clothing and body hair, body moisture, and increased body temperature. After calibration, the athlete is properly prepared, and minimal clothing is worn (e.g., swimsuits, compression shorts, sport bras, and swim caps). The athlete's mass is determined via the digital scale. The athlete enters the chamber and sits quietly during testing while a minimum of two measurements (within 150 milliliters) are taken to determine body volume. Corrected body volume (thoracic gas volume subtracted from raw body volume) is calculated, body density is determined, and percent body fat is calculated using prediction equations.

Bioelectrical Impedance Analysis Bioelectrical impedance analysis (BIA) is an easy, noninvasive tool for determining body composition. The underlying principle is that electrical conductivity is proportional to the fat-free tissue of the body. A small electrical current is sent through the body, and the impedance to that current is measured. Lean tissue (mostly water and electrolytes) is a good electrical conductor, whereas fat is a poor conductor and impedes an electrical current. Bioelectrical impedance analysis can measure percent body fat and total body water. Accuracy among BIA devices varies greatly. Athletes should not have eaten or consumed a beverage within 4 hours of the test, exercised within 12 hours, or consumed alcohol or diuretics. The athlete should have completely voided the bladder within 30 minutes of the test. Many current BIA analyzers function similarly to scales that the athlete stands on with moistened bare feet to determine body composition. Also, some facilities may have handheld devices for BIA analysis.

Somatotyping *Somatotyping* involves categorizing athletes into variations of physique types using anthropometric and photoscopic measures. The basic physique types include (1) *endomorph* (round physique, high fat), (2) *mesomorph* (muscular), and (3) *ectomorph* (lean body build). Ten anthropometric measures are taken to calculate the anthropometric somatotype for endomorphy, mesomorphy, and ectomorphy: stature, body mass, four skinfolds (triceps, subscapular, suprailiac, medial calf), two breadths (biepicondylar humerus and femur), and two limb girths (arm flexed and tensed, and calf) (Carter and Heath 1990). A Heath-Carter somatotype rating form is completed by filling in the data obtained from the anthropometric assessments. Calculations can be done manually or with a software program. For a manual calculation, follow these steps:

- The endomorphy rating is calculated by recording and summing the four skinfolds and correcting for height by taking the sum $\times$ (170.18 divided by height in centimeters).

The value is circled from the table, and the corresponding value below it in the endomorphy row is circled.

- The mesomorphy rating is calculated by recording height and breadth values. Skinfolds are corrected before recording the girths of the biceps and calf by converting the triceps skinfold to centimeters by dividing by 10. The converted triceps skinfold is subtracted from the biceps girth. The calf skinfold is converted to centimeters and subtracted from the calf girth. Height is circled, as is each breadth and girth. The average deviation of the circled values is found for breadths and girths from the circled value in the height column.
  - Column deviations to the right of the height column are positive, and the left is negative. (Circled values directly under the height column have deviations of zero and are ignored.)
  - The algebraic sum of the ± deviations (D) is calculated with the following formula: mesomorphy = (D divided by 8) + 4.0 rounded to the nearest one-half (½) rating unit. This value is circled in the mesomorphy row.
- Ectomorphy rating is calculated by recording mass (weight) in kilograms. The height divided by the cube root of mass (weight) is calculated, recorded, and circled in the table. The value directly below in the ectomorphy row is circled and used as a score.

Ratings are given for each somatotype, plotted, and athletes are placed into one of 13 categories, including *balanced mesomorph, mesomorph-endomorph, mesomorphic endomorph,* and *endomorphic mesomorph*. Rankings of 0.5 to 2.5 are considered low, 3 to 5 are moderate, 5.5 to 7.0 is high, and greater than 7 is very high. Somatotype scoring and profiles can be seen in Carter and Heath, 1990.

Muscular Strength

Maximal strength testing is critical to the assessment of the athlete. It comes in different forms depending on the type of strength measured, including dynamic concentric (CON) and eccentric (ECC), isometric (ISOM), and isokinetic (ISOK). The gold standard of dynamic strength testing is the *one-repetition maximum* or 1RM—that is, the maximal amount of weight that can be lifted once for a specific exercise at a given velocity—performed with free weights and machines. Although other RMs (greater number of repetitions) may be used, the 1RM is highly reliable and provides the most accurate dynamic strength assessment when performed properly. The key for rests between efforts is that they represent a minimal recovery time; the coach wants the athlete to feel ready for the next given repetition. The biggest mistake is to overshoot the athlete's capability. Still, one can estimate with a prediction equation (e.g., the Epley equation) the athlete's approximate 1RM from training logs and plan who to move up to this number or surpass it. Strength testing is an art as well as a science. The 1RMs of athletes are most commonly assessed using multiple-joint exercises like the squat, bench press, deadlift, and power clean. Although many strength testing protocols are effective, one we have used successfully is as follows (Kraemer et al. 2006; Ratamess 2022):

1. General warm-up and specific warm-up: selected dynamic flexibility or calisthenic exercises, foam rolling, core facilitation and potentiation exercises, and unloaded bar.
2. Perform a light warm-up of 5 to 10 reps at 40% to 60% of the estimated 1RM.
3. Rest for 1 minute. For very strong athletes attempting heavy weights, 1 to 3 additional warm-up sets may be needed.
4. Perform 3 to 5 fast reps at 60% to 80% of the estimated 1RM.
5. Rest 1 to 2 minutes and perform a set for 1 rep with approximately 90% to 95% of the estimated 1RM.
6. Step 5 will take the athlete close to the 1RM. A conservative increase in weight is made, and another 1RM is attempted.
7. Rest approximately 3 minutes or more if the attempt is successful. It is important to allow enough rest before the next 1RM attempt.
8. Obtain a 1RM within 3 to 5 sets to avoid excessive fatigue. The process of increasing the weight up to a true 1RM can be

enhanced by prior familiarization of the athlete and effective coaching of the tester. This process continues until a failed attempt occurs, at which point the weight is adjusted accordingly.

9. Record the 1RM as the weight of the last successfully completed attempt.

If a multiple RM is determined, the following protocol targeting a 6RM (after completing the general and specific warm-up) may be used:

1. Warm up with 5 to 10 reps with 50% of the estimated 6RM.
2. Rest for 1 minute.
3. Perform 6 reps at 70% of the estimated 6RM.
4. Rest for at least 2 to 3 minutes.
5. Repeat step 3 at 90% of the estimated 6RM for 3 to 6 reps.
6. Rest at least 2 to 3 minutes or more.
7. Perform 6 reps with 100% to 105% of the estimated 6RM.
8. After at least 3 to 5 minutes of rest, if step 7 is successful, increase the resistance by 2.5% to 5% for another 6RM attempt. If 6 reps were not completed in step 7, subtract 2.5% to 5% of the resistance used and attempt another 6RM following 3 to 5 minutes of rest.
9. The maximum weight lifted for 6 reps is the 6RM. If not determined within a few sets and fatigue is noticeable, it is better to retest 2 to 3 days later with adjusted attempts.

Figure 3.1 depicts a checklist that may be used for strength testing (Kraemer et al. 2006; Ratamess 2022). This list can guide coaches and athletes because it describes specific issues to consider before and during strength testing. Communication and proper spotting must take place between the athlete and testing staff. Trained staff can recognize an athlete's capacity and determine a properly progressed loading scheme. Feedback from the athlete is critical to determining the loading progressions, especially if the athlete has experience and a general idea of the perceived 1RM. Training logs help determine a narrow range of what the expected 1RM may be. A *trial-and-error approach* may be used initially with novice athletes with limited resistance training experience; however, an experienced coach may be able to look at an athlete and come up with a specific loading scheme. "How do you feel?" "Are you ready to go?" "How close to your 1RM do you think you are?" "Can you lift five more pounds?" These types of questions are vital to interacting with the athletes as they attempt to exert maximal force. The rest interval length and the number of preliminary warm-up repetitions are important. It is essential that there are enough repetitions for a proper warm-up but not so many as to fatigue the athlete. These factors must be individualized; athletes lifting very heavy weights will require more warm-up sets and longer rest intervals than those lifting lighter weights. Some individuals may require at least 5 minutes of rest between attempts, whereas some individuals need only 1 to 2 minutes of rest, depending on the loading relative to their eventual maximum. If a greater number of repetitions are performed (5RM-10RM), fewer warm-up sets are suggested. The general and specific warm-ups should not be overlooked. Other than the basic physiological benefits of warming up, the facilitation or potentiation associated with the warm-up can help the athlete attain a higher 1RM than what would be observed following an inadequate warm-up.

Isometric strength tests are performed while the athlete is in a static position. The evaluation angle, standardization between athletes, feedback (visual and from coaches), and motivation all make ISOM testing demanding. Remember that muscular strength varies throughout joint range of motion (ROM); therefore, careful consideration is needed for standardizing joint angles and body position. Some ISOM equipment has been used considerably over the years, such as the hip and back dynamometer (used to examine ISOM deadlift strength) and the handgrip dynamometer (used for measuring ISOM grip strength). In addition, ISOK machines may be used to measure peak torque at 0°/sec. A calibrated force plate can be used with an immovable resistance for several free weight or Smith machine exercises to measure peak force, rate of ISOM force development, and

Strength Testing Checklist

- [ ] Has the individual been medically cleared to resistance train, and can this individual safely perform strength testing?
- [ ] Does this individual require any special accommodations?
- [ ] Is the time of day similar between multiple testing sessions?
- [ ] Is a 1RM or multiple RM to be tested?
- [ ] Was the individual thoroughly familiarized with the testing protocol? How many familiarization sessions were performed?
- [ ] Was proper technique explained and demonstrated (including range of motion, grip, stances, body position, and so on)?
- [ ] Was test-retest reliability of the equipment and protocol performed?
- [ ] What is the individual's training history?
- [ ] Was adequate nutrition intake (and hydration) consumed before testing?
- [ ] Was ambient temperature controlled for?
- [ ] If the individual is experienced, what is his or her perceived or expected RM?
- [ ] What type of muscle action is to be tested?
- [ ] Concentric?
- [ ] Eccentric?
- [ ] Isometric?
- [ ] For isometric testing, what joint angles will be examined?
- [ ] What type of resistance is to be used?
- [ ] Dynamic constant external resistance?
- [ ] Variable resistance?
- [ ] Isokinetic?
- [ ] Isometric?
- [ ] For machine-based exercise, what are the appropriate machine settings and starting position of the resistance?
- [ ] Was the individual properly positioned, and does the equipment accurately accommodate the individual?
- [ ] What is the velocity of movement?
- [ ] Are knowledgeable spotters present?
- [ ] Was the equipment calibrated according to manufacturer's guidelines?
- [ ] Test specificity:
- [ ] Were the movement patterns tested similar to those performed during training?
- [ ] Is there metabolic (energy system) specificity?
- [ ] Were adequate instructions given?
- [ ] Was a proper warm-up performed? Did it include submaximal practice repetitions for the testing exercises?
- [ ] Did the individual use proper technique, and did spotters assist in lifting the weight?
- [ ] Was adequate rest given between repetitions and sets?
- [ ] Were proper breathing patterns used?
- [ ] Was the individual verbally encouraged throughout the testing protocol, and was a proper lifting environment set for testing?
- [ ] Was visual feedback given for isokinetic testing?
- [ ] Were the proper units of measurement used?
- [ ] What was the individual's 1RM or multiple RM?
- [ ] Did the individual give 100% effort?
- [ ] Were there any other factors that may have affected the test (e.g., illness, injury)? Were ergogenics controlled for? What types (if any) were used?
- [ ] Lifting accessories and apparel?
- [ ] Nutrition supplements?
- [ ] Drugs?

FIGURE 3.1 Strength testing checklist.

Reprinted by permission from W.J. Kraemer, A.C. Fry, N.A. Ratamess, and D.N. French, "Strength Testing: Development and Evaluation of Methodology," in *Physiological Assessments of Human Performance*, 2nd ed., edited by P.J. Maud and C. Foster (Champaign, IL: Human Kinetics, 2006).

fatigue rates. In addition, some ISOM tests are used to subjectively assess core stability, such as the supine bridge, plank, and side plank. Many protocols can be used for ISOM testing. The following is one example:

1. General warm-up and specific warm-up: selected dynamic flexibility or calisthenic exercises, foam rolling, core facilitation and potentiation exercises.
2. Perform 1 to 3 practice trials with submaximal progressive effort (50% to 75% of maximal voluntary contraction).
3. Maximal trials require only 2 to 3 maximal voluntary efforts of 3 to 6 seconds with 1 to 5 minutes of rest between trials. Additional trials may be necessary if the athlete is still increasing strength output.
4. The peak force for the highest trial is recorded.

Multiple-joint ISOM strength testing has greater applicability to specific athletic movements and is highly related to 1RM strength. Common exercises tested (in addition to the hip and back dynamometer) include the ISOM squat, leg press, bench press (elbow angles of 90° to 135°), and mid-thigh pull at various ROM positions (i.e., knee angles of 90° to 140° for the squat and 120° to 145° for the mid-thigh pull). These are often assessed during maximal efforts of 3 to 6 seconds with 2 to 5 minutes rest intervals between trials. The peak force, impulse, and rate of force development for the ISOM mid-thigh pull correlate with change of direction and agility performance time, jump height and reactive strength index, throwing ability, weightlifting (e.g., snatch and clean and jerk) performance, sprint speed and power, and maximal strength (e.g., squat and deadlift), which makes it a very effective assessment tool for athletes. It is performed on top of a force plate, in a power rack or related device, with an immovable barbell placed in a position corresponding to the second pull in Olympic weightlifting. Often the data are expressed and analyzed in time windows (e.g., the first 30, 50, 90, 100, 150, 200, and 250 milliseconds). It is important to note that equipment use should be as specific as possible and standardized for multiple testing points. For example, athletes should be tested on one force plate consistently if a facility has multiple force plates. Different force plates yield different values making comparison difficult if not impossible.

Isokinetic strength testing is performed with a dynamometer that maintains the lever arm at a constant angular or linear velocity. Isokinetic machines control velocity; thus, the strength evaluation accounts for CON and ECC velocity of movement, which is not the case with free weights and machines. The cost of ISOK equipment can be prohibitive, but many laboratories, training rooms, and clinical facilities use them extensively. Often, single-joint exercises are tested for ISOK strength but have given valid data, especially when examining strength ratios and relationships to injury (e.g., ACL tears, hamstring strains, and rotator cuff injuries). There are devices on the market that use multiple-joint movements as well. ISOK testing should match the training velocity, or a spectrum of slow, moderate, and fast CON and ECC velocities can be assessed. Remember from our previous discussions of the force–velocity relationship that higher levels of force will be seen at slower CON velocities and lower levels at faster CON velocities. Three to five repetitions are recommended with rest intervals of 1 to 3 minutes between sets to attain peak torque or force. Other testing considerations include ensuring a standardized ROM; standardized test position and proper postural stabilization; equipment calibration; gravity compensation; and feedback, instruction, and familiarization. Test–retest reliability for ISOK testing is high when the position is standardized, equipment is calibrated, and the athletes give maximal effort.

Another option in certain circumstances is estimating a 1RM or multiple RM from prediction equations or a table. Each equation is exercise-specific, and the error rate increases when equations are applied to different exercises. However, the most accurate results are obtained from true RM testing. Estimation is typically used for multiple-joint exercises and may help assess athletes during specific training phases where max testing could influence the workout schedule. It can also be used to predict maximal strength and provide the coach and athlete with a targeted value for maximal strength testing (e.g., targeting a weight may reduce the number of sets needed to obtain the 1RM). The load used typically ranges from 55%

to 95% of the 1RM (for 2 to 20 repetitions), but accuracy is greater when fewer than 10 repetitions (especially 2 to 3 repetitions) are performed using nonlinear equations. Prediction is attractive from an administrative standpoint, but its validity is questionable. It should be noted that the number of repetitions performed relative to the 1RM for different exercises is highly variable, an observation dating back to the research of Hoeger et al. (Hoeger et al. 1987; Hoeger et al. 1990; Kraemer et al. 1999) and others who showed, for example, that at 80% of the 1RM, double the number of repetitions could be performed for the leg press than for the leg curl. This remains consistent for other exercises as well. Table 3.1 depicts some equations (Kraemer et al. 2006) used to predict 1RM strength, and figure 3.2 depicts a nomogram for predicting 1RM strength for the bench press, squat, and leg press from 5RM and 10RM data (Fukuda 2019).

Muscular Endurance

Local muscular endurance tests measure the ability of selected muscles to perform repeated contractions over time. The contractions can be low to moderate in intensity (*submaximal endurance*) or high in intensity (*high-intensity endurance*). Muscular endurance tests for athletes usually involve performing body weight exercises for a maximal number of repetitions or the maximal number of repetitions in a specified time, repetitions for a resistance training exercise at an absolute percentage of the 1RM, and sustained maximal duration tests. Power endurance can be measured if appropriate technology is available (force plates, linear position transducers, or related technology).

Body weight exercises may be performed for maximal numbers of repetitions or maximal repetitions in a measured time interval (e.g., 1 or 2 minutes) using standardized procedures (Kraemer et al. 2006; Ratamess 2022). The exercises chosen should match the training program's demands and the athlete's needs for the sport. Many exercises can be selected. The coach only needs to choose a few to assess the athlete's muscular endurance accurately. Test performance will improve if the athlete trains for the tests as well. Not only has training focused on sport-related KPIs; it has also been adapted to target performance tests (e.g., training for the NFL combine). The most common exercises assessed include the following:

- Partial curl-up
- Sit-up
- Push-up
- Pull-up
- Dip
- Squat
- Inverted row
- Burpee

TABLE 3.1 Formulas Used to Estimate 1RMs

Reference	Equation
Brzycki (1993)	1RM = Wt./1.0278 − 0.0278(# reps) %1RM = 102.78 − 2.78(# reps)
Epley (1985)	1RM = 0.033(Wt.)(# reps) + Wt.
Lander (1985)	1RM = Wt./1.013 − 0.02671(# reps) %1RM = 101.3 − 2.67123(# reps)
Mayhew et al. (1999)	1RM (lb) = 226.7 + 7.1(# reps w/225) (used for college American football players)
Cummings & Finn (1998)	1RM = Wt.(1.149) + 0.7119 1RM = Wt.(1.175) + # reps(0.839) − 4.2978 (used for untrained women)
Mayhew et al. (1992)	1RM = Wt./([52.2 + 41.9$e^{-0.055(\# reps)}$]/100) %1RM = 52.2 + 41.9$e^{-0.055(\# reps)}$
O'Connor et al. (1989)	1RM = Wt. (1 + 0.025 × # reps)
Wathen (1994)	1RM = 100 × Wt./[48.8 + 53.8$e^{-0.075(\# reps)}$]
Abadie, Altorfer, & Schuler (1999)	1RM = 8.8147 + 1.1828(7RM-10RM)

Reprinted by permission from W.J. Kraemer, A.C. Fry, N.A. Ratamess, and D.N. French, "Strength Testing: Development and Evaluation of Methodology," in *Physiological Assessments of Human Performance*, 2nd ed., edited by P.J. Maud and C. Foster (Champaign, IL: Human Kinetics, 2006).

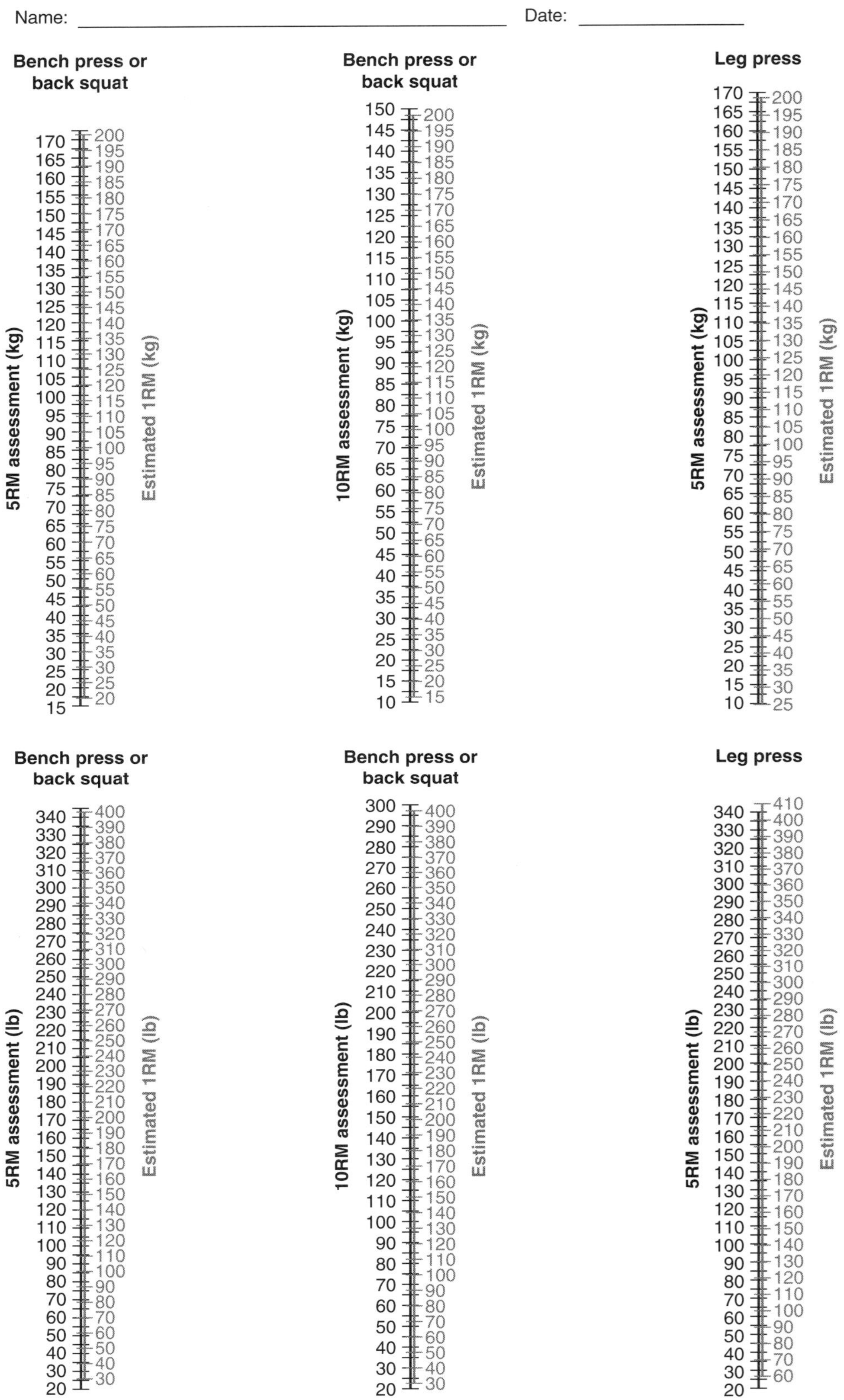

FIGURE 3.2 Conversion nomograms for predicting 1RM strength for the bench press, squat, and leg press.
Reprinted by permission from D.H. Fukuda, *Assessments for Sport and Athletic Performance* (Champaign, IL: Human Kinetics, 2019).

Power endurance is the athlete's ability to maintain maximal or high levels of power over time. As with muscular strength, power declines over time as the exercise continues. Thus, power endurance can be assessed with maximal repetition tests used in tandem with force plates or linear position transducers. The power (force or velocity) data obtained with each repetition can be compared over time. One example is the 30-second vertical jump test. After proper general and specific warm-ups, the athlete performs maximal vertical jumps in succession with standardized technique (e.g., hands on hips) for 30 seconds. Several variables may be calculated and recorded, including maximal and mean jump heights, maximal and mean power per jump, mean jump height or power for selected intervals (e.g., first 5 seconds versus last 5 seconds), the number of total jumps, and a measure of the *fatigue index* (highest − lowest / highest × 100 or a similar point such as the first rep versus the last rep or the mean of first few reps versus the mean of the last few reps). In addition, we have used the 20-repetition jump squat test performed on a Smith machine using 30% of the individual's pretraining 1RM squat to calculate the fatigue index (Ratamess et al. 2003). Athletes are instructed to jump as high as possible for each repetition while maintaining proper exercise technique and standardized ROM. A maximal effort is required; otherwise, the curves may flatten and yield inaccurate data. Other variations may be used, such as using a hex bar, weighted vest, dumbbells, or kettlebells for external loading instead of the Smith machine. High test–retest reliability is seen when the procedures are standardized and the same coach performs the tests. As discussed in subsequent sections, it is essential to note that a coach cannot compare force, velocity, or power data obtained from different pieces of equipment because each model and company product will yield significantly different values. Comparisons can be made when the same equipment is used over time under standardized conditions.

Muscular endurance can be assessed in the weight room via using resistance training exercises for a maximum number of repetitions with a standard load. An important consideration is the loading to use. *Relative loading* is based on a percentage of the individual's RM capability, whereas *absolute loading* has the same load for all athletes and all tests. Relative muscular endurance performance may not change, but absolute muscular endurance will, so using a standard load for measuring is a good idea. The relationship between strength and absolute muscular endurance is positive, whereas the relationship between strength and relative muscular endurance is negative. Thus, absolute testing may provide better indicators of athletic performance. A common test, especially in American football players, is the *225-pound maximum repetition bench press test*. Although considered a strength test by some (only if the athlete's max is near 225 pounds!), it is a test of absolute muscular endurance for most athletes. Following a general and specific warm-up, the athlete performs as many repetitions as possible using standardized procedures, ROM, and cadence. Any exercise can be used for muscular endurance testing (preferably multiple-joint basic resistance training exercises), and coaches may even be able to establish their own norms over time if less-commonly used exercises are included in the testing battery.

Sustained maximal duration trials usually involve an ISOM exercise held for maximal time. Many variations can be performed. We have used muscular endurance tests, including maximal ISOM elbow flexion (90°) against a standard load, and a grip test in which individuals hold or maintain a position against a load for maximal time. The ISOM wall squat test at various depths as well as the flexed-arm hang, which measures the amount of time an athlete can maintain the final ISOM pull-up position, have been used over the years. Failure to maintain position is the criterion for test termination, and these latter tests are greatly affected by strength and body weight. ISOM measures of *core stability and endurance* have been used increasingly in athletes, given the importance of core strength and endurance to health and performance and the dedication of using a segment of the training program to increase core strength and endurance. Collectively, these tests involve holding an ISOM position targeting anterior, posterior, and lateral regions of core musculature for the maximal time while maintaining proper position. Some of the more commonly used body weight ISOM trunk muscular endurance tests include the following (Ratamess 2022):

- Biering-Sorensen test and modified versions
- Prone ISOM chest raise
- Prone double straight leg raise
- Trunk flexor test (various positions)
- Plank
- Side plank

Aerobic Endurance or Capacity

Aerobic endurance or capacity assessments involve the direct measurement or estimate of $\dot{V}O_2$max or $\dot{V}O_2$peak. The difference in terms lies in the test itself, meaning the final result of the test is the $\dot{V}O_2$peak, which may or may not be the true $\dot{V}O_2$max. Nevertheless, we will use the term $\dot{V}O_2$max here with the understanding of this critical point. Different modes of exercise yield different values (e.g., treadmill tests yield higher $\dot{V}O_2$max values than cycle and rowing ergometers and arm cycle ergometry). Coaches should select modes similar to the athlete's sport. Depending on the test, aerobic capacity testing may also allow the coach to assess lactate threshold and other critical variables that can be used in interval training exercise prescription, such as velocity and power at $\dot{V}O_2$max. Some field tests that assess aerobic capacity may also be used to estimate $\dot{V}O_2$max. Several lab-based progressive treadmill and cycle ergometer graded exercise testing protocols have been used over the years for direct measurement via indirect calorimetry with a metabolic cart (i.e., Åstrand, Bruce, and Balke protocols). These protocols used in tandem with a metabolic cart provide the gold standard for $\dot{V}O_2$max assessment against which other maximal and submaximal tests are validated against. Many protocols for $\dot{V}O_2$max testing have been developed. For example, one treadmill test (a variation of Åstrand) we have used to assess the $\dot{V}O_2$max of athletes is a progressive, multistage ramp protocol consisting of 2-minute stages at a running speed of 6.0 mph (9.7 kph) with increments in percent grade of 2.5% per stage (Ratamess et al. 2016). The UFC Performance Institute uses multiple maximal aerobic capacity tests. One is performed on an AirBike Elite ergometer with a metabolic cart. The protocol starts after a 1-minute warm-up at a targeted rpm based on the athlete's weight. The UFC test comprises 1-minute stages; at each stage there is an increase in rpm by five until the test is terminated (French 2017). Upper-body cycle ergometry testing may have practical applications, especially in assessing upper-body aerobic performance improvements. We have used a progressive, multistage ramp protocol (with metabolic cart and following a standard warm-up) that consists of 1-minute stages beginning at 60 rpm and 12 watts with increments in the power of 12 watts at each stage until test termination. During maximal aerobic testing, the athlete continues until exhaustion or until the test is terminated based on the following criteria:

- $\dot{V}O_2$ plateau
- Heart rate max within 10 beats of age-predicted max heart rate
- Respiratory exchange ratio value of ≥ 1.15
- Rate of perceived exertion ≥ 17
- Blood lactate ≥ 8.0 mmol/L

$\dot{V}O_2$max prediction from field tests is the most practical because most athletes and coaches may not have access to expensive metabolic carts. These tests have been validated and typically require variables such as heart rate or test time to predict $\dot{V}O_2$max. For some tests, several athletes can be tested simultaneously, making it easier for the coaching staff to collect data and save time in the process. Athlete performance effort needs to be maximal because aerobic capacity can be underestimated if the athlete does not put forth the maximal effort. Thus, proper familiarization is critical to accurate results. In some cases, coaches may require athletes to complete a certain distance within a certain amount of time rather than predicting $\dot{V}O_2$max. For example, as a preseason screening tool, a sports team may be required to complete the 1.5-mile (2.4 km) run in less than 12 minutes (or a similar time depending on position, body size, age, or other factors). In addition, time trials (especially for aerobic endurance athletes) offer another practical means of assessment, especially since they help athletes determine appropriate race paces. Tests should be selected based on the major modes used by the athlete (e.g., running, cycling, or swimming). Many tests have been developed and used to test the aerobic capacity of athletes.

Single-stage or multistage submaximal tests—such as the Åstrand-Rhyming cycle ergometer test, YMCA submaximal cycle ergometer test, and the Queens College and YMCA step tests—have been used chiefly in fitness and lab settings but also had limited use for athletes as well. Several continuous and intermittent field tests that require athletes to put forth maximal or near maximal effort serve as better performance indicators.

Field tests include running assessments of fixed length, a specified time, or a combination of fixed distance and progressive reductions in time, such as a 1.5-mile run (2.4 km), 12-minute walk or run, multistage 20-meter (22 yd) shuttle run (PACER or beep test), Yo-Yo test, and 30-15 Intermittent Fitness Tests. Variations have been developed to target other modes such as swimming, ice skating, cycling, and rowing, as well as sport-specific tests. The procedures are as follows:

- *1.5-Mile (2.4 km) Run:* A quarter-mile track is needed. Following a proper warm-up, the athletes begin at the starting line and run as rapidly as possible (at a steady pace) for six laps while timed by staff until they cross the finish line. The time is recorded. The following equation can estimate $\dot{V}O_2$max:

$$\dot{V}O_2\text{max (mL/kg/min)} = 3.5 + (483 \text{ divided by the run time in minutes})$$

or

Men: $\dot{V}O_2$max (mL/kg/min) = 91.736 − (0.1656 × body mass in kg) − (2.767 × run time in min)

Women: $\dot{V}O_2$max (mL/kg/min) = 88.020 − (0.1656 × body mass in kg) − (2.767 × run time in min)

- *Cooper 12-Minute Walk or Run:* A running track, markers, and measuring device or marked areas on track are needed. Athletes run for 12 minutes, and the total distance covered is recorded. Walking may be allowed, but the maximal effort is strongly encouraged. Similar tests have been used for swimming and cycling. From running or walking, $\dot{V}O_2$max (ml/kg/min) may be estimated by the following equations:

$$\dot{V}O_2\text{max (mL/kg/min)} = (35.971 \times \text{distance in miles}) − 11.288$$

$$\dot{V}O_2\text{max (mL/kg/min)} = (22.351 \times \text{distance in km}) − 11.288$$

- *Multistage 20-Meter (22 yd) Shuttle Run—Beep Test or Progressive Aerobic Endurance Run (PACER) Test and Variations* (Leger and Lambert 1982): A flat, stable area marked with parallel lines or cones separated by precisely 20 meters (22 yd) and the beep test CD or multimedia package are needed for this field test. A coach is used to record completed laps or shuttles. Audio cues (beeps) are used to allow the athlete to set a running pace while continuously running between the two lines or cones at a pace based on the stage of the test. A beep begins the test, the athlete runs 20 meters (22 yd) and returns 20 meters (22 yd) upon the next beep, and so forth. The test is progressive, where the beeps come in shorter intervals with each successive stage, forcing a faster running pace until the athlete can no longer maintain it. There are approximately 21 levels, each lasting a minute; most athletes complete between 6 and 15. The test ends when athletes can no longer keep pace with the beeps on two successive trials. Proper practice should be used prior to testing for familiarization. The final score is the level (indicated by the number or corresponding velocity) or the number of laps attained. The validity and test–retest reliability of the test is good. $\dot{V}O_2$max can be estimated using the following equations:

Adults (mean age = 26 years):
$$\dot{V}O_2\text{max (mL/kg/min)} = 5.857 \text{ (speed in km/h)} − 19.458$$

Adults and children (8 to 19 years):
$\dot{V}O_2$max (mL/kg/min) = 31.025 + 3.238 (speed in km/h) − 3.248 (age in years) + 0.1536 (age in years × speed in km/h) where speed begins at 8.0 + 0.5 (stage number)

Adults and children (19 to 36 years):
$$\dot{V}O_2\text{max (mL/kg/min)} = 14.4 + 3.48 \text{ (level completed)}$$

- *Yo-Yo Intermittent Recovery Tests:* These tests are designed to measure repeated interval performance and recovery ability and may be used to estimate $\dot{V}O_2$max. The YY1R1 is used for individuals with lower fitness levels, whereas the YY1R2 test is used for fit individuals (Bangsbo, Iaia, and Krustrup 2008). The YY1R1 starts at a lower speed with moderate increases in speed (lasting 10 to 20 minutes), while the YY1R2 starts faster (lasting 5 to 15 minutes) with larger speed increases. Cones measured 20 meters (22 yd) and 5 meters (5.5 yd) apart are needed, plus the auditory system for timing signal cues. The athletes begin aligned with the starting cone, run (upon the start signal) to the finish cone, and immediately return to the start cone before the next audio signal (figure 3.3).

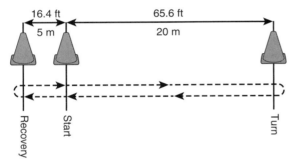

FIGURE 3.3 Yo-Yo setup.

Reprinted by permission from D.H. Fukuda, *Assessments for Sport and Athletic Performance* (Champaign, IL: Human Kinetics, 2019).

Once the start cone is reached, athletes have a 10-second recovery period in which they must jog or walk in between the cones set 5 meters (5.5 yd) apart to prepare for the next shuttle. The shuttles are repeated while the speed increases via the increased tempo of the audio signals. Athletes are only allowed two consecutive fail attempts before the test is terminated. Distance is calculated by recording the number of shuttles completed, multiplied by 40 (each shuttle is 2 × 20 meters). The distance completed is used as an assessment tool for anaerobic capacity and the top speed attained during the last successful shuttle can be used for interval exercise prescription, as can the following equation:

Yo-Yo speed = speed attained (in km/h) in next to last stage + 0.5 × (n divided by 8)

where n is the number of runs completed during the last stage and 8 represents the number of runs in each stage.

The following equations may estimate $\dot{V}O_2$max:

Yo-Yo IR1 test: $\dot{V}O_2$max (mL/kg/min) = (distance in meters × 0.0084) + 36.4

Yo-Yo IR2 test: $\dot{V}O_2$max (mL/kg/min) = (distance in meters × 0.0136) + 45.3

Figure 3.4*a* depicts a sample data sheet showing speeds per stage completed for the YY1R2, and figure 3.4*b* is a nomogram that can be used to estimate $\dot{V}O_2$max from YY1R1 and YY1R2 data (Fukuda 2019).

- *30-15 Intermittent Fitness Test (30-15IFT):* This test is a reliable measure of anaerobic capacity and estimate of $\dot{V}O_2$max (Buchheit 2008). It consists of 30-second shuttle runs interspersed with 15-second walking intervals (figure 3.5). Velocity is set at 8 km/h to start for the first 30-second run and then increased to 0.5 km/h every stage thereafter. The athletes are required to run back and forth between two lines set 40 meters (44 yd) apart, and audio beeps control speed. The 3-meter (3.3 yd) zones in the middle allow the athlete to gauge running speeds and serve as start points for subsequent stages after the 15-second recovery intervals. The test is terminated when the athlete can no longer maintain the required running speed or cannot reach a 3-meter (3.3 yd) zone by the beep three consecutive times. The final velocity attained may be used for interval training. The following equation may estimate $\dot{V}O_2$max:

$\dot{V}O_2$max (mL/kg/min) = 28.3 − (2.15 × S) − (0.741 × age) − (0.0357 × body mass (kg)) + (0.0586 × age × final speed) + (1.03 × final speed)

S = 1 for male; 2 for female; final speed in km/h

Lactate Threshold Measurement of lactate threshold (LT) provides the athlete with a specific intensity that can be trained at specific intervals. The simplest way to assess LT is to use a portable calibrated lactate analyzer with strips, lancets, and alcohol wipes. Testing should be as specific to the

Stage	Speed (km/h)	Pace (min/km)	Speed (mph)	Pace (min/mi)	Time per 20 m lap (sec)	Number of shuttles (2 × 20 m laps)	Shuttles completed
S1	13	4.6	8.1	7.4	5.54	①②③④⑤⑥⑦⑧	
S2	15	4.0	9.3	6.5	4.80	①	
S3	16	3.8	9.9	6.1	4.50	①②	
S4	16.5	3.6	10.3	5.8	4.36	①②③	
S5	17	3.5	10.6	5.7	4.24	①②③④	
S6	17.5	3.4	10.9	5.5	4.11	①②③④⑤⑥⑦⑧	
S7	18	3.3	11.2	5.4	4.00	①②③④⑤⑥⑦⑧	
S8	18.5	3.2	11.5	5.2	3.89	①②③④⑤⑥⑦⑧	
S9	19	3.2	11.8	5.1	3.79	①②③④⑤⑥⑦⑧	
S10	19.5	3.1	12.1	5.0	3.69	①②③④⑤⑥⑦⑧	
S11	20	3.0	12.4	4.8	3.60	①②③④⑤⑥⑦⑧	
S12	20.5	2.93	12.7	4.7	3.51	①②③④⑤⑥⑦⑧	
S13	21	2.86	13.0	4.6	3.43	①②③④⑤⑥⑦⑧	
S14	21.5	2.8	13.4	4.5	3.35	①②③④⑤⑥⑦⑧	
S15	22	2.7	13.7	4.4	3.27	①②③④⑤⑥⑦⑧	
						Total shuttles	

a

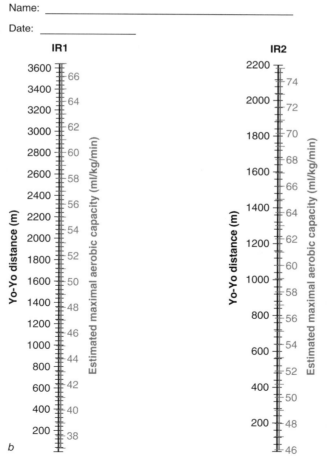

b

FIGURE 3.4 *(a)* Data collection sheet for the Yo-Yo intermittent recovery level 2 (IR2). *(b)* Conversion nomogram for estimating maximal aerobic capacity from the Yo-Yo intermittent recovery level 1 (IR1) and level 2 (IR2).

Reprinted by permission from D.H. Fukuda, *Assessments for Sport and Athletic Performance* (Champaign, IL: Human Kinetics, 2019).

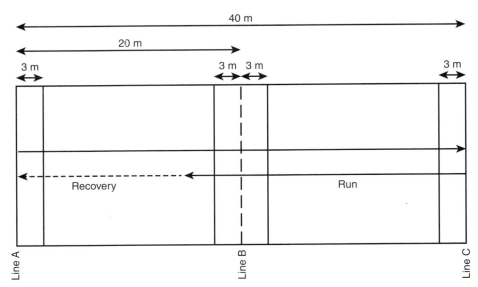

FIGURE 3.5 Intermittent Fitness Test (30-15IFT): A reliable measure of anaerobic capacity and estimate of $\dot{V}O_2$max (Buchheit 2008). It consists of 30-second shuttle runs interspersed with 15-second walking intervals.

training program as possible. Progressive ramp protocols in stages of 2 to 3 minutes are recommended (with intensity increases of 5% to 15% per stage) so that a sample can be taken near the end of a stage or at regular time intervals. Blood lactate data can be plotted versus speed or power output. The deflection point where blood lactate increases beyond a resting level is the LT. Another way to determine LT is from data obtained with a metabolic cart during a progressive ramp protocol. VCO_2 may be plotted against $\dot{V}O_2$ throughout the test. Lines of best fit for each segment can be plotted, and the intersection represents the LT (known as the *V-slope method*). The time of that intersecting point or $\dot{V}O_2$ data point can be traced back to the protocol stage to determine the intensity. This method is more costly than the use of a portable lactate analyzer.

Flexibility, Muscle Length, and Posture

Flexibility depends on several factors, including tendon and ligament stiffness, muscle viscosity and bulk, distensibility of the joint capsule, pain tolerance, and muscle temperature. Joint flexibility can be measured in multiple planes and may isolate a joint, or tests may be used to assess multiple areas simultaneously. Often, the shoulder, spine, and hip regions of athletes may be targeted with routine flexibility assessment, although some sports may require other areas of emphasis. Basic equipment used for testing flexibility includes goniometers, electrogoniometers, inclinometers, and tape measures. Visualizing anatomical landmarks may be sufficient for some tests to determine a certain level of flexibility on a pass-fail basis. The following are a few basic flexibility tests:

- *Trunk rotation test:* This test is performed with no equipment or specialized device. A vertical line is marked on a wall. The athlete stands, back to the wall, with a shoulder-width stance, and at approximately arm's length away. The athlete then rotates to the right as far as possible (with arms straight in front and parallel to the floor) and touches the wall. This position is marked, and the process is repeated to the left. The feet must remain stationary, but the trunk, shoulders, and knees are free to move. The distance from the line is measured. A positive score indicates that the mark passes the vertical line, whereas a negative score indicates failure to surpass the vertical line.

- *Shoulder elevation test:* This measures the flexibility of the shoulder and pectoral areas but also requires some muscular strength to elevate the arms against gravity. It has great applicability to assessing the flexibility needed for overhead lifting and the overhead squat. The athlete grasps a stick in front of the body using a pronated grip. The arm length is determined by measuring the distance from the acromion process to the top of the stick.

The athlete then assumes a lying-prone position on a mat where the chin touches the floor and extends the arms straight overhead while holding the stick. The athlete slowly raises the stick upward as high as possible while maintaining chin contact with the mat and keeping the elbows fully extended. The highest position is held for 1 to 2 seconds while a coach takes a measurement from the stick position to the floor. Three trials should be used. Either recording scores the highest length attained from the floor or uses the following formula: shoulder elevation score = arm length (inches) – best height attained (inches).

- *Modified sit-and-reach test:* This test assesses lower back, gluteal, and hamstring muscle flexibility but is also affected by abdominal girth and limb and torso lengths. The modified sit-and-reach test establishes a zero-point based on limb and torso lengths. A sit-and-reach box, tape measure, or stick is needed. Following a proper warm-up, the athlete sits shoeless with feet against the sit-and-reach box. The athlete's starting position is determined by having the athlete place the arms together with the right hand over the left hand, feet flat against the box with the knees fully extended, and the back against the wall. The athlete reaches forward by protracting only the shoulder girdle to determine the starting position. This calibrates the starting point and limits limb and torso length bias. While keeping the knees extended, the athlete slowly flexes forward at the waist as far as possible (without bouncing) and pushes the sliding device forward to achieve the greatest ROM possible. This final position is held momentarily. The score is obtained, and the best of three trials is recorded.

Pass-Fail Tests Visualization for a number of ROM tests can be done without special equipment. These subjective tests provide the coach with information that could be used to target weak areas or muscular imbalances. These tests assess what could be potential problem areas for athletes; for example, the physiotherapist Vladimir Janda characterized postural distortions linked to pain and dysfunction in areas leading to major postural issues, including *upper cross* (sloped shoulders) and *lower cross* (rotated pelvis) *syndromes* and *pronator distortion syndrome* (excessive foot pronation, knee flexion, internal rotation, and knee valgus torque) (Clark and Lucett S.C. 2011). Several of these tests are helpful in looking at imbalances or mobility issues that may predispose athletes to undue stress or injuries over time via overuse. Some of these potentially nonquantitative tests have been described in more detail elsewhere (Ratamess 2022) and include the following assessments:

- Prone and supine transversus abdominis muscle activation
- Pectoralis minor length
- Shoulder flexion ROM
- Internal and external rotation ROM
- Supine straight leg raise test
- The FABER (flexion, abduction, and external rotation) Test (assesses ROM of the hip)
- Thomas test (assesses the flexibility of the hip flexor and the abductor and adductor muscles)
- Ober test (evaluates tightness in the tensor fascia latae, iliotibial [IT] band, gluteus medius and minimus muscles)
- Supine hip abduction and adduction
- Wall angel (assesses thoracic spine immobility, latissimus dorsi, and pectoral muscle tightness)
- Supine lat ROM
- Seated and prone hip external and internal rotation

Posture and Mobility *Posture* relates to the alignment and function of all human body segments at rest and during motion. Postural assessment allows the coach to determine potential muscular imbalances and weaknesses and can be applied to specific areas in the training program. Just as a house must be built on a strong foundation, increasing muscular strength, hypertrophy, endurance, and power in athletes can only be optimized if the athlete's foundational posture can withstand the load. Posture may be assessed statically and dynamically, and it is relatively easy to assess. It is important to stress posture and mobility screening early in the athlete's career to identify and train weaknesses early. Many postural assessments have been developed. One popular and often studied screening assessment is the functional movement screen (FMS) (Cook et al. 2014). It consists of applying a score from 0 to 3 (0 = pain during movement, 1 = unable to perform the prescribed movement, 2 = can perform movement but needs to compensate and has difficulty, and 3 = good performance of skill) to selected movements (see figure 3.6). The coach may use the measuring device, hurdle, and measuring dowel that come with the kit. The maximum score is 21; there are seven tests (with three additional clearance tests not scored) with an optimal score of 3 points. For tests of asymmetry involving separate performance and scoring of right and left sides, the lower score of the two (if there is a difference between right and left sides) is used for calculating the total number of points. The coaching staff needs to be effectively trained in the application of the tests for high inter- and intra-rater reliabilities because there is

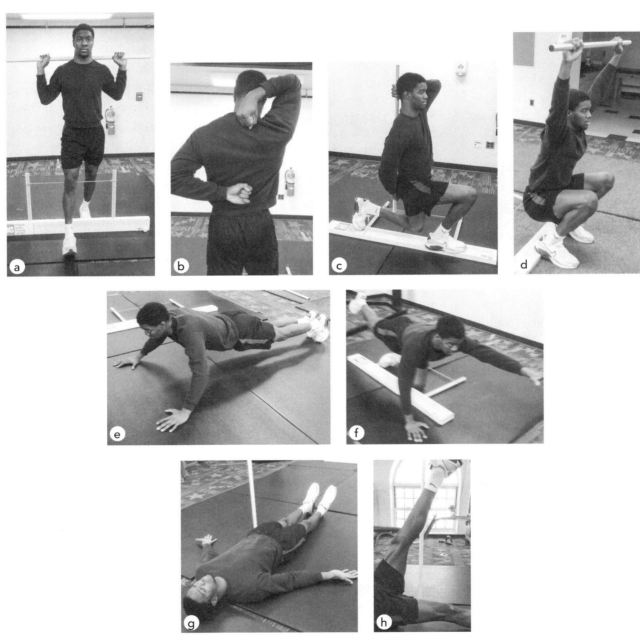

FIGURE 3.6 Selected movements of the functional movement screen used in the assessment of an athlete.

Photos courtesy of Justin Dominique and Dr. Nicholas Ratamess.

a significant subjective component to it. The same coach should test the same athlete on repeated occasions to increase the accuracy of the assessment. The FMS has been shown to have poor to high inter-rater reliability and good test–retest reliability, with higher values seen when coaches are trained to use this assessment. Some studies have shown higher injury rates in athletes who score low on the FMS (e.g., 14 or less) and those with notable asymmetries. The movements assessed (shown in figure 3.6) include the following:

- The overhead (deep) squat
- Hurdle step
- In-line lunge
- Shoulder mobility
- Active straight leg raise
- Trunk stability push-up
- Rotary stability

Assessment of Skill-Related Fitness Components

Testing several skill-related fitness components is paramount to a comprehensive testing battery for athletes. These include power, anaerobic capacity, speed, agility, reaction time, and balance.

Power

Power testing is critical to assessing anaerobic athletes. *Power* is the rate of performing work and is the product of force and velocity. Peak power tests are explosive, short in duration (a few seconds), predominantly stress the ATP-PC system, and are commonly reported in watts (W). Some peak power tests include 1RM Olympic lifts (strength and power), jump tests, jump squat on a force plate or transducer, medicine ball throw, and rate of force development (RFD) tests. Power tests may be adapted to reflect greater sport specificity.

Vertical Jump A tape measure, chalk, or special device like the *Vertec* is needed. If using a wall, chalk may be used to mark the measured location. When using a Vertec, the athlete sets the starting position. The Vertec is adjustable and has color-coded vanes. The very first vane marks the reading. A red vane is placed every 6 inches (15 cm), and blue and white vanes are placed 1-inch (2.5 cm) apart, marking whole- and half-inch (1.3 cm) measures, respectively. The athlete stands with the dominant arm flexed vertically as high as possible and touches the corresponding vanes to demarcate the starting height. Stance width should be standardized at approximately hip width. The athlete performs a countermovement and then jumps (CMJ) as high as possible (touching the highest possible vane) to demarcate the attained height. Starting height is subtracted from the achieved height to determine the vertical jump-height difference. The best of three to five trials is recorded. Several equations have been developed to estimate peak and mean power during the vertical jump. Below are peak power equations:

- Sayers et al. (Sayers et al. 1999) developed the following equation:

$$\text{Peak power (W)} = 60.7 \,(\text{jump height in centimeters}) + 45.3 \,(\text{mass in kilograms}) - 2{,}055$$

- These are some additional equations (Amonette et al. 2012):

$$\text{Peak power (W) for 12 to 15 years} = (61.9 \times \text{VJ height (cm)}) + (40.8 \times \text{BM (kg)}) - 1{,}680.7$$

$$\text{Peak power (W) for 16 to 18 years} = (63.6 \times \text{VJ height (cm)}) + (46.2 \times \text{BM (kg)}) - 2{,}108.2$$

$$\text{Peak power (W) for 19 to 24 years} = (83.0 \times \text{VJ height (cm)}) + (54.5 \times \text{BM (kg)}) - 3{,}436.8$$

$$\text{Peak power (W) overall} = (63.6 \times \text{VJ height (cm)}) + (42.7 \times \text{BM (kg)}) - 1{,}846.5$$

Variations of the basic vertical jump test can be used. A *squat jump* (SJ) may be used. The difference is that the bottom position is held statically to minimize stretch-shortening cycle (SSC) activity, or no countermovement is used. The CMJ should yield ~15-30% greater height if the athlete efficiently uses their SSC during the explosive movement. Sport-specific strength and power training can increase both SJ and CMJ performance significantly (French et al., 2004). This was shown in a previous study where we tracked Division I female gymnasts over their collegiate careers. Initially, little separation was shown between CMJ and SJ peak power during their first year where they participated in machine-based resistance training in addition to gymnastics training. After implementing a periodized strength and power program, both SJ (43%) and CMJ (46%) peak power increased over the remainder of their collegiate careers, showing greater targeting of SSC function (French et al., 2004). The improved power capabilities were translated to the various events (e.g., floor, vault,) and improved scoring was also achieved. This was due to the ability greater arial heights attained from greater whole-body kinetic control and power. Another example is the *one-step vertical jump test*, commonly used in sports like basketball in which jumping off of a single leg is common. Multiple steps may be used for athletes where running precedes a jump. Another variation for water polo players involves performing a jump in the pool while treading water. Jump height can be determined from other types of jumps in addition to the squat, counter-movement, and one-step (or multiple-step) jumps. A single-leg jump without the step can be used to assess unilateral power. Versions involving hands on the hips (on a force plate) measure lower-body power by eliminating the effects of arm swing. Arm swing is critical to jump performance and may contribute up to 10% to takeoff velocity. It helps keep the torso upright, increases the center of gravity at takeoff, increases downward force (and subsequent ground reaction force), and increases torque produced by lower-body musculature during propulsion in which the combined effects of these actions augment jump performance. In addition, using the arms relates to greater specificity of the sport (e.g., rebounding in basketball, spiking in volleyball), as it closely matches the technique used. The *depth jump* may be used and serves multiple purposes. It is especially useful when determining the appropriate height of the box used during plyometric training. It may also help determine jumping parameters of interest to the coach, such as the *reactive strength index*, because the depth jump represents a fast SSC activity exercise (less than 250 milliseconds). Several other essential data may be generated if the jumps are performed on a force plate, especially if dual force plates allow the measurement of right and left sides. It is important to note that each variation should be treated as a distinctly different test. Coaches should not directly conflate results from different jumps (i.e., arm swing versus no arm swing) or data obtained from different equipment. Other measures that can be used based on jump height (or power from a force plate) include the following:

- Prestretch augmentation % (PSA): [(CMJ − SJ) divided by SJ] × 100 (approximately 0.5% to 6.8% if peak power is used; approximately 12.5% to 25% if peak jump height is used)
- Eccentric utilization ratio (EUR): CMJ divided by SJ (approximately 1.12 to 1.25 if peak jump height is used; approximately 1.01 to 1.06 if peak power is used)
- Reaction strength (RS): CMJ − SJ
- Reactive strength index-modified: Jump height and ground contact time to takeoff (could use CMJ for slow SSC or depth jumps for fast SSC) (top 90% greater than or equal to 0.547 in male NCAA Division I athletes; greater than or equal to 0.434 in female NCAA Division I athletes (Sole, Suchomel, and Stone 2018)

Broad Jump The broad jump assesses horizontal power development. Other variations, including the two-jump or three-jump tests (or more), involve the performance of consecutive repetitions of broad jumps emphasizing the landing and subsequent SSC activation prior to the next subsequent jump. Here, the total length covered by two or three jumps is recorded. For a single-repetition broad jump, a flat area (at least 15 ft [4.6 m] in length) (e.g., grass field or gym floor), a tape measure, and masking tape are needed. The tape serves as a start marker, and the athlete starts with toes just behind the starting line. Using a countermovement with arm swing, the athlete jumps forward as far as possible, landing on both feet. A point at the athlete's rearmost heel is marked, and the distance is measured. The best of three to five trials is recorded.

Force and Power Testing with Force Plates, Linear Position Transducers, and IMUs There have been advances in technology to assess power over the years, including force plates, linear position transducers, accelerometers, gyroscopes, magnetometers, video or optical analysis (e.g., *motion analysis*), and timing mats. *Force plates* (single and dual) and linear position transducers can be used for a number of different exercises and movements. Force plates contain strain gauges or load cells that directly measure ground reaction force from the athlete. Force output (and torques or moments) can be measured in three planes of motion. Force–time data and velocity–time data are generated such that impulse, momentum, the center of pressure, velocity, power, and flight time can be determined. RFD data can be generated directly (per phase of movement) from the force–time curves and software calculations. Force and power data can be expressed in absolute or relative terms. For example, relative propulsion impulse is a good metric to use for determining jump performance and movement velocity. Power data normalized to body weight can provide the coach with additional data for those athletes who require a high strength- or power-to-mass ratio. Relative power measures allow for comparisons among athletes of different body weights. There is a variety of force plates: They can be set in the floor, portable, single, and dual (i.e., measures right and left sides). Several unilateral and bilateral exercises can be performed on force plates: running, jumping, ground-based resistance training, plyometrics, and sport-specific exercises (e.g., jumping to spike a volleyball or rebound in basketball and pushing off during pitching in baseball). Upper-body power can be measured via the plyo push-up (Wang et al. 2017). Unilateral tests can be used to assess potential imbalances; for example, right-to-left differences of more than 15% may increase the risk of injury in athletes. A major advance has been to use dual force plates to measure potential asymmetry. Prior to this, unilateral movements had to be performed on a single plate. Dual plates allow for a measure of asymmetry during bilateral and unilateral jumps and other exercises. Figure 3.7*a* depicts force curves for a CMJ. Eccentric or braking (unloading, yielding, and deceleration), CON (propulsive), flight, and landing (loading and attenuation) phases are shown. Displacement curves may overlay changes in force, velocity, and power during each phase as well. Figure 3.7*b* depicts numerous variables of interest the coach can acquire from force plate software.

There are several ways to measure RFD, which is a variable composed of both strength and power performance. Force plates generate RFD data during power testing, which may be used for comparison via the slope of the rise in force. Another common RFD assessment involves ISOM testing. An ISOM squat (performed on a force plate), mid-thigh pull (discussed earlier in this chapter), or leg press (when a force plate or strain gauge is built into the sled) can be used. The bar or sled is fixed at a specific position where it cannot move (e.g., with stoppers, with pins in a rack, or via ultra-heavy weights). Other ISOM tests, such as the athletic shoulder test (from the prone I, Y, and T extended arm positions on the plate) (Ashworth et al., 2018), may be helpful in testing athletes. The athlete is instructed to produce as much force as possible in the shortest amount of time. Several variables of interest can be used from the data generated, such as the peak force produced, the time to produce 100% of peak force, and the time to produce a specific intensity (e.g., 80% of peak force). A reduction in the time to produce a specific level of force indicates an increased RFD. In addition, the force developed during specific time windows may be identified (e.g., 0 to 50, 0 to 100, and 100 to 200 milliseconds). Lastly, some coaches have used force plates to calculate the *dynamic strength index*, which is a ratio of ballistic peak force to ISOM peak force (e.g., CMJ peak force and ISOM mid-thigh pull peak force). A low score (≤ 0.6) indicates the athlete needs to improve ballistic exercise performance, whereas an athlete with a high score (≥ 0.8) will benefit from increasing maximal strength (Suchomel et al. 2020).

The technology used in force plates can be incorporated into sport-specific equipment. Force transducers may be strategically placed in sport-specific training equipment to measure force and power. Force and pressure transducers can be placed into footwear to measure forces produced during various tasks. They have been placed within treadmills to measure force and velocity during sprinting (Ross et al. 2009). Placing force

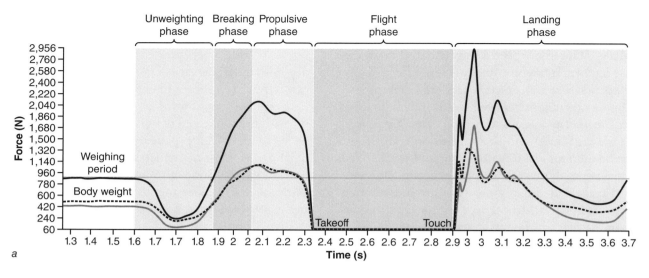

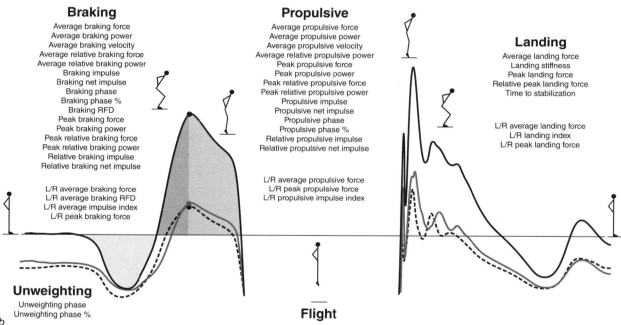

FIGURE 3.7 (*a*) Countermovement jump. (*b*) Various force plate parameters. Key measures we have used include jump height, mRSI, peak propulsive power, peak relative propulsive power, peak relative braking power, and relative peak landing force (e.g., <500% or 5X body weight). The L/R braking force can be used to see if this is exaggerated on one leg, e.g., > 10% asymmetry.

Courtesy of HAWKIN Dynamics.

transducers into a blocking sled can measure sport-specific force and power for an American football player. Boxing and striking dynamometers have been developed to measure force during punches in boxers and MMA athletes. Different models are available, each showing good validity and reliability. This technology has been essential to the training and assessment of combat and striking athletes because data generated in real time allows the athlete to gauge output and adjust accordingly. The most critical element of sport-specific tests is their ability to measure athletic performance accurately during direct motor skill applications. Coaches may collect data over time, analyze it, and find the *minimal detectable change* for each piece of equipment and technique used so that higher values obtained can be interpreted as changes and not just occurring within the margin of error. In chapter 5, we discuss the role of technology in monitoring athletes during training.

Linear position transducers and *inertial measurement units* (IMU) have become more practical and affordable for coaches to use. Inertial measurement units are generic sensors that integrate information from accelerometers, gyroscopes, and magnetometers into displacement, velocity, and acceleration data. They are linked with an app that can display real-time data. Given the popularity of *velocity-based resistance training*, their use has dramatically increased for testing and monitoring athletes. They may be attached to the athlete's belt (for jumping) or mounted to a barbell to measure displacement, power, and velocity. They have been shown to be valid and reliable during testing, although IMUs are susceptible to error depending on environmental conditions. Instant feedback is provided, so athletes know their subsequent effort for each repetition. We have used this technology for over 20 years, particularly with ballistic exercise testing. Ballistic exercises eliminate the deceleration phase of traditional exercise performance and provide a better indicator of power development. We have used linear position transducers to measure velocity and power during loaded ballistic exercises such as the *bench press throw* and *jump squat* (Ratamess et al. 2003). Our protocol consisted of loading a Smith-machine-like device (Plyo Power System) with 30% of the squat and bench press 1RM, respectively, after a proper warm-up. It is important to use a system that has an electromagnetic or hydraulic braking system to catch the released weight by the athlete (or at least slow the descent of the bar). Otherwise, a barbell, weighted vest, or hex bar could be used for the jump squat, but caution is needed, especially during landing or when a barbell is used and the bar separates from the shoulders and resets. Each athlete is given three to five maximal trials with 2 minutes of rest between sets. The best trial is recorded for analysis. Another option is to perform two to three repetitions per set, given that some athletes may hit their peak power on the second or third repetition. Here, two to three consecutive repetitions are performed, followed by a 2-to-3-minute rest interval. The highest value is recorded. The process is repeated for the second exercise in sequence. Selecting a load that can yield high power output is crucial, although any standard load or relative percentage may be used. Meta-analytical data showed 0% to 30% of the 1RM to be the optimal loading for peak power during the jump squat and bench press throw (Soriano et al. 2015; Soriano, Suchomel, and Marin 2017). The coach can use this loading scheme for successive power assessments. It is important to note that power output generated from ballistic assessments is variable when comparing data from one study to others, so establishing norms can be challenging. The coach must develop the norms based on power data generated from one device.

Transducers enable power assessment for any resistance exercise, traditional or ballistic, although ballistic exercises are preferred (e.g., jump squat, bench press throw, and Olympic lifts). For example, the UFC Performance Institute uses linear position transducers with the loaded *landmine punch throw test* to measure power specificity for striking. The National Hockey League uses a bench press test with 50% of the athlete's body weight for three repetitions performed as fast as possible using a linear position transducer. We have used them for traditional exercises to measure peak and average power and velocity changes over traditional sets of resistance training for the high pull, back squat, bench press, incline bench press, bent-over barbell row, deadlift, seated shoulder press, and push press exercises (Ratamess et al. 2012; Ratamess et al. 2016). Technology has advanced to where we now see optical systems in power racks or IMUs placed in watches to monitor velocity and power during each repetition of any exercise. As cost decreases and these devices are shown to be valid and reliable, more coaches will use them for monitoring athletes and periodic power testing.

Medicine Ball Throws Several different medicine ball (MB) throws (side throws, overhead throws, rear scoop throws, rotation throws, and underhand throws) can be used in standing, seated, or kneeling positions and have shown to be valid and reliable measures. The distance the ball is thrown relates highly to upper-body (or total-body) power. Each throw is unique, so coaches can pick one that matches the demands of the sport. For example, overhead throws are more specific to athletes like basketball players and soccer players who regularly use this motion in the sport. Rotational throws apply to athletes who require rotational power. Rear scoop throws have a greater lower-body component, whereas side throws test rotational power. Direct upper-body power has been assessed using the MB chest pass from a standing or seated position. A seated throw isolates the upper body to a greater extent. Medicine balls vary, but one standard size can be used (approximately 2% to 5% of the athlete's body weight). When standing, a shoulder-width stance is used. Back support (e.g., a belt or a wall) is helpful for the seated position because the athlete needs to maintain contact with the support during the throw. The toes should be aligned with a tape marker to set the starting line. The athlete throws the MB as far as possible at an angle of less than 45°. The center of the ball is marked, and its distance from the starting line is measured upon landing. Chalk may be used to mark the landing spot. The best of three to five throws is recorded.

Anaerobic Capacity Tests

Anaerobic capacity tests measure power endurance and typically last 15 to 90 seconds. They stress the anaerobic systems of athletes and the buffering capacity enabling athletes to perform during high levels of acidosis. Tests include specific all-out duration tests (where the goal is to complete the distance in the shortest time possible), timed shuttle tests, and timed multiple-repetition repeated sprints or shuttle runs. Coaches can use shuttle tests to compare the total time completed over time, or they can use pass-fail tests in which the athletes complete the entire shuttle or one repetition of the shuttle within a specified period of time. Aerobic endurance athletes are commonly assessed with time trials. For runners, the amount of time needed to complete the desired distance can be used to assess anaerobic capacity. For some tests, a desired or goal time is used, and the distance covered in that time is recorded. We have previously discussed the 30-second vertical jump test and the 20-repetition jump squat test performed on a Smith machine using 30% of the 1RM squat tests and the calculation of the fatigue index. Those tests could be included here as well. A few other common tests of anaerobic capacity are the Wingate anaerobic power, the 300-yard (274 m) shuttle, and line drill tests.

Wingate Anaerobic Power Test The Wingate anaerobic power test is an all-out maximal cycle ergometry test lasting 30 seconds (although shorter and longer variations have been used). Cycling is performed against a resistance relative to the athlete's body mass (e.g., 0.075 kilograms per kilogram of body mass on a Monark cycle ergometer) and with it several valuable variables can be determined, including absolute and relative peak power, average power, minimum power, time to peak power, total work, and the fatigue index. A mechanically braked cycle ergometer is needed with a sensor attached to the frame. This can measure flywheel revolutions per minute and interfaces with a computer and software program that performs all of the calculations. The athlete sits comfortably on the cycle and warms up for approximately 5 minutes at a comfortable pace (60 to 70 rpm) against a light resistance or approximately 20% of the test resistance. A couple of short sprints are performed as part of the warm-up. Upon the signal "go," the athlete pedals as fast as possible (against zero resistance to overcome inertia), and the resistance is applied to the flywheel at the onset (0.075 kilograms per kilogram of body mass). The athlete pedals as fast as possible throughout the 30-second test while using good technique. The duration of the test may be modified depending on the athletes. We have adapted the test to 1 minute for wrestlers to assess further anaerobic capacity and power endurance (Ratamess et al. 2013).

The Wingate test can be applied to upper-body anaerobic power with an arm cycle ergometer. For the upper-body Wingate test, the athlete grasps the handles of the arm cycle ergometer while seated on the bench positioned with a slight bend of the elbows at the farthest distance. The arm cycle ergometer wheel axle is aligned with the athlete's shoulder joint. Following a 5-minute warm-up (60 rpms at approximately 25 to 35 W) with all-out sprints at the end of each minute, the tester counts down from five to zero while the athlete pedals at the fastest speed with no load, says "go," applies the resistance (approximately 4% to 5% of body weight), and the athlete continues to pedal with maximum effort for 30 seconds. Repeated upper-body Wingate tests (i.e., 3 to 5 maximal 30-second bouts) may be used to assess power endurance.

300-Yard (274 m) Shuttle This test requires a stopwatch and two parallel lines 25 yards (23 m) apart (on a flat surface). The athlete assumes a starting position at one line (after a proper warm-up). Upon the signal "go," the athlete sprints as fast as possible to the other line 25 yards (23 m) away, making foot contact with it. The athlete immediately sprints back to the starting line, and this process is repeated for six continuous round trips totaling 300 yards (274 m). Time is kept from the "go" signal until the athlete touches the final line. After the first trial and 5 minutes of rest, a second trial is performed. The average of both trials is calculated and recorded.

Shuttle tests are common for assessing anaerobic capacity. The length (total and repetition lengths) and the number of direction changes are variable and can be altered to meet the demands of the athlete's sport. The following are some examples of other shuttle tests used by athletes:

- 300-yard (274 m) shuttle variation: 5 sprints × 60 yards (55 m); player rests 3 minutes and repeats. The times of both trials are averaged.
- 100-yard (91 m) shuttle: 10 sprints × 10 yards (9.1 m); total time is recorded.
- 60-yard (55 m) shuttle: preferably on the marked American football field; player sprints 5 yards (4.6 m) and back, 10 yards (9.1 m) and back, and 15 yards (14 m) and back; total time is recorded, best of 3 trials.
- Baltimore Ravens Shuttle Test: 900 yards (823 m) in total; 6 sets of 6 × 25 yards (23 m) shuttle sprints; rest 64 seconds in between sets and repeat; players have to complete each repetition within 27 to 32 seconds to pass the test.

The Running-Based Anaerobic Sprint Test This test requires a track, stopwatches, speed trap, and cones set 35 meters (38 yd) apart (Draper and Whyute 1997). The athlete sprints 35 meters (38 yd) and rests for 10 seconds (following a proper warm-up). Six sprints are performed in total and each one is timed. Sprint times and body mass are used to calculate maximal, minimal, and average power outputs along with the fatigue index. For each sprint, power is calculated with the following formula: power = body mass (kilograms) × 1,225 meters divided by time^3 (in seconds). Minimum and maximum power are calculated from the best and worst repetitions, and average power can be determined by summing the six repetitions and dividing them by six. The fatigue index can be calculated by subtracting the minimum power from the maximum power and dividing the result by the total time for the six sprints.

Repeated 40s Test The repeated 40s test developed by the National Association of Speed and Explosion (NASE) measures repeated sprint ability and anaerobic capacity (Dintiman, Ward, and Tellez 1998). The test requires a track or measured area of 40 yards (37 m) and a speed trap or stopwatch. The athletes perform a proper warm-up and then sprint for 40 yards (37 m). There is a 15- to 30-second (depending on the sport) rest interval in between sprints. Ten sprints are performed altogether, and each sprint time is recorded. The best and worst times are compared, and to pass the test there should not be a difference of more than 0.2 to 0.3 seconds. There have been other repeated sprint ability tests where the number of repetitions, length, or rest interval differed. For example, some coaches have used ten 30-meter (33 yd) sprints (with a 30-second rest), ten 20-meter (22 yd) sprints (with a 20-second rest), and other variations. Each requires all sprints to be timed and recorded, although the criteria may differ for passing the test or require the calculation of fatigue rate or percent decrement score.

Line Drill The line drill is performed on a basketball court and involves four back-and-forth sprints to all lines on a basketball court. The athlete begins on the baseline and sprints to the foul line and back. The athlete then sprints from the baseline to the half-court line and back, then sprints from the baseline to the far foul line and back. Lastly, the athlete sprints from the baseline to the far baseline and back, touching each line. The stopwatch begins on "go" and stops when the athlete touches the final baseline. Two minutes of rest are given between trials, and the average score is calculated.

Speed

Assessments of speed involve maximal linear movement. Short sprint tests assess the maximal speed and acceleration ability, whereas long sprint tests assess speed endurance. Speed tests can be performed for many modes, including swimming, cycling, rowing, skiing, and skating. The length of the test varies; for example, speed may be assessed at any distance from 5 yards or meters to more than 100 yards or meters. Sprint assessments discussed are the 10-yard (9.1 m) dash, 40-yard (37 m) dash, and 120-yard (110 m) sprint. Technological advances have made speed determination easier. The rise in global positioning system (GPS) and local positioning system (LPS) technology has made it easier for coaches and player development staff to track and monitor speed. This technology has shown good validity and reliability, especially when the system measures at a high sampling rate (10 Hz). Technology such as GPS and LPS is useful for tracking player speed, distance, acceleration and deceleration, change of direction, impact, jumps, and speed thresholds, and for quantifying player load. This section discusses traditional speed assessment with electronic timing devices or stopwatches. In chapter 5 we discuss how speed is monitored with GPS and LPS technology.

10-Yard (9.1 m) Dash The 10-yard (9.1 m) dash is a measure of acceleration. A 10-yard (9.1 m) marked area (with room for deceleration) and a stopwatch or electronic timing device are needed. Electronic timing devices are more accurate because stopwatches contain more human errors. The same coach should time each athlete if a stopwatch is used. Following a proper warm-up, the athlete assumes a starting position using either a three- or four-point stance at the starting line. On the "go" signal, the athlete sprints as fast as possible through the 10-yard (9.1 m) marker. A coach begins the stopwatch on "go" and stops timing once the first segment of the athlete's body crosses the finish line. If an electronic timer is used, infrared sensors are placed at the finish line to stop timing. A start switch is used at the starting line, and timing begins once the athlete lifts off during acceleration. Three to four trials can be used with 3 to 5 minutes of rest in between.

40-Yard (37 m) Dash A 40-yard (37 m) marked area (with room for deceleration) and a stopwatch or electronic timing device are needed for this assessment. Following a proper warm-up, the athlete assumes a starting position using either a three- or four-point stance at the starting line. On the "go" signal, the athlete sprints as fast as possible through the 40-yard (37 m) marker. The time is recorded. Following a rest period of at least 3 minutes, a second and third trial are run. Deceleration should be assessed since it has been suggested that athletes decelerate within seven to eight steps following a maximal sprint (Dintiman, Ward, and Tellez 1998).

120-Yard (110 m) Dash This assessment is conducted similarly to the 40-yard (37 m) dash, but it is three times the distance. It allows more relevant information to be determined by the coach. Each 40-yard (37 m) interval is measured separately, giving the coach information on all three phases of sprinting (Dintiman, Ward, and Tellez 1998). Three timers are needed: one to start the test and conclude at the 40-yard (37 m) mark, one to begin timing at the 40-yard (37 m) mark and conclude at the 80-yard (73 m) mark, and one to start at the 80-yard (73 m) mark and conclude at the 120-yard (110 m) mark. A variation is to have all three timers begin timing on "go" and stop on completion of the three marks. The interval times are determined by subtracting the 40-yard (37 m) time from the 80-yard (73 m) time and the 80-yard (73 m) time from the 120-yard (110 m) time. An electronic timing device can be used and is preferred, but three sets of infrared sensors would be needed for each 40-yard (37 m) interval. The athlete begins in a three- or four-point stance and sprints as fast as possible throughout the 120-yard (110 m) distance. The initial 40 yards (37 m) are the *stationary 40-yard (37 m) dash*, and the recorded times relate similarly to the performance of a normal 40-yard dash. The second segment is the *flying 40-yard (37 m) dash* because it begins with the athlete at full speed. Acceleration can be assessed by subtracting each flying 40 time from the corresponding stationary 40 time. Acceleration is good if the athlete's difference is less than 0.7 seconds. The third segment is known as the *speed endurance 40 segments* because it measures the athlete's ability to maintain maximal speed. It is determined by subtracting each speed endurance 40 time from the corresponding flying 40 time. Speed endurance is good if the difference is less than 0.2 seconds.

Agility and Change-of-Direction Ability

Agility tests assess the athlete's ability to accelerate rapidly, decelerate, and change direction in a controlled manner using forward, backward, and side shuffling types of movements. They test an athlete's change-of-direction (COD) ability and reactive ability. Cones, lines, or other markers, as well as stopwatches (or more accurate timing devices) are used for agility testing. Tape and tape measures are needed to measure and mark off appropriate distances. The same coach must measure every test for the same athlete to increase consistency and reduce errors in timing. Coaches should select drills for movements that are highly specific to the sport. Any line or cone agility drill, COD drill, or ladder drill can be timed and used to assess or monitor athletes. Some drills have been used extensively and shown to be valid and reliable. Although a multitude of drills can be used for assessment, the 505 COD test (and COD deficit), *t*-test, hexagon test, pro agility, three-cone drill, and Edgren sidestep tests are discussed.

505 COD Test The 505 COD test involves a 15-meter (16 yd) sprint, COD 180° turn, and subsequent 5-meter (5.5 yd) sprint (figure 3.8). The 505 COD test may help distinguish between dominant and nondominant limb performance differences because it uses one single 180° turn. A marked area, tape measure, and timing devices are needed. After a warm-up, the athlete stands on the starting line with a two-point split stance. On "go," the athlete accelerates maximally for 15 meters (16 yd) to the third line marker, touches the line with the foot, turns 180° quickly on the right or left leg, and sprints maximally for 5 meters (5.5 yd) to the second line marker (or finish). Timing begins at the 10-meter (11 m) marker and stops after the athlete crosses the finish line marker. The test should be repeated for the opposite limb. At least 2 to 3 minutes of rest should be used between trials. Multiple trials should be performed for each leg and the times recorded. It has been recommended that the *COD deficit* be calculated from the 505 test by subtracting the 10-meter (11 yd) sprint time from the 505 test time to better represent the COD time (Nimphius et al. 2016).

T-Test Four cones and a stopwatch are needed. Three cones are aligned in a straight line, 5 yards (4.6 m) apart, and a fourth cone is aligned with the second cone, 10 yards (9.1 m) apart, forming a "T" shape. Following a warm-up, the athlete sprints forward 10 yards (9.1 m), shuffles to the left 5 yards (4.6 m) to the cone, shuffles back to the

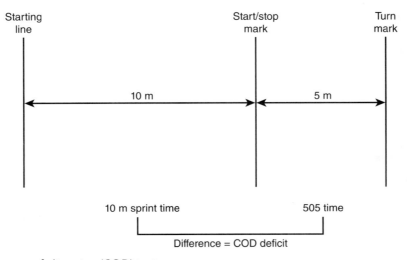

FIGURE 3.8 505 change-of-direction (COD) test.

right 10 yards (9.1 m) to the other cone, shuffles left to the middle cone, and backpedals back to the starting cone (figure 3.9). The athlete faces forward at all times and does not cross the feet. Cones are touched at each marker. The athlete begins on "go," and timing stops when the athlete backpedals past the starting cone at the end.

Pro Agility Test This test, also called the 20-yard (18 m) shuttle run, can be performed on an American football field with parallel lines 5 yards (4.6 m) apart or on another marked area. A stopwatch is needed. The athlete begins by straddling the center line in a three-point stance.

On "go," the athlete sprints 5 yards (4.6 m) to the line on the right (touching the line with hand and foot), then sprints left for 10 yards (9.1 m) to the farthest line (touching the line), then sprints right for 5 yards (4.6 m) through the center line (figure 3.10). Timing ends when the athlete passes the center line. The best time of two to three trials is recorded.

Three-Cone Drill Three cones are placed in an upside-down "L" configuration, with each cone separated by 5 yards (4.6 m). A stopwatch is needed for timing. The athlete begins behind the starting line at cone A, sprints to cone B and back to cone A, then sprints to the outside of cone B, rounds cone B and sprints to cone C, rounds cone C, sprints back to cone B, and then sprints back to cone A at the finish point (figure 3.11). Timing begins on "go" and finishes when the athlete crosses the finish line. The best of three trials is recorded.

Hexagon Test This test requires adhesive tape, a tape measure, and a stopwatch. A hexagon is formed, each side measuring 24 inches (61 cm) to form angles of 120°. Following a proper warm-up, the athlete begins by standing in the middle of the hexagon. On "go," the athlete begins double-leg hopping from the center of the hexagon to each side and back to the center. The athlete starts with the side directly in front and continues clockwise until the drill is complete (which requires three revolutions), for a total of 18 jumps outward and 18 back to the center (figure 3.12). The trial is stopped

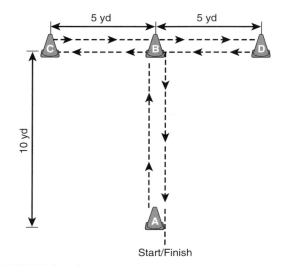

FIGURE 3.9 The standard t-test.

Reprinted by permission from D.H. Fukuda, *Assessments for Sport and Athletic Performance* (Champaign, IL: Human Kinetics, 2019).

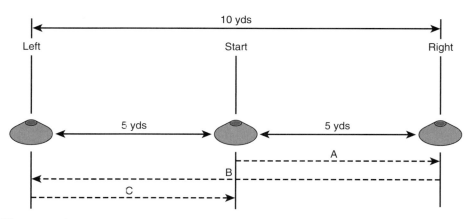

FIGURE 3.10 The pro agility test.

Reprinted by permission from D.H. Fukuda, *Assessments for Sport and Athletic Performance* (Champaign, IL: Human Kinetics, 2019).

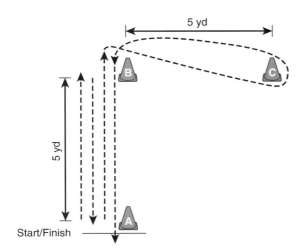

FIGURE 3.11 The three-cone drill.

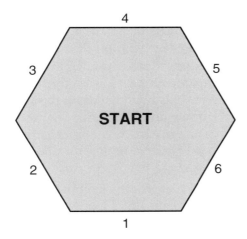

FIGURE 3.12 The hexagon test.

Reprinted by permission from D.H. Fukuda, *Assessments for Sport and Athletic Performance* (Champaign, IL: Human Kinetics, 2019).

for violations, including landing on the line (rather than over it), loss of balance, and taking extra steps. The best of three trials is recorded.

Edgren Side Step Test   A 12-foot (3.7 m) area is needed where lines (or tape) are placed 3 feet (0.9 m) apart. Five taped lines are needed altogether on a gym floor. Following a proper warm-up, the athlete begins the test by straddling the center line. On "go," the athlete performs side steps to the right to the outside line, then left to the farthest line, and then performs side shuffles back and forth for 10 seconds (figure 3.13). A tester counts the number of lines crossed during the 10-second period.

Balance

Balance is the ability to maintain static and dynamic equilibrium and to control the center of gravity relative to the base support. Assessing balance can be of great value to the athlete because poor balance is related to an increased risk of ankle and knee injuries. Balance training embodies a combination of all training modalities in addition to specific balance exercises. Balance can be tested in different ways, including with timed static standing tests (eyes closed or on one leg), dynamic unilateral standing tests that involve a measurable movement with opposite limb or upper extremities, balance tests using unstable surfaces (*stabilometers*, wobble board, BOSU, pads, foam rollers, stability balls), standing tests on force plates (to measure

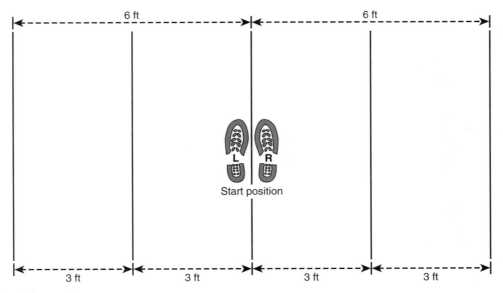

FIGURE 3.13 Edgren side step test.

postural sway or total shifts of the center of pressure during a prescribed time), and specialized balance testing equipment. Some examples of balance tests include the following:

- *Single-leg squat:* The athlete stands with hands on hips, a shoulder-width stance, eyes focused straight ahead, and feet positioned forward. The athlete squats on one leg while the opposite leg is elevated. The ROM depends on strength and body size. The coach looks at posture (erect torso), hip position, and knee movement. Inward movement of the knee (*valgus stress*) is an issue for female athletes who are at greater risk for ACL injuries than men. Coaches should make sure the shoulders and pelvic girdle remain level and the tested knee aligns with the foot. Excellent single-leg squat assessment would be indicated by hip flexion greater than 65°, less than 10° of hip abduction or adduction, and more than 10° of knee valgus motion. A similar test for single-leg balance and strength is the *anterior reach*, in which the athlete extends a leg out as far as possible (while balancing on the opposite leg), keeping the front foot close to the floor without touching it. The farthest distance reached out of three to four trials with the front leg is measured.

- *The star excursion balance test (SEBT) and Y balance test:* The athlete stands in the center with eight lines extending out at 45° increments. The eight lines represent the anterolateral, anterior, anteromedial, medial, posteromedial, posterior, posterolateral, and lateral directions. The athlete maintains a single-leg stance while reaching with the contralateral leg as far as possible for each taped line, lightly touching the farthest point, and then returns to a bilateral stance. The distance is measured from the center to the contact point. The best or average of three trials (using 15-second rest intervals) is recorded and repeated for the opposite side. Reach distances are normalized to leg length. Trials are discarded if the athlete does not touch the line, lifts the stance foot from the center, loses balance, or does not maintain start and return positions for 1 full second. The Y balance test (YBT) (figure 3.14) was developed to reduce the length of the SEBT by including only three movements (anterior, posterolateral, and posteromedial). The score is calculated by summing the three directions and normalizing the quantity to leg length. After a warm-up and practice trials, the athlete performs at least three trials (with hands on hips) for each leg in each direction while sliding the guide piece as far as possible in each direction using the Y balance kit. Loss of balance results in a failed attempt.

- *Landing tests:* These involve either stepping off of an elevation or jumping and landing bilaterally or unilaterally. They examine postural control and balance during landing, which is important for optimizing technique (by teaching a soft landing) during power movements, especially

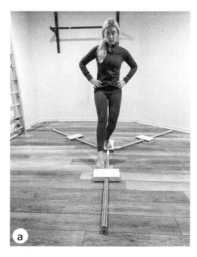 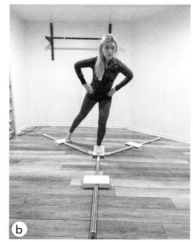 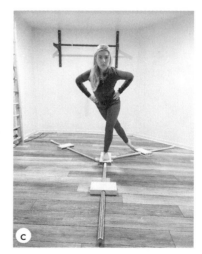

FIGURE 3.14 The Y balance test.

Photos courtesy of Dr. Tamara Rial Rebullido and Dr. Avery Faigenbaum.

when prescreening athletes for potential injuries. Soft landing involves greater hip and knee ROM, and less ground reaction force. Single-leg tests involving drop landings, vertical jumps, hops, and side-step cutting have been used to assess injury risk factors. Single-leg hops may be assessed by distance covered or the time needed to cover a specified distance. The *Klatt test* assesses balance and stability during a single-leg landing after the athlete steps off of a small box. Likewise, coaches should look for knee valgus motion, internal rotation, and degree of flexion, in addition to balance, stability, and posture. One bilateral landing test is the *landing error scoring system* (LESS). The LESS test involves standing on a 12-inch (30 cm) box, jumping forward and landing bilaterally on a marked line on the floor, and maximally jumping vertically as high as possible. Two cameras are placed approximately 10 feet (3 m) away in front and to the right of the landing area. At least three trials are performed after a warm-up and practice repetitions. Scoring is based on errors that occur through a 17-point subjective technical grading sheet for at least two of the three trials recorded.

- *Balance error scoring system (BESS):* This requires a foam pad (approximately 2.5 inches [6.4 cm] thick), stopwatch, and score card. Testing consists of six separate 20-second balance tests performed with no shoes: (1) single-leg, (2) double-leg, and (3) tandem stances performed on the floor and on the foam pad. The athlete stands with hands on hips and eyes closed for all tests. For a double-leg stance, feet are kept side-by-side and touching. For a single-leg stance, the athlete stands on the nondominant foot, the opposite hip is flexed 30°, and the knee is flexed approximately 45°. For tandem stance, the athlete stands heel-to-toe with the nondominant foot in the back (the heel of the dominant foot should be touching the toe of the nondominant foot). A spotter can assist if an athlete loses balance. Errors are recorded for each trial when the athlete: (1) moves hands off of the hips, (2) opens eyes, (3) loses balance or falls, (4) abducts or flexes hip more than 30°, (5) lifts forefoot or heel off of the surface, and (6) remains out of proper testing position for more than 5 seconds. The maximum number of errors per trial is 10; therefore, the worst possible score attained would be 60. The lower the score, the better the balance.

Reaction Time

Reaction time is the time that elapses from when an athlete perceives a stimulus until the response begins, while *response time* includes reaction time and movement time (the amount of time it takes to complete the movement). Reaction and response times involve a complex, sequential synapsing coordination pattern between the central and peripheral nervous systems and skeletal muscle (figure 3.15). Because reaction and response times depend on many factors, training and testing reaction time are multimodal. They depend on the comprehensive physiologic response of the body's motor, neural, metabolic, hormonal, and cardiorespiratory systems to stimuli (discussed in chapter 4), but fast reaction time also requires visual acuity, contrast sensitivity, depth perception, general perception, and cognitive skills (i.e., decision-making, anticipation, pattern recognition, and situational probability) (Hadlow et al. 2018). Reaction and response times are trained by general strength and conditioning, sport participation, and perceptual training. Modified perceptual training involves on- and off-field tasks, such as sport vision training and perceptual-cognitive training, implemented with conventional training and practice to improve the athlete's ability to transfer anticipation and decision-making skills to sport-specific movements (although, unfortunately, empirical evidence linking modified perceptual training to improved decision-making is sparse). Sport vision training targets the lens and extraocular muscles of the eyes through the occipital lobe's visual cortex and association area (Hadlow et al. 2018). Perceptual-cognitive training involves video-based systems (e.g., console, TV, and computer), virtual reality and gaming, field-based systems (e.g., stroboscopic lights and glasses), handheld device apps, touch screen tools, and LED lighting systems. Although any training tool can be used for assessment, this section discusses a few reaction and response tests that target hand–eye coordination and physical mobility.

Testing an athlete's reaction and response times involves measuring the interval it takes to react to an open stimulus or the number of accurate hits within a specific period. The stimuli supplied by the testing device can be altered to accommodate novice to elite abilities. One test we have used in

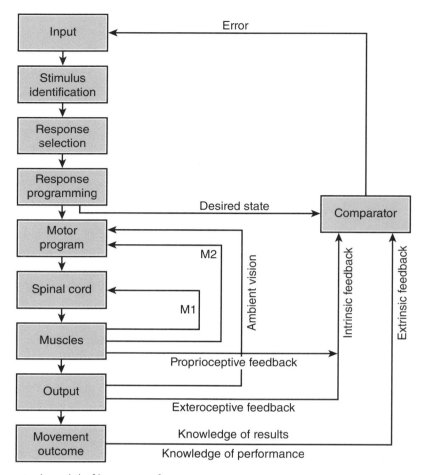

FIGURE 3.15 Conceptual model of human performance.

Reprinted by permission from R.A. Schmidt and C.A. Wrisberg, *Motor Learning and Performance*, 3rd ed. (Champaign, IL: Human Kinetics, 2004).

testing is the Makoto light system test (Hoffman et al. 2009). It is triangular shaped (8 feet [2.4 m] from base to apex), consists of three steel towers 6 feet (1.8 m) in height, and each tower contains 10 targets that light up and make sound during the test. The athlete begins in the middle of the base, holding a padded stick or wearing gloves (whatever is relevant to the sport). Each test lasts 2 minutes and consists of random lights and sounds that the athlete must respond to by striking the appropriate target before the lights and sounds cease. This device has 12 levels of difficulty, so it is essential to record the level used for each athlete. Scoring calculates the total number of successful direct strikes (i.e., ones that count), divided by the total number of possible hits in the 2-minute period. Multiple trials may be used and the best is recorded.

Light board tests have been used especially for boxers, MMA fighters, and other combat striking athletes. A light board or similar device is needed for displaying a target light that moves randomly. The athlete stands on the floor or on an instability device such as a BOSU ball, faces the light board, and attempts to press as many active lights as possible. The total number of lights pressed is recorded. A number of light systems are available that give the athlete random targets for multiple levels, heights, and bodily positions. Some lighting systems are portable and can be placed on cones used in an agility circuit for an open drill.

Sport-Specific

Sport-specific tests can be used as part of the testing battery. They are strictly related to the sport's movements and often test multiple fitness components. For example, in baseball and softball, coaches can measure the specific time it takes to sprint from home to first base, bat swing velocity, batted ball exit velocity, throwing velocity, pick-off time for pitchers, and home-to-second base throw time for catchers. Boxers can be assessed for punching velocity, punching power, and punching speed (for a variety of punches). MMA athletes can be tested for the same as well as kicking power, velocity, and takedown speed. A number of specific aerobic tests, tests for agility and speed, and sandbag throw tests have been developed for boxers, wrestlers, striking athletes (e.g., karate, judo, and taekwondo), and fencing athletes (Chaabene et al. 2018). Basketball players may be assessed with tests such as the three-quarter court sprint, lane agility drill, and reactive shuttle run. Sport-specific tests can be used in every sport to determine the translation of the strength and conditioning program to a sport-specific task (figure 3.16) (Kraemer et al. 2003; Doan et al. 2006). Thus, the testing battery of athletes should include a mix of tests that target specific fitness components as well as sport-specific tests that can be used to assess the transfer effects of training to the sport.

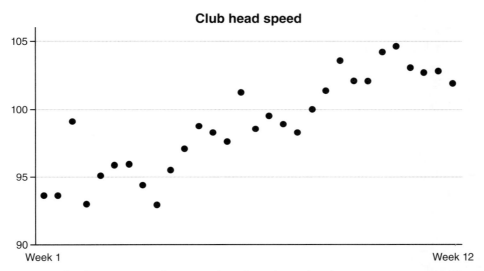

FIGURE 3.16 An example of a sport-specific test to directly evaluate the changes in a sport-specific task (club speed in golf).

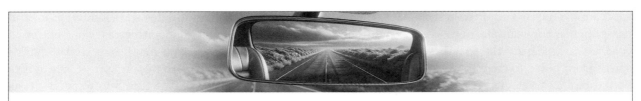

LOOKING IN THE REARVIEW MIRROR

- Developing a testing battery and preparing the staff for appropriate testing procedures are priorities. The staff must adopt scientific and standardized procedures to determine the most accurate data during testing. Testing must be valid and reliable.
- Preparing the athlete for testing (e.g., medical clearance, familiarization, nutrition and hydration, and procedural practices) is paramount.
- Health-related fitness components to be tested include body composition and anthropometry, muscular strength, muscular endurance, aerobic endurance, and flexibility and posture. The player development team should pick one to three tests per component, depending on the athlete, and implement them with high levels of standardization.
- Skill-related fitness components to be tested include power, anaerobic capacity, speed and acceleration, agility, change of direction, mobility, balance, and reaction time. The player development team should pick one to three tests per component, depending on the athlete, and implement them with high levels of standardization.
- Developing sport-specific tests for the athletes helps the player development team bridge the gap between transfer of performance from the strength and conditioning program to performance in a specific sport.

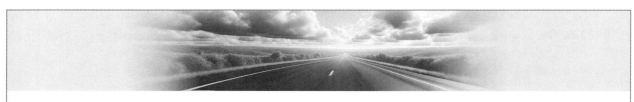

LOOKING AT THE ROAD AHEAD

Development of the athlete composite depends on understanding the exercise stimuli used to bring about adaptive changes. Basic principles must be understood if conditioning programs are to be based on scientific foundations. Fundamental guidelines for exercise prescriptions are vital to developing workout and training routines. The variations in workouts, defined by the different approaches to periodization, are critical to optimizing training quality and recovery. The training adaptations that lead to performance improvements occur over a given time frame. Individualization is also important for addressing the needs of the different athletes.

4

Understanding the Workout Stimuli: Impact on the Athlete Composite

The movements performed in a workout, practice session, or competition create a unique demand for muscle force and power, which in turn create a specific need for motor units. One motor unit comprises an alpha motor neuron and its associated muscle fibers. When the demands of a movement are processed in the brain, especially in the sensory and premotor cortices, the aggregate of information interacts with the brain's primary motor cortex to create action potentials or electrical charges of different strengths (expressed in hertz) to produce the desired body movements. These action potentials are sent from the brain down the spine (i.e., central nervous system) and out into the periphery (i.e., peripheral nervous system) via the motor neuron to recruit muscle fibers to produce the exact amount of force or power in each muscle demanded by the activity (for a review see Kraemer, Fleck, and Deschenes 2021; Ratamess 2022).

The movements or exercise demands of the muscles require the support of the different physiological systems (see chapter 1) for acute performance but even more for the recovery process on completion. Thus, the exercise stimulus is critical to understanding the exercise demands, recovery responses, and resulting training effects. This is where complex interactions of different exercises, practices, and competitions can create exercise incompatibilities and therefore disruptors that negate proper recovery or adaptive training progress. This is one of the most important considerations the player development team must be aware of in their assessments, monitoring, and evaluations of workouts, practices, and competition for each athlete (see chapter 5).

Size Principle: Understanding Is Crucial to Practice

The player development team must understand *Henneman's size principle* to have a common language for the demands placed on the neuromuscular system. This principle is named after Elwood Henneman (1915 to 1996) of Harvard University, who built upon discoveries from the early days of neuroscience and studied the recruitment of motor units. Motor units are homogeneous, consisting of all type I (slow twitch) or all type II (fast twitch) muscle fibers. The term "size" comes from the fact that one can recruit motor units based on a sizing factor to activate more skeletal muscle (e.g., recruit more motor units or recruit motor units with larger fibers) to achieve the needed force. His research showed in various studies that motor units are recruited from smallest to largest, whether during concentric or eccentric muscle actions. Recruitment depends on the external activity demands (e.g., light or heavy resistance). Each motor unit has its electrical activation threshold (in hertz) that must be met to recruit the associated fibers before activation. As the exercise demands increase, more and more motor units must be recruited to meet the force demands. This is accomplished by sending action potentials with higher and higher electrical signals from the brain down the line. As my wife Joan (WJK) explained, using her elementary school background, "it is like turning on a conventional stove's burner to get the heat; you start at zero, and then you have to continue to turn the knob up to higher numbers on the dial to get the exact amount of heat you want." Thus, motor units are recruited in all of the different muscles associated with the activity (e.g., it takes 244 different muscles activated in various ways to perform a squat exercise). Each activity (e.g., a jump or a power clean) requires different levels of force and power for different muscular actions (i.e., concentric, eccentric, or isometric) to perform the activity using the proper technique. A resistance exercise loading example for the recruitment of motor units is shown in figure 4.1. The complexity of movement is centered in the brain's ability to activate the neuromuscular system effectively and repetitively in response to the activity's or skill's external demands.

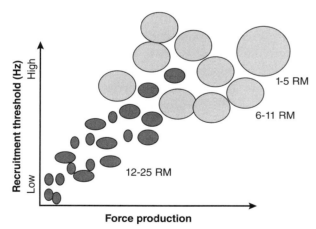

FIGURE 4.1 The dark-colored circles represent type I motor units with different amounts of muscle fibers based on the circle's size. The lighter circles represent the type II motor units with larger or more muscle fibers. In this example of resistance exercise intensity, as the repetition maximum (RM) intensity increases, more and larger motor units must be recruited to provide the needed force. The recruitment threshold (Y-axis) needed for each RM load requires a different electrical charge to activate the motor unit and produce the required force (X-axis).

The Exercise Stimuli Create an Exercise Drug

The analogy has often been made that exercise is like a drug. The American College of Sports Medicine uses the phrase *exercise is medicine*, which implies that an exercise stimulates physiological systems as if it were a drug. The elevations in physiological systems in response to exercise, however, far exceed what any typical drug is capable of producing. The player development team needs to view exercise as a physician views medicine when diagnosing illness and prescribing the right kind and dose using evidence-based practices to point them in the right direction. Activating the body's neuromuscular system to produce a specific movement awakens all physiological systems. The mechanical and physiological characteristics of that movement will determine the magnitude of involvement for each physiological system in meeting the demands of the exercise. Exercise workouts are not trivial in player development—exercise can be very potent. As with any medication, exercise can be underdosed or overdosed in its prescription, so the exercise prescribed must be carefully designed according to the various intensities and volumes needed at different points in the training cycle for altering the athlete's composite.

Safety for the Athlete Is Priority One

The athlete's safety has to be a priority for the player development team. This must be communicated to everyone involved with the athlete, including athletic and sport administrators, friends, family, and the community. Administrators often betray this principle with hiring practices that do not follow the three Cs noted in chapter 3—"credentials, competence, and commitment."

Inter-Association Guidelines for Workouts

Over the last 10 to 15 years, safety in athletics has come to the forefront as many different organizations have arrived at guidelines for competent and accepted practices to prevent sudden death in athletics. The legal responsibilities related to such practices are also significant. These guidelines have covered everything from practice to environmental conditions to optimize high school and collegiate athletics safety. Much of this was initiated after the tragic and preventable death of Korey Stringer, an offensive tackle for the Minnesota Vikings, on August 1, 2001, from heatstroke. The Korey Stringer Institute was developed by Dr. Douglas Casa, a professor at the University of Connecticut (https://ksi.uconn.edu), and it continues to be a tremendous free resource for questions and answers on safety and prevention of sudden death in athletics. Administrators and all involved with athletes, including emergency medical personnel, should read and be aware of these fundamental concepts and practices for preventing sudden death in sports (Cools et al. 2022; Hosokawa et al. 2021; Casa et al. 2012; Yeargin et al. 2016; Szymanski et al. 2020).

While documented in great detail in the suggested readings referenced earlier, some of the major areas that must be addressed for workout safety include the following (Casa et al. 2012):

1. Progressive acclimatization for utmost safety
2. Gradual introduction of new conditioning activities
3. Prohibition of exercise and conditioning activities as punishment
4. Proper education, experience, and credentialing of strength and conditioning professionals
5. Appropriate medical coverage
6. Development and practice of emergency action protocols
7. Cognizance of medical conditions
8. Administration of strength and conditioning programs
9. Partnerships with recognized professional organizations
10. Adequate continuing education for the entire coaching and medical teams

Importance of Having a Policy and Standards Manual

One of the first things that happen when there is an adverse event in a player development program is that administrators and legal counsel want to know where the policy manual and standards of practice guides are housed in the facility. Documentation is vital for demonstrating the safety and prudent care of the athlete. It will be covered further in chapter 5 (e.g., monitoring of workouts, injuries, and pre-workout injury checks). Ideally, the player development team should have a legal consultant to vet practices and questions. The NSCA has detailed ideas on this topic (Haff and Triplett 2016). Additionally, the NSCA's standards of practice document is essential for supporting the program's approach (NSCA 2017; Haff and Triplett 2016). Communicating these practices with the program's administrators and legal counsel is vital. Specialty areas (e.g., nutrition and athletic training) beyond conditioning also need to support and define their practices as part of the player development team, as discussed in chapter 1. Have proper forms and templates for the program; for a reference, see the following resource and its associated web reference templates (Lopiano and Zotos 2014).

The Stimulus–Response–Adaptation Cycle

The stimulus for developing the athlete's composite comes from the movement demands the athlete is exposed to in sport competitions, practices, and conditioning. The recruitment of motor units in specific ways dictates the physiological demands that result in any adaptive progress in the athlete's composite. This is called the *stimulus-response-adaptation cycle*. When a stimulus for recruitment of motor units to produce movement occurs, all systems are activated, only differing in the magnitude of priority as to what system is needed more to meet the acute demands (e.g., walking versus sprinting or biceps curl versus squat).

The *adaptation* phase of the cycle is achieved during the recovery time after the *stimulus and response*. As training progresses in any mutable characteristic, this cycle will also differ as more work becomes possible, system responses become more efficient, and structural morphologies of the body advance. But this takes time, and while some adaptive progressions can be observed in a few workouts, others take weeks, months, or years.

As noted in chapter 1, adaptation is a stepwise progression: The cycle repeats itself over time until the genetic ceiling for a mutable characteristic flattens out any progression, or until the target level or training goal is met. The stimulus for the cycle then becomes one of maintenance. Thus, acute responses and chronic adaptations both have time scales associated with them. A critical response will occur no matter the level of the adaptive state (e.g., three months of training experience versus five years). Still, that acute response may differ depending on the evaluated variable. For example, with training, the athlete's body learns how to respond to an exercise or competitive stress and modulate itself to meet the exact demands. Conversely, novice athletes or athletes with little training background must learn how to modulate their physiological responses, and they typically overshoot what is required. Their bodies have little left when the athletes need them most for maximal exercise challenges. We see this in the response of the adrenal glands to exercise (Kraemer et al. 1985). Trained athletes do not secrete as much adrenaline (i.e., epinephrine) in response to submaximal exercise because they know how to respond to low-level demands. They save a big response when they need it most for an extreme or maximal exercise challenge when it helps produce higher muscle force and power. Modulating adrenaline is related to the concept of being "in the zone," where, physiologically, one has all systems in tune with what is needed for the optimal neuromuscular performance of skills in the sport.

Logistical Comfort and Peak Performance: A Symbiosis

Achieving peak performance necessitates transcending logistical comfort zones to formulate and implement optimal programming. This pursuit is defined not merely by high standards but also by harmoniously marrying scientific acumen with artistic innovation. It is an intricate balance that requires scrutiny of key questions:

1. What is the ultimate program for my athletes, grounded in the most credible research and anecdotal wisdom?

2. Does the staff possess the requisite skill and quality control to meticulously administer the program, ensuring the level of compliance and execution necessary to induce the desired adaptation?

3. Is the program's execution logistically viable, given the available human and physical resources?

The pursuit of peak performance requires an unceasing commitment to education, innovation, and iteration. Staff should be inspired to venture beyond their comfort zones, mirroring the zone of proximal development used to encourage growth in athletes. Embrace a culture of constant evolution, driving the team to deliver unmatched results.

The paramount goal is to architect programs that resonate with athletes, striking a precise equilibrium between ideal programming and the realistic capacities of staff and resources. This balance ensures adherence, challenging both the logistical boundaries and the athletes' potential without overstepping the feasible limits.

By meticulously weaving this intricate tapestry, coaches enable athletes, clients, and operators to advance swiftly toward their fullest potential. It's an approach that demands more than mere technical mastery; it's an art form where precision, creativity, and adaptability coalesce to unlock performance like never before. In this landscape, logistical comfort is not a boundary but a steppingstone toward an unexplored realm of excellence.

Program Variables in Training Program Design

The acute program variables describe any workout in a resistance training program. As one adds variables for other components to the program, the toolbox grows even bigger. The player development team needs professionals in the areas with the three Cs to optimize the training program designs and then individually modulate them over time in an effective and integrated program of monitoring and assessments. This will be discussed further in the next chapters. Each of the elements in the player development program must be integrated daily based on a plan.

Acute Program Variables in Resistance Workout Designs

For many years, the acute program design variable domains for choices in designing resistance training workouts have been documented. While these domains have been extensively written about and studied, they still require the art of the strength and conditioning professional to choose correctly, just as a skilled physician would choose and titrate a drug. The variable domains consist of the following:

- Choice of exercise
- Order of exercise
- Intensity of exercise
- Volume (number of sets × repetitions × intensity) and velocity (or duration)
- Rest period lengths
- Frequency of exercise

Other Conditioning Programs

In addition to resistance training, the athlete composite is affected by a host of other conditioning programs, which have also been extensively described and studied. They include the following:

- Anaerobic programs related to
  - Speed
  - Anaerobic capacity endurance (i.e., buffering mechanisms of H^+ and pH changes)
  - Plyometric drills augmenting weight room power training
  - Agility and change-of-direction drills
- Aerobic endurance
- Flexibility

Compatibility of Exercise Programs

These different training stimuli must be integrated so as not to interfere with each other. Interference can occur because of the volume or intensities of simultaneous exercises, potentially from acute nonfunctional overreaching, or because of struggles between different stimuli (e.g., aerobic versus high force) for adaptational changes (e.g., muscle fiber hypertrophy). This has been most dramatically observed in high–intensity, long duration, and aerobic endurance training using concurrent running modality and heavy resistance training for maximal strength and power. The impact appears to reduce the hypertrophic capabilities of the type I units when both exercise stimuli recruit fibers. Thus, the type I muscle fibers do not demonstrate as much cellular hypertrophy when both are used simultaneously with high intensity and volume (Kraemer et al. 1995). This may limit the total hypertrophic response of the lower-body muscle used in locomotion.

Recovery

One of the primary concerns in a player development program is the importance of recovery. Workouts can differ in how much stress is placed on physiological systems. Stress results in fatigue, which depresses the different systems to various extents but most apparently the neuromuscular system. It is a challenge for the body to bring everything back to resting homeostasis, but if training is effective, structures and functions will improve to a new level to adapt to the imposed demands. This is classically called the *SAID principle* (specific adaptations to imposed demands). A lack of recovery can lead to *nonfunctional overreaching* without a plan for supercompensation after a sequence of workouts. *Functional overreaching* is designed with a sequence of workouts to suppress recovery, followed by a timed relaxation of workout demands (or taper) to produce a dramatic supercompensation or rebound to higher performance levels (*planned functional overreaching*). This is often part of peaking programs in different sports (e.g., swimming, cycling, and distance running) and workout approaches in resistance training. However, it has been observed that such workout sequences produce highly individual response patterns, and it takes a fundamental understanding of each athlete's response pattern to optimize functional overreaching sequencing. Thus, *functional overloading* is challenging and only possible when serious monitoring and accounting practices are in place, especially in more advanced athletes.

Recovery can also involve multiple interventions postworkout to enhance the body's physiological system's adaptive mechanisms. While beyond the scope of this text, it is well known that a host of different interventions exist, and care is needed to ensure that they conform to the legality of the sport's governing bodies (e.g., USADA, WADA, and NCAA). Each element of the player performance team needs to address recovery in all its physical and psychological dimensions. A comprehensive program is required and can vary for each athlete. While global recovery interventions (e.g., nutrition, sleep, and cooldown interventions) are put in place by each element of the player development team, each athlete may still have additional specific recovery needs.

Before individual recovery interventions are implemented, the player development team should go back and assess the different variables that are part of the monitoring and assessment program. What is going on with the athlete's normative status? What is the difference (e.g., nutrition, performance, psychology, and injury statuses)? Unknowns constantly threaten optimal recovery, usually from a lack of regular assessments or missing assessments. Differential problems can exist because of undocumented injury, soreness, nutritional deficiencies in caloric intake, vitamin deficiencies (e.g., in vitamin D), sleep, and alcohol or drug abuse. In each case, a variable that is "out of whack" can be individually corrected if properly assessed and analyzed before, as they say, "throwing everything but the kitchen sink" at the athlete in the hope of something working. Such problems can become evident if workouts are carefully assessed in real time or within 24 hours. If this is not done, it is typically because of the number of athletes, a lack of technology, time constraints, and a limited number of professionals working on the team. Solutions to these issues need to be addressed by the athletic administrative units. The performance development team must continually educate administrators on the scope of their professional duties and ethical responsibilities toward the care and safety of the athletes whom they manage daily. These assessments will help individualize the recovery interventions needed. If the program eventually finds something that was not assessed, then such assessments must be added to the existing player development monitoring and assessment program. Thus, the evolution of a player development program for each sport, and as a total program, is a building process. Some aspects are universal for every sport (e.g., sleep and nutritional basics).

Some common interventions successfully used are protein and creatine monohydrate supplementation, compression and cryocompression, mindfulness, flotation-restricted environmental therapy, foam rollers, and contrast hydrotherapy. However, assessing workout and practice demands and sequences sit at the core of stress and recovery demands.

Variation in Training Programs Mediating Recovery and Performance

Further training theory and programming discussions will be addressed in chapters 6 and 7. For more than 100 years, many training theorists have tried to look at the optimal progression of the training stimulus, leading to many concepts in resistance training and other conditioning modalities. Periodization has evolved as a global training concept that, at its core, involves variation in supporting recovery or supercompensation of the different performance variables. Another concept arising from training theory is the need for variation in the exercise stimuli. This construct of variation has led to the term *periodization*, whether for a resistance training program, other conditioning modalities, practices, or game and match schedules. Periodization is highly specific to a sport and its needs for enhancing the athlete composite with various conditioning tools. The athlete composite must be optimized in the sequence of training phases that are designed to lead to success at the time of competition.

Still, one of the most crucial recovery elements is the proper sequencing of resistance training workouts and their integration with other sport activities. This has been the holy grail in sport training for centuries. Classical training sequences developed with early periodization models can thrive when disruptors do not exist, but in today's academic, club, and professional sports, disruptors come from all dimensions of the athlete's world. Some of the different topical domains for disruptors include the following:

- Sport practices
- Competitions and travel
- Available weekly training opportunities and time
- Facilities
- Numbers of athletes
- Athlete training experience
- Number of performance professionals
- Sport coach's philosophies
- Academic demands
- Work demands
- Athlete behavioral patterns (e.g., nutrition and sleep)
- Social and behavioral choices
- Psychological challenges
- Injury and rehabilitation

We know from training theory that the classical concept of periodization evolved from the use of different segments that broke up the training year or Olympic training cycle into smaller parts. The well-known standard terms of the macrocycle, mesocycle, and microcycle evolved from this and were often given different operational periods. The classical periodization model typically started with a macrocycle of 1 year, a mesocycle from 12 to 16 weeks, and a microcycle from 2 to 4 weeks. The intensity and volume progressed similarly, from high volume and lower intensity to lower volume and higher intensity, leading to the peaking of performance. These approaches have been extensively written about in books, papers, Internet articles, blogs, and social media. Many models within this primary genre of periodization were developed for specific sports. Furthermore, various terms—besides the standard terms of intensity, frequency, volume, and load—were coined for different classical periodization models to describe the different program elements, which often led to more confusion.

The constancy of using the same intensity and volume over one microcycle in classical periodization stimulated others to experiment with more dramatic variations over a week to 10 days. Other associated changes in acute program variables, including rest period lengths and choice of exercises, were integrated into this novel approach to periodization. This created a completely different sequence of daily workouts, which evolved into a daily microcycle. This approach was at first called an *undulating* approach to periodization, with its three-day cycling of heavy, moderate, and light intensities, but it soon came to be called *nonlinear* to differentiate it from what was perceived to be a linear model in the so-called classic periodization microcycle duration for intensity and volume over time. Early undulating protocols did not vary the intensity and volume over the week's schedule as dramatically as later models did (Rhea et al. 2002; Poliquin 1988).

While arguments and controversy exist, choosing the best approach is somewhat irrelevant when working with athletes in different sports and with various disruptors that must be addressed daily. The nonlinear approach and the prioritizing of quality, rather than just getting it done, supported the needs of recovery. Even the first undulating or nonlinear periodization model used a predetermined sequence of workouts. If the sequence could not be performed, the athlete defaulted to another workout style or rested a day. It became apparent to many who worked in sports that even this was too rigid to address the need for optimization on each available training day. Skipping to the next workout or doing the missed work next could reduce exposure to the required stimuli over the mesocycle. Available training time in many sports only allowed about 6 to 12 weeks for target goals to be achieved.

Flexible Nonlinear Periodization

The development of the *flexible nonlinear* periodization model, which is a "chameleon" approach to periodization because of its ability to use any sequential pattern of workouts, was needed to stimulate targeted adaptive changes in the available time period. The evolution to the flexible nonlinear model was driven by the notion of capitalizing on an athlete's training schedule. This approach involved strategically sequencing workouts to focus on the specific goals of each training phase (mesocycle). Even if it meant performing consecutive workouts with no variation, such as back-to-back strength or power sessions, the aim was to ensure high-quality training without interruptions or disruptions. The primary objective was to optimize training outcomes by aligning the training regimen with the athlete's schedule and objectives for each training phase.

On a given day, a decision for that day would be made based on various readiness markers. This approach could mimic any periodization model and use multiple models at different times of the yearly macrocycle. Many programs began to use linear and nonlinear methods over the macrocycle based on the sport schedule, available training times, and control of disruptors.

The flexible nonlinear periodization approach is the most effective way to deal with the various disruptors in a typical player development program. Nonlinear programming was introduced in the 1990s in resistance training, but it was more structured, using different intensities and volumes of workouts on different days in a cycle of 7 to 10 days. This approach soon evolved to become flexible enough that any acute program variable could be changed to optimize the quality of the workout. Any sequencing during the 7-to-10-day microcycle and over a 6-to-12-week mesocycle was done to respond to the disruptors and emphasize quality rather than just to go through the motions. However, as we will see in chapter 5, this approach takes a great deal of effort; it involves real-time monitoring and postworkout accounting.

Defaults in Nonlinear Periodization Models

Defaults in training in the nonlinear approach to periodization became a hallmark of this training theory. This was primarily due to the regular disruptors in the academic worlds of strength and conditioning from high school to collegiate levels. This is where the art and monitoring technology used by strength and conditioning professionals comes into play. One could default to the workout, after some preworkout testing and evaluations, or after the workout starts, with the primary exercise routine. If target intensities and repetitions for sets were not met, conventional nonlinear periodization decisions could be made to go to a lighter resistance or to rest for a day. The athletes and coaches needed to be aware of what was happening with the programs and have intentionality for each workout's quality. Most of the time, defaults were observed with heavy and power days. Defaults after preworkout evaluations usually occur for the following reasons:

- Prior injury
- High levels of soreness
- Poor vertical jump performance before a power day
- Poor sleep and high fatigue
- Psychological or personal issues making concentration difficult

Each workout must be evaluated, but during the workout a default mechanism must be in place so that if the athlete does not hit the target goal, the workout can default to a lower intensity or less volume or the workout can be stopped, and a rest day taken. This concept of a default was developed in the early evolution of the nonlinear workout when dramatically different workouts in sequence were used. A default meant going to the next workout in line at the time of the next scheduled training day. This method changed when the flexible nonlinear approach was taken. No longer did a default mean skipping to the next workout in the sequence, but instead it meant getting in the missed workout the next time in order not to miss the stimuli needed to achieve the goals of the mesocycle (i.e., maximal strength, power, general preparation, etc.). Each mesocycle sequence would take advantage of the time frame to meet the training target for that mesocycle. Defaults or a reduction in a specific workout stimulus needed to achieve the goals of that mesocycle indicated that the mesocycle had failed to achieve its goals because of disruptors. Hence the need for highly individualized workouts and monitoring. The goal of each mesocycle in a flexible nonlinear program was to achieve the goals by limiting the effects of disruptors and the potential for nonfunctional overreaching. The challenge for the player development team is to deal with program disruptors on a daily basis and to work around them to attain the targeted goals of the mesocycle.

The Acute Exercise Response

Exercise stress poses the critical stimulus affecting acute performance and is the initial step in mediating chronic adaptations. As mentioned previously, the interaction of intensity, volume (or duration), contraction velocity, muscle mass involvement, and rest intervals govern exercise stress. Exercise stimulates several physiological systems that simultaneously prepare the human body for stress. The two significant control systems are the *nervous* and *endocrine* systems. In combination, these systems control the acute exercise responses and recovery. The nervous system consists of the brain, the spinal cord (*central nervous system*), and all the nerves that regulate tissue function (*peripheral nervous system*). The nervous system exemplifies the true definition of a control system: It receives input (sensory information), integrates or translates the information (CNS), and then coordinates the output response, which may be control of skeletal muscle (motor system) or other glands and organs (autonomic nervous system). The movement originates in the brain in a complex manner that involves many parts. Communication between nerves and tissues is critical to coordination, movement efficiency and technique, and all aspects of muscle function. The line of communication is electrical, and the total electrical activity, initiating in the brain and then stimulating skeletal muscle, is termed *neural drive*. The patterns of neural drive networking and the magnitude of the neural drive are key factors in determining how muscles will function. Likewise, all areas in this neuromuscular chain (and signaling map), from crucial brain segments to the connection with skeletal muscle (known as the *neuromuscular junction*), play vital roles in muscle activation but also are critical areas of adaptation over time with training.

The nervous system responses to aerobic and anaerobic exercise differ. Anaerobic exercise requires the maximal and optimal recruitment of fast-twitch (type II, strength and power) muscle fibers, whereas aerobic exercise requires mostly the recruitment of slow-twitch (type I, endurance) muscle fibers. The acute expression of strength, power, and speed can only be maximized when the neural drive to skeletal muscle is maximal. That means that high-intensity exercise requires the recruitment of maximal numbers of muscle fibers (*motor units*). Resistance exercise involves heavy loading and fast lifting velocities. The size principle (discussed earlier in this chapter) states that larger, stronger motor units are recruited when the intensity increases. Thus, optimizing recruitment is a significant goal for any strength and power training stimulus. Besides recruitment, faster rates of stimulation and coordinated activation of muscle fibers (as well as limiting the activity of other muscles that may impede motion) assist in producing greater force, power, and rates of force development. Motor unit recruitment is critical because only recruited muscle fibers adapt to training. Aerobic exercise primarily targets slow-twitch fibers because, as the intensity of exercise increases, eventually the stimulus becomes anaerobic, and recruitment of slow-twitch muscle fibers governs the acute response to aerobic exercise. As a result, the neural response to anaerobic exercise is more complex due to the systematic activation of these high-force and high-threshold motor units.

The nervous system also prepares the human body for the stress of exercise by stimulating nonskeletal muscle tissue and organs. The term *fight-or-flight* is commonly used to describe the response of the *sympathetic nervous system* (a branch of the autonomic system) to stress. Here, tissues such as cardiac and smooth muscle, eyes, and organs like the heart and lungs are stimulated to increase heart rate and breathing rate, regulate blood pressure and flow, increase fuel (glucose and fat) mobilization, and dilate the pupils for enhanced performance. Of course, once exercise ceases, this system response is reduced, and the opposing system (e.g., the *parasympathetic nervous system*) predominates, returning the body to normal (i.e., *homeostasis*) during the initial recovery period.

The other key system of control is the endocrine system (i.e., hormones). The endocrine system releases hormones (chemical messengers), transports hormones to specific target tissues, and elicits a chain of intracellular signaling events leading to the desired function. Hormones come in various types and perform a multitude of functions. Most hormones are released from glands, although some are released from the nerve, muscle, cardiac, fat, and other tissues. Hormone signaling is part of a complex system involving thousands of molecules and is almost analogous to playing a team sport in that cohesion is needed at each step for the function to occur correctly. All stages, including production, release, transportation, tissue uptake, and intracellular signaling, must be considered in an integrative way to accurately portray the hormone's effects. Hormones bind to receptors, which leads to cell signaling, and all elements involved are crucial to the response. Some of the essential hormones that are important for preparing the body for the stress of exercise include testosterone, the growth hormone superfamily, insulin and IGF-1, cortisol, thyroid hormones, glucagon, catecholamines, β-endorphins, and atrial peptide and other fluid regulatory hormones (Ratamess 2022; Kraemer, Ratamess, and Vingren 2019). For example, catecholamines enhance the fight-or-flight response and help increase the athlete's arousal. These hormones help liberate fuel for energy, stimulate neuromuscular function, improve psychological focus, and help mediate the cardiovascular and respiratory responses to enhance oxygen delivery to working muscles. In addition, several of these hormones help begin the recovery process once exercise has stopped.

Skeletal muscles contract to produce force and movement. The size of a skeletal muscle is determined mainly by the number and size of its individual muscle fibers. Muscle fibers must be recruited as part of a motor unit during exercise to contribute to performance. Muscle fiber number is mostly nonmutable, but the size and composition (fiber type) are mutable during training. The slow-twitch units have high endurance capacity and lower force and power, whereas the fast-twitch fibers have great strength and power potential but lack endurance. Thus, slow-twitch fibers are recruited for low-to-moderate intensity exercise, especially aerobic exercise. Fast-twitch fibers are needed to achieve high levels of force, power, and speed, so they are highly recruited during anaerobic exercise. Intense contractions and warm-ups potentiate acute muscle force. Systemic factors (e.g., hormones) and neural recruitment facilitate muscle function primarily by increasing sensitivity to calcium and promoting better interaction of contractile and structural proteins. As a result, the athlete is capable of producing force and power at higher levels than during resting conditions. Lastly, some muscles control motion at one joint while others control multiple joints. Human movement is predicated on a complex recruitment strategy for muscle activation to allow the best and most efficient movement patterns to occur during exercise.

Skeletal muscles require energy to fuel muscle contraction. All cells contain metabolic mechanisms that help liberate energy for performance while helping to reduce fatigue. Skeletal muscle can only store enough energy to last 1 to 2 seconds, but humans possess three major energy systems, two anaerobic and one aerobic, that replenish energy during exercise. All energy systems are always engaged and contributing to energy production, but one or two may predominate depending on the demands of the exercise stimulus. For example, the *ATP–phosphocreatine (ATP–PC) system* is a high-energy system that provides energy for high-intensity activities lasting 5 to 10 seconds. It is engaged initially during low-intensity activities but resynthesizes quickly and is still an essential energy source during intermittent high-intensity exercise. Its concentration within the skeletal muscle is more prominent in fast-twitch fibers than it is in slow-twitch fibers. The second anaerobic system is *glycolysis*, which involves the breakdown of carbohydrates to form energy. It provides energy for high-intensity exercise for up to 2 minutes. Sources include stored glucose (glycogen) and glucose in circulation. However, its by-products induce acidosis and the formation of blood lactate, which is why certain athletes need a high buffer capacity to delay fatigue. *Buffering capacity* is the ability to resist changes in pH; many intracellular and extracellular factors contribute to improved skeletal muscle buffer capacity. The third system is the *aerobic system*, which is highly engaged when adequate oxygen is available. The majority of energy derived aerobically comes from carbohydrates and fats. The aerobic system provides the primary energy source at rest and during low to moderate steady-state exercise. As exercise intensity increases, so does the percentage of energy from carbohydrates. Having a well-developed aerobic system helps with ATP–PC recovery during rest intervals, which demonstrates how aerobic fitness can improve anaerobic energy metabolism.

Skeletal muscle takes in nutrients and oxygen while also eliminating waste products, so the respiratory and cardiovascular (CV) systems must be engaged to supplement acute exercise. The cardiovascular system consists of three major components: the heart (pump), the blood vessels (transport portals), and the blood (fluid medium). All other systems depend on the CV system, including the lungs, which are essential for blood oxygenation and removal of CO_2, a process that occurs during breathing. During exercise, several CV variables increase to meet the CV demands, such as heart rate, the heart's force of contraction, blood pressure (although some differential responses may be noted with systolic and diastolic values), *stroke volume* (amount of blood pumped per beat), and *cardiac output* (amount of blood pumped per minute). During exercise, blood flow to skeletal muscle may increase to more than 80% of total flow via redistribution to meet the metabolic demands in a dose–response manner. Blood flow also increases to the skin to help heat escape from the body (i.e., thermoregulation). The respiratory system introduces oxygen into the body and removes CO_2. Respiration includes breathing, pulmonary diffusion, oxygen transport, and gas exchange. Similar to the CV system, breathing rate and volume increases during exercise to supply as much oxygen as possible and remove carbon dioxide. More substantial increases are seen during aerobic exercise than anaerobic exercise.

The acute exercise response is primarily catabolic, which means it involves some degree of breakdown. For example, energy liberation is a catabolic process to break down energy stores for use. Skeletal muscle undergoes catabolism during exercise in a dose–response manner in which proteins are broken down and must be repaired during the recovery process. Thus, the adaptation cycle includes acute breakdown, which leads to supercompensation during recovery. The postexercise period of 24 to 48 hours is critical to recovery. Macronutrients must be consumed at levels that meet the needs of the athletes. Studies have consistently shown that muscle protein synthesis is elevated during this time. Proteins serve many functions, so not only is replacing proteins in skeletal muscle necessary for muscle growth but replacing other proteins (e.g., those that act as enzymes and buffers) is also critical to recovery. Aerobic and anaerobic exercise, especially with a large eccentric component, can produce significant muscular damage in the athlete when the stimulus is novel or unaccustomed and of considerable volume and intensity. The damage response is initially greatest but then lessened over time as an adaptation. Repairing damaged muscle and possibly forming new muscle fibers are critical to normal muscle function.

The immune system plays a crucial role during exercise. It is critical to health and prevention of disease, and it is involved in inflammation and repair of damaged muscle fibers. The primary type of immune cell is the white blood cell (leukocyte). White blood cells are elevated during exercise, with some showing dependency on intensity and volume of the exercise. The elevation persists for several hours following exercise, except among lymphocytes, which belong to one of the white blood cell types. Immune system modulator cells known as *cytokines* are also released during exercise, where pro-inflammatory cytokines are increased. Some anti-inflammatory cytokines are released postexercise, demonstrating that exercise poses a pro-inflammatory response initially but is countered after the workout. Skeletal muscle takes some immune cells, which helps initiate the repair process. The immune system's response plays a significant role in recovery via the inflammation of muscle fibers, damage, and the repair cycle following exercise.

The Role of Genes in Exercise and Adaptation

Genes are specific segments of deoxyribonucleic acid (DNA) that contain the instructions or "blueprint" that determine the athlete's makeup. Genes are organized within 22 paired chromosomes, plus the X and Y sex chromosomes. DNA is replicated and transcribed into messenger ribonucleic acid (mRNA), which ultimately produces proteins. The human genome contains more than 25,000 genes that encode a host of proteins. Although humans share these genes, they are expressed differently, making everyone unique. For example, different forms of the same gene are called *alleles* or *polymorphisms*. These variations create the protein but will be expressed differently. Athletes typically have unique combinations of gene variants that enable them to perform at higher levels. This also helps explain why some athletes respond to certain training stimuli better than others, often discussed in terms of responders versus nonresponders. Genes are responsible for all of the mutable and largely nonmutable characteristics. Several genes, known as *candidate genes*, encode proteins that directly affect athletic performance. One gene does not make or break an athlete; instead, a composite of candidate genes strongly influences specific fitness components and overall athleticism, including the athlete's level of susceptibility to injuries. Research has shown that more than 200 genetic variations exist that affect athletic performance (Puthucheary et al. 2011). The heritability status for athletic performance (independent of the sport) has been estimated to be approximately 66% (Guth and Roth 2013). In addition, the athlete's profile reflects not only genetics but also the influence of environmental factors (e.g., *epigenetics*). Here, gene expression can be increased or decreased by aging, diet, exercise, disease, drugs, and environmental chemicals. Many training adaptations are mediated by gene expression. Aerobic and anaerobic exercise can alter the expression of several genes as part of the adaptation process. The acute workout stimulus will target specific genes, these genes will encode proteins, and the protein expression will change over time to match the training program's demands. These changes lead to chronic adaptations associated with all forms of training.

Chronic Training Adaptations

The workout provides acute stress to the athlete, stimulating major physiological responses and subsequent recovery and adaptation (figure 4.2). The stimulus targets tissues at the genetic level, and subsequent changes in gene transcription help mediate recovery and adaptations (figure 4.3). Acute exercise elicits responses that remain throughout the workout and up to several hours into recovery. Within 48 to 72 hours following a workout, the body returns to normal homeostasis. The stimulus must be repeated to keep the cellular responses primed. Thus, sporadic workouts do little to accomplish a specific goal. *Training* is the systematic pattern of using exercise to target specific fitness and performance goals. When structured, consistent workouts lead to rapid adaptations for some measures, but other measures may take a substantial period of time to incur noticeable improvements. Chronic physiological adaptations enable improvements in all health- and skill-related fitness components.

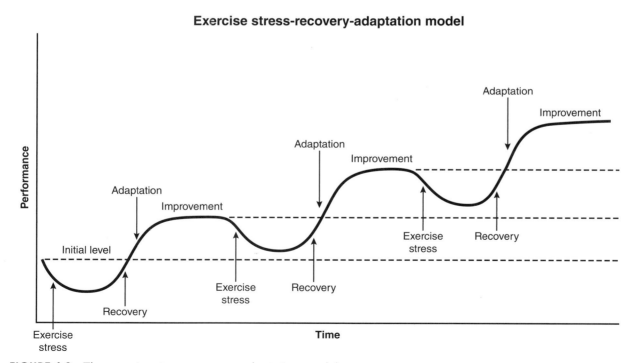

FIGURE 4.2 The exercise stress-recovery-adaptation model.

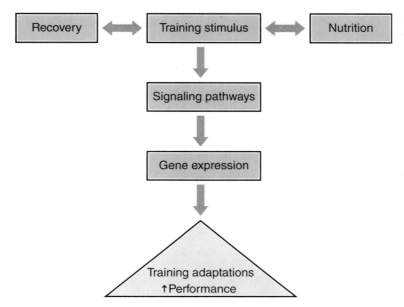

FIGURE 4.3 The stimulus-response pattern.

The nervous system adapts to training rapidly, typically within a few workouts. Neural drive increases as a function of training. This means better communication between nerves in the brain, greater neural drive, and subsequent recruitment of skeletal muscle. Aerobic and anaerobic training increase cognition, memory, blood flow, and overall function of the brain. Exercise causes muscles to produce and release messengers (in a dose–response manner) known as *growth factors*, which can improve brain function. This is an acute exercise phenomenon because it only occurs during and after a workout. Acute elevations do not persist, so there is a need for consistent workouts. Chronic training via strength and conditioning and sport skill practice improves motor learning, coordination, skill acquisition, strength, power, and speed. This results in a more efficient pattern of neural drive to muscles, meaning that pathway stimulation improves while muscular noninvolvement is reduced. This type of adaptation takes place when athletes are training sport-specific skills or when they are exposed to new exercises or training modalities.

The ultimate goal of the increased neural drive is to recruit muscle fibers maximally. An untrained person cannot recruit all of their muscle fibers, especially in large locomotor muscles, but training can significantly reduce this deficit. Training helps improve the function of the human sensory nervous system, reduces inherent inhibition that limits neuromuscular performance, and increases the neural activation of muscle fibers. Heavy resistance training provides a neural stimulus that is unique and cannot be mimicked by other forms of training. High force and power activities such as plyometric, speed, and agility exercises require maximal recruitment of fast-twitch fibers. Aerobic and anaerobic training leads to neural drive improvements. However, since anaerobic training requires greater activation of fast-twitch motor units, neural drive increases are far more comprehensive during anaerobic training. Neural improvements occur in the form of improved coordination and muscle fiber activation—that is, motor nerves can recruit more muscle fibers, activate them faster, alter the timing of their activation, and recruit fast-twitch muscle fibers earlier in sequence during ballistic exercise. Thus, progressive overload increases neural drive, but athletes also undergo improved neural adaptations when learning new exercises or techniques. The key factors that influence neural drive adaptations are as follows:

- Intensity of contraction and high-intensity muscle loading maximizes stimulus
- Rate of force development, power, and high-velocity actions

- Muscle actions trained (concentric, eccentric, and isometric)
- Exercise complexity
- Unilateral and bilateral training
- Fatigue

How long improvements take depends on the training program. Large increases in the neural drive are seen during anaerobic training over the first 12 to 24 weeks of training. Many of the muscle's motor units can be recruited by this point, so less dramatic increases may occur. However, muscle adaptations (i.e., strength and endurance) lessen the need to recruit as many muscle fibers as possible to perform a specific task. For example, fewer motor units are needed to produce a threshold level of force when individual muscle fibers get stronger. Progressive overload in training is needed to keep stoking the neural drive primer, forcing more motor unit recruitment after muscle fiber adaptation. This is accomplished via heavy resistance training and explosive exercise (ballistics, plyometrics, speed, and agility training). Thus, there appears to be a constant interplay between changes in neural drive and muscle fiber adaptations that occur throughout an athlete's career. Changes in a neural drive lead to changes in muscle fiber morphology, and neural improvements occur when athletes are exposed to new exercises or training modalities. Nervous system changes are key to driving adaptations at the muscle fiber level.

Skeletal muscle is a fast-adapting soft tissue capable of rapid and long-term adaptations to progressive exercise. Any human biological tissue capable of adapting to overload must be able to couple mechanical stimuli to biochemical signaling (a process known as *mechanotransduction*). As discussed previously, overload comes in many forms via aerobic and anaerobic stimuli and lengthening. The overload stimulus creates tissue deformation of several muscle proteins and structures in response to the intensity and volume of loading. Skeletal muscle, in turn, senses the magnitude of the stimulus, integrates the stimulus with appropriate pathway activation, and increases intracellular signaling leading to the anticipated outcome. The response is mediated by several systems or pathways communicating with each other and is proportional to the overload level. Thus, skeletal muscle adapts to exercise in specific ways. Training upregulates the activity of numerous genes that enhance muscular function. Skeletal muscle can become enlarged (hypertrophied) when stress demands greater force production. Fiber-type and architectural transitions can occur, increasing strength, power, and endurance. Changes in skeletal muscle enzyme activity, substrate content, receptor content, capillary and mitochondrial density, and protein content also enhance athletic performance. These latter changes reflect metabolic, hormonal, and cardiovascular changes for skeletal muscle.

One potential type of muscle fiber adaptation consists of the transitions within each fiber type. Landmark studies from the 1960s and 1970s showed that skeletal muscle fiber types reflect the type and pattern of stimulation they receive from the nervous system. Muscle fiber types reflect a combination of heritability and activity level. As mentioned, the two general types are type I slow-twitch (ST, endurance) and type II fast-twitch (FT, strength and power), each having distinct characteristics leading to its own force and endurance profile. Every muscle in the human body contains a mosaic of fiber types that exist on a continuum, hybrid variations existing within each type. Fiber transitions occur within the first few weeks of training, while changes in protein expression occur within the first few workouts. Simply put, the level of stimulation (i.e., strength and power versus endurance) targets specific intracellular signaling pathways (i.e., anabolic and oxidative) that ultimately lead to protein isoforms and organelle expression characteristic of the fiber type that relates to the force, speed, power, and endurance qualities of the motor unit. Although the proportions of type I and II fibers are genetically determined to a large extent, transitions occur based on the pattern of muscle stimulation. The most common pattern is the type IIX to IIA transition, which occurs across multiple training modalities (e.g., resistance, sprint, plyometric, and aerobic endurance training). Although type IIX fibers are strong, fast, and powerful, their fatigue may limit their true potential, so transitioning to more oxidative FT types appears beneficial for certain strength and power performances. Intense exercise (based on the size principle) is needed to recruit these fiber types. Once activated consistently, the fibers transition to another type II and ultimately to IIA fibers. Moderate-to-high-intensity aerobic training produces similar transitions but not to the same extent as anaerobic training. Detraining results in an increase in type IIX fibers and a reduction in type IIA fibers, with half of the benefits lost within 16 weeks (Bickel, Cross, and Bamman 2011).

A key chronic skeletal muscle adaptation is the ability to hypertrophy to progressive overload and proper resistance training prescription. There is a positive relationship between a muscle's size and its force potential—a larger muscle is stronger. Hypertrophy results from increased protein synthesis, decreased protein breakdown, or a combination of both. Acute exercise is catabolic; however, protein synthesis rates exceed breakdown to the point that net protein balance favors growth for 24 to 48 hours following a workout. Hypertrophy is a complex process involving many factors and pathways (see figure 4.4). Although neural adaptations predominate early, hypertrophy becomes increasingly important as resistance training continues. Both fiber types respond to training, but larger absolute muscle size increases in FT fibers. Changes in muscle proteins occur within a couple of workouts, although it takes a longer period (at least two weeks or more) to show measurable muscle growth. It has been suggested that 8 to 12 workouts may elicit modest hypertrophy of 3% to 4%, and more than 18 workouts (over the course of 6 to 10 weeks) may lead to higher levels of hypertrophy (approximately 7% to 10%) (Damas et al., 2018). Men and women may experience similar relative hypertrophy during training; however, male athletes display greater absolute hypertrophy mostly due to higher testosterone concentrations. Hypertrophy occurs nonuniformly at a higher magnitude along the muscle belly, where highly activated muscle segments may experience higher growth levels. Intensities greater than or equal to 60% of the 1RM produce greater rates of hypertrophy in trained individuals (Wernbom, Augustsson, and Thomee 2007). Fry (Fry 2004) showed that intensity accounted for 18% to 35% of the variance in fiber hypertrophy induced by resistance training and suggested that 80% to 95% of the 1RM may be an ideal range for long-term hypertrophy in competitive lifters.

Structural changes also occur in skeletal muscle that help increase strength, power, and endurance performance. Structures involved in neural propa-

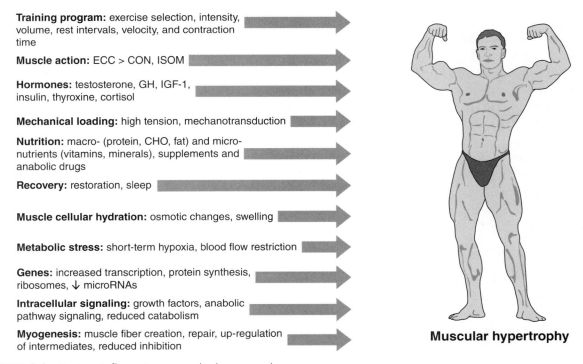

FIGURE 4.4 Factors influencing muscular hypertrophy.

gation, muscle contraction, and calcium mobility are enhanced. Anaerobic training increases anaerobic substrate content (i.e., phosphagens and glycogen), alters enzyme activity, and increases a muscle's buffer capacity. Aerobic training increases the activity of aerobic enzymes and the number of muscle substrates (i.e., glycogen and fat). There is upregulation of hormone receptors and other intermediates, which improves the signaling pathways and enhances function. Aerobic training increases the mitochondrial and capillary number and density (expressed relative to muscle fiber area); however, anaerobic training may increase the capillary and mitochondrial number but decrease density when sufficient hypertrophy occurs. These improvements help the muscles extract more oxygen from circulation, improve blood flow, and increase endurance capacity. Aerobic training also allows the athlete to rely more on fat as a fuel source, enabling easier weight loss and body fat reduction. Adding lean body mass resulting from resistance training allows the athlete to burn more kilocalories per day, making weight control and fat reduction more likely. These two adaptations increase the athlete's metabolism and result in greater kilocalorie expenditure. Connective tissue within skeletal muscle increases in capacity, which helps support strength development and hypertrophy. The length of groups of muscle fibers (*fascicles*) and muscle fiber orientation may change in response to anaerobic training, which favors force production and power.

Changes in muscular performance must also be accompanied by the strengthening of connective tissue. Connective tissue (CT) enhancement refers to strengthening of bones, tendons, ligaments, fascia, and cartilage. Adaptations in training-induced connective tissue adaptations are critical for transmitting muscle force to the bone, joint stability, and injury prevention. Compared to skeletal muscle, connective tissue adaptations are slower (and heal more slowly) because these structures are much more rigid. This could be a concern early in training since muscular adaptations occur before CT and too much stress could increase the risk of injury. Much like skeletal muscle, connective tissue strengthening is governed by mechanotransduction and can only adapt when it is progressively overloaded by increasing mechanical stress. CT structures require a minimal stimulus threshold to force adaptations; otherwise, there would be no need for CT structures in athletes to get stronger.

Bones undergo normal remodeling when packets of old bone are broken down and replaced by new bone. However, the term *bone modeling* is more appropriate here as it refers to the process by which bone adapts to mechanical loading. Bones are strengthened by aerobic and anaerobic training. Higher levels of adaptation are seen with anaerobic training because the bone is sensitive to the magnitude and rate of loading, which both reflect the high-intensity nature of anaerobic training. Training must be of sufficient intensity and volume to elicit increases in bone mass, bone mineral content, and *bone mineral density* (BMD). Compared to muscle adaptations, BMD increases at a much smaller relative percentage, but one should not be deceived—an increase in BMD of 5% may increase bone strength by 65% (Burr, Robling, and Turner 2002). Classic studies showed that measurable BMD increases were primarily seen after 6 months of training (Ratamess 2008) and only if the athlete trained beyond the current minimal essential strain, which is why most bone studies last one year. However, some studies have shown small increases in BMD within 9 weeks of resistance training and plyometric training (Guadalupe-Grau et al. 2009). A higher stimulus magnitude may elicit increased BMD in a shorter period compared to programs that use slow training progression rates. Stronger athletes tend to have higher BMD values than individuals who are less fit. Collectively, strong anaerobic athletes have shown BMD values 9% to 42% higher than control subjects, with some of the largest percent differences seen in powerlifters and Olympic weightlifters (Ratamess 2022). A case study examining a male powerlifter, who at the time held the world record for the squat, showed the highest recorded lumbar spine BMD (Dickerman, Pertusi, and Smith 2000). We examined the BMD of some of the world's strongest men and found that overall BMD was 1.80 g/cm^2, the highest reported for male athletes (Kraemer, Caldwell et al. 2020). Aerobic endurance athletes (e.g., runners) have higher BMD than controls, especially in the lower body. Weight-bearing exercise is most effective for increasing BMD, and lifting and contact sports as well as sports and activities requiring explosive running and jumping ground reaction forces (e.g., plyometrics, sprint, and agility) are excellent means of increasing BMD. Swimming is less effective because water buoyancy decreases stress on the skeletal system. Although the quantitative adaptation of bone is a long process, the initial bone growth processes begin after the first few workouts, as evidenced by the release into the blood of what is known as *bone biomarkers* (proteins involved in either anabolic or catabolic reactions relating to bone metabolism). These bone biomarkers can be measured to determine if the current stimulus can lead to long-term BMD increases. The keys to training to increase BMD include:

- Multijoint exercises (e.g., squat, power clean, deadlift, and bench press) for resistance training, and speed, agility, and plyometric exercises for comprehensive anaerobic training.
- Heavy loading (10 reps and less) with multiple (at least 2 to 3) sets per exercise.
- Fast contraction velocities.
- Rest intervals should be moderate-to-long in length (at least 2 to 3 minutes) to allow more recovery and accommodate more significant loading during each set.
- Training frequency of at least 2 to 3 days per week and up to 6 days per week for resistance training, plyometrics, speed and agility, or combined training.
- Variation in training is important for altering the stimuli.

The major stimulus for the growth of tendons, ligaments, and fascia is mechanical loading (mechanotransduction), which brings about a cascade of events leading to changes in the CT cytoskeleton, structure, and protein (several proteins but especially collagen) content. Tendons are stronger than ligaments because they connect muscles to bones, and ligaments need to be more pliable because they assist in establishing a joint's ROM. Tendons are unique in that they become stiffer before increasing in size; several hormones control their metabolism to a certain extent. This is critical because muscle adapts quickly, so changes in *stiffness* help accommodate improved muscle performance. Acute exercise (aerobic and anaerobic) initially results in collagen breakdown; however, in the days following, the collagen synthesis rate increases. Greater collagen deposition initially aids in increasing the stiffness of the tendon due to organizational restructuring by 9% to 83% during the initial 2 to 3 months of training (Ratamess 2022). Stiffness means resistance to a change in length. Therefore, a stiffer tendon is a stronger tendon. Collagen synthesis remains elevated during chronic training (Kjaer et al. 2005). Prolonged training ultimately increases tendon size; for example, tendons may hypertrophy in as little as 12 weeks of resistance training (Kongsgaard et al. 2007). Aerobic endurance athletes such as runners have larger Achilles tendon sizes than untrained controls. Thus, aerobic and anaerobic athletes possess larger and stronger tendons, but a dose–response pattern (within a limit to avoid overtraining) is also seen here. For example, data show that resistance training with an intensity greater than or equal to 70% is sufficient to increase tendon stiffness and size (McCrum et al. 2018). Progressive overload is needed to keep tendons adapting positively over time. Heavy and ECC resistance training have been used effectively to treat tendinopathies. These positive effects only last a short time because detraining reduces tendon stiffness and size in as little as a few weeks to one month.

Cartilage adaptations are less clear. *Articular cartilage* covers the ends of long bones at joints to provide a smooth surface for joint motion and act as a shock absorber. It is known to degenerate as one ages, especially in individuals with low activity levels. Moderate, regular exercise is thought to preserve cartilage volume and thickness up to a certain point; however, it is unclear if training can increase adult cartilage thickness or restore lost cartilage thickness. It appears that training may help maintain cartilage thickness or possibly produce structural changes at the surfaces that assist in improving joint stability and load absorption over time, but joint injuries, excessive mechanical stress, and highly repetitive intense exercise upon injured joints may together facilitate joint degeneration. Athletes from sports requiring great impact loading may be more susceptible to degeneration. It has been suggested that the athletes who are most susceptible to joint degeneration are those with abnormal joint anatomy, previous joint injury and surgery, joint instability, heavy body weight, inadequate muscular strength, or altered muscle innervations (Buckwalter and Martin 2004).

The endocrine system helps the body maintain normal function, prepares the body for exercise, mediates several adaptations, and is involved in every physiological system. Hormonal signaling is part of a complex system involving thousands of molecules that involves many cellular actions. We previously mentioned that hormones are released or elevated in response to exercise. This change in the circulating levels of a hormone help mediate a slew of activities and intracellular signaling cascades (especially since blood flow is increased to working skeletal muscles) that either help the body perform acutely or help mediate the recovery process over the next 48 to 72 hours. The acute responses of several hormones appear significant for immediate performance and subsequent adaptations. This is particularly true for several hormones, such as catecholamines and fluid-regulatory hormones. The endocrine system works predominately on negative feedback response, meaning that a hormone's systemic concentration will be lowered if it is high or elevated if it is too low. Several hormone concentrations in the blood quickly return to homeostasis within 30 minutes of a workout, with some lingering effects. The concentration of the hormone in the blood is determined by several factors, including the amount of hormone released, the pattern of release (*pulsatility*), the rate of metabolism, the quantity of transport proteins, the time of day, fluid volume shifts, genetics, sex, menstrual cycle, age, diet, and various stimuli (in addition to regulation from other hormones). Exercise poses a small perturbation in the circulatory hormone profile until normal homeostatic values are re-engaged. Because hormones work through receptors, this communication pattern is essential to keeping receptors primed and preventing unwanted desensitization effects in signaling. Resting concentrations of most hormones do not change much as a function of training, but the acute response may be enhanced in some cases for some hormones. For example, some aerobic endurance athletes produce a more substantial catecholamine response to exercise than untrained individuals, a concept known as the *sports adrenal medulla*. The hormone action must be viewed within the context of a signaling cascade. Thus, signaling elements may show longer-term effects (i.e., receptor upregulation following a workout). For example, testosterone may be elevated during a workout and 15 to 30 minutes postexercise before returning to normal circadian concentrations; however, the *androgen receptor* (the protein that binds to testosterone mediating intracellular signaling) may be upregulated for 24 to 48 hours following the workout (Kraemer, Ratamess et al. 2020; Kraemer, Ratamess, and Nindl 2017). This course of events is consistent with a key recovery period following exercise.

The importance of hormones to chronic adaptations must not be viewed simplistically by only looking at the concentrations in the blood—the whole signaling apparatus must be taken into consideration. Some hormones are very complex, and some may function more locally than systemically. For example, growth hormone (GH) has been described as a mixture of several different forms or a superfamily because more than 100 isoforms of GH exist at various levels in the anterior pituitary and the blood. Studies have shown some changes in some resting concentrations of hormones, but often blood sampling may coincide with the recovery period. In some cases, changes in resting concentrations may occur due to a major change to the training stimulus, but these may be somewhat transient. One exception is the catabolic hormone cortisol: A stressed, overtrained athlete may show consistent elevations of cortisol in the blood and possible reductions in testosterone. Another example is insulin, which is highly related to nutrition (i.e., carbohydrates and protein) intake. Thus, hormones govern the recovery and adaptation processes in a complex manner, acting at many levels of control. The best example of the effects of low hormone responses may be seen during aging as men and women lose muscular strength, power, muscle mass, BMD, and increase fat mass due in part to reduced levels of hormones such as testosterone, GH, thyroid hormones, and estrogen.

Long-term adaptations over time of the cardiovascular and respiratory systems are common. Although aerobic and anaerobic training lead to various chronic improvements in cardiorespiratory function, aerobic training leads to more substantial and comprehensive improvements. For example, the heart responds to both pressure (increased blood pressure and intrathoracic pressure) and volume (increased blood flow to the heart) overload. Pressure overload increases the heart's muscle mass, whereas volume overload increases the heart's chamber size. Although the heart has four chambers, the left ventricle is most adaptable to training, while smaller changes occur in other parts. Anaerobic and aerobic training produces adaptations in the heart related to pressure overload. However, aerobic training is superior for volume overload due to the higher level of continuity. Several measures of cardiorespiratory function are improved with both forms of training. Improvements in CV function occur as chronic changes at rest and in the acute response to exercise.

Table 4.1 depicts some of the key CV and respiratory changes that occur with consistent aerobic and anaerobic training. Several of these variable changes are more substantial following aerobic training. On the whole, aerobic training increases cardiac musculature, which makes the heart stronger in its contraction and helps it tolerate stress. Chamber size increases as well, which allows more blood to flow into the heart and then to be pumped to the rest of the body. In addition, cardiac workload decreases, as evidenced by reduced heart rate at rest and during submaximal exercise, blood pressure, arterial stiffness, increased stroke volume, blood volume, and heart rate variability. $\dot{V}O_2$max improvements also occur, which improve pulmonary ventilation. Anaerobic training produces several of these adaptations but at a lower level; aerobic training produces more comprehensive and substantial improvements in CV function.

TABLE 4.1 Cardiorespiratory Changes Following Training

Variable	Aerobic	Anaerobic
Left ventricular mass and wall thickness	↑	↑
Right ventricular mass and wall thickness	↑	↑
Interventricular septal wall thickness	↑	↑
Left ventricular cavity size	↑	↔ or small ↑
Cardiac output at rest	↔	↔
Cardiac output during exercise	↑	Slight ↑
Heart rate at rest	↓	↔ or slight ↓
Heart rate during submaximal exercise	↓	↓
Heart rate variability at rest	↑	↔ or slight ↑
Stroke volume at rest	↑	↔ or small ↑
Stroke volume during exercise	↑	↑
Ejection fraction at rest	↑	↔ or slight ↑
Ejection fraction during exercise	↑	Slight ↑
Blood volume	↑	↔ or slight ↑
$\dot{V}O_2$max	↑	↔ or small ↑
Systolic blood pressure at rest	↓	↔ or ↓
Diastolic blood pressure at rest	↓	↔ or ↓
Arterial stiffness	↓	↔, ↑
Muscle blood flow during exercise	↑	↑
Pulmonary ventilation during maximal exercise	↑	↔, small ↑
Lung volumes	↔, ↑	↔, ↑
Lung capacities	↔, ↑	↔, ↑

Time Course of Adaptations

The adaptive progress for structural morphology (bone, glands, muscle, etc.) or cybernetic changes in the molecular flow of molecules (e.g., hormones) in response to stress all occur on different timelines over the athlete's development. The chronic adaptations previously mentioned ultimately lead to improvements in health- and skill-related fitness components as well as improvements in sport-specific performance. The time course of adaptations is highly related to the athlete's training status regarding that specific fitness component as well as to the quality of the training program. Training status ranges on a continuum from novice to elite in strength, power, and endurance, but there are also hybrid athletes. Factors to consider include the athlete's history of strength and conditioning practice (months and years of experience), level of conditioning (magnitude of strength, power, endurance, and hypertrophy), genetic endowment, and sport participation experience. Training status and whether the athlete is a responder or a nonresponder are culminations of these factors and can be difficult for the coach to determine in some cases. Nevertheless, progression in any fitness component tends to follow a similar pattern: The most significant improvements are seen early in training, and progress slows from that point on. The largest window of adaptation is when an athlete begins to train the component. For example, aerobic endurance training leads to $\dot{V}O_2$max increases of 10% to 30% during the first 6 months, but the rate of progress is reduced beyond that (Brawner, Keteyian, and Saval 2010). The player development team must be cognizant of this for all fitness components and design proper periodized training programs that train the athlete at or above the threshold level of adaptation to allow the athlete to keep progressing.

Another example of time course adaptations occurs in relation to maximal muscular strength. Figure 4.5a depicts the theoretical strength curve and the interplay between neural and hypertrophic factors contributing to the strength gains. This curve shows that more substantial strength gains are made early in training, while progress becomes more and more difficult over time. In fact, in the position stand we coauthored in 2002 (and revised in 2009), we compared strength gains observed in several studies based on the author's classification of training status (American College of Sports 2002, 2009). A continuum was shown where progression lessened with advancing training status. For example, average (across all exercises tested) strength increases of approximately 40% were seen in untrained individuals, 20% in moderately trained (e.g., at least 4 to 6 months of training experience and having attained notable improvements), 16% in trained (e.g., at least 1 year of consistent training and having experienced a substantial level of adaptation), 10% in advanced (e.g., several years of experience with a high level of adaptation), and 2% in elite (e.g., top 1 to 2 percentile of trait, found in high-level competitions) over training periods ranging from 4 weeks to 2 years (American College of Sports 2002). Although strength continually increases (as long as the workouts are progressive), the rate of that increase decreases over time. Some spurts may be seen throughout, such as after puberty in young male athletes, during program changes, and when using some supplements or other ergogenic aids. Nevertheless, continual program modifications that become more specific to a precise element of the fitness component (i.e., strength) are necessary. Figure 4.5b depicts the contributions of maturation to strength development in male youth athletes through adulthood.

To address the slower rate of progress, the training paradigm must begin with a simple program design to build a foundation and progress with more specificity over time. This is referred to as a *general-to-specific model of progression* (American College of Sports 2002, 2009; Ratamess 2022), meaning that low-to-moderate training complexity is needed from novice to intermediate (INT) training, but high training complexity is needed in program design for advanced athletes. Simple programs with little variation work well during the initial stages of training when the athlete should be focused on building a foundation and learning the proper technique for each modality. This general phase is characterized by low-to-moderate training in intensity and volume; enhancing technique and establishing a conditioning base are primary goals. However, more variation and detail to specific components is needed with progression to a more advanced training status. Training cycles are designed to target specific components of fitness.

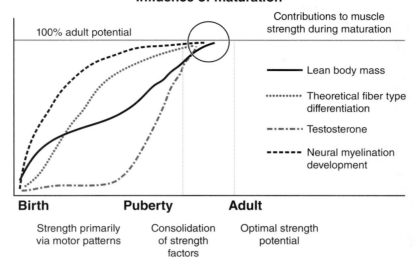

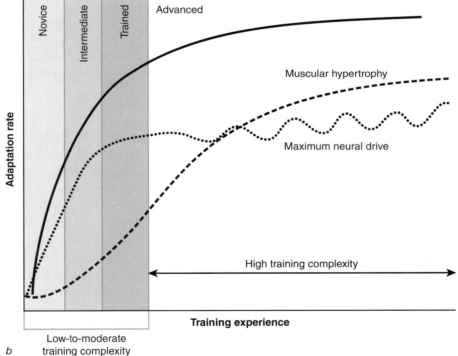

FIGURE 4.5 (a) Theoretical maximal strength adaptation curve. (b) Contributions of maturation to strength development in male youth athletes through adulthood.

Figure 4.5a Adapted from N.A. Ratamess, *Foundations of Strength Training and Conditioning*, 2nd ed. (Philadelphia, PA: Wolters Kluwer, 2022). Figure 4.5b Reprinted by permission from W.J. Kraemer, A.C. Fry, P.N. Frykman, B. Conroy, and J. Hoffman, "Resistance Training and Youth," *Pediatric Exercise Science* 1 (1989): 336-350.

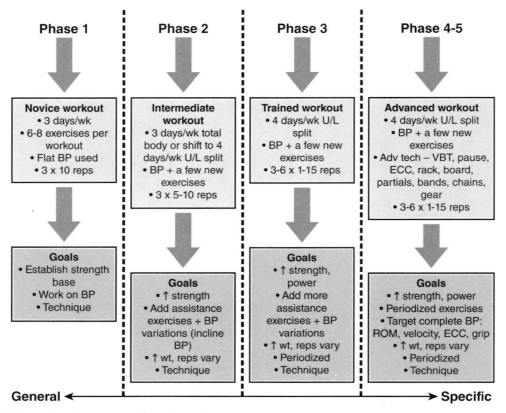

FIGURE 4.6 Example of sequence of workout phases.

Figure 4.6 depicts an example of a 5-phase general-to-specific model of progression for an athlete who strives to compete in the sport of powerlifting from novice to advanced training status. This figure only focuses on the bench press exercise, one of the three competition lifts. In Phase 1, the goals are to establish a strength base and work on good technique. A very general novice program of 3 days per week for six to eight exercises (3 × 10 repetitions) targeting all major muscle groups, including the flat bench press (BP), is a good place to start. In phase 2, the athlete progresses in loading but expands the repetitions range to 5 to 10 to start increasing the loading needed to maximize strength. Several powerlifters are known to split workouts into upper and lower-body splits to target each exercise specifically. Here, the athlete may continue from phase 1 or switch to the split. More exercises are added to the workouts, stressing muscles involved in the BP, including a few BP variations that use different postures or hand and grip positions (i.e., incline, decline, reverse, and close-grip). In phase 3, the loading and volume are periodized to target specific phases, such as hypertrophy, strength, and strength/power. The goal is to increase muscle size and have these increases translate into strength gains while continuing to target the nervous system through heavy loading and fast repetition velocities (or at least having the intent to move the weight fast). Focus can shift to other variations of the BP to maximize strength with the hope of carryover to the flat BP. Loading can increase in assistance exercises (e.g., triceps extension) to help strengthen BP musculature. Athletes may also alter exercises by including unilateral or alternating exercises in the predominately bilateral program. Phases 4 and 5 progress to train and target all facets of the bench press. Specific training cycles are included that target maximum strength, power gains, and muscle size. Periodization of intensity and volume are used within each cycle, as is *exercise periodization* (or the rotation of exercises in 4-to-6-week phases to increase muscular development at different angles). Advanced training techniques may be introduced here (or in the previous phase, depending on the athlete's progression). Advanced techniques target all elements of the BP by using different grip widths and positions, ROM specificity, bar trajectories, velocity, and power, as well as by pausing between ECC and CON phases, maximizing ECC and ISOM strength, and by varying assistance exercises to directly affect the BP. Some examples include heavy negatives (ECC), functional BP isometrics, rack work with partial ROM BP at different positions, floor presses, board presses, grip variations, use of specialty bars (e.g., Tsunami and vibration), bands, chains, ballistic BP, rest-pause, clusters, lockouts or overloads, and pause presses (the pause being used in competition). In addition, the athlete should incorporate some BP work using competition gear, including bench shirts or even a SlingShot® in the final preparations for a competition. We can refer to these last phases as specific because BP improvements may only occur at this advanced stage when specific elements are directly targeted in various training cycles.

The development of an athlete is a complex and nuanced process, one that demands careful attention to the varying stages of adaptation. It is an ongoing journey, from the early days of beginner training to the pinnacle of elite performance and requires a specialized understanding of the individual athlete's composite and context over time.

1. *Early phase beginner training:* In the initial stages, player development and strength and conditioning professionals must recognize that exercise prescriptions need to be tailored to the athlete's foundational needs. Goals are set, targets are met, and new objectives are created to broaden the athlete's capabilities.
2. *Intermediate training:* As the athlete progresses, intermediate training must be sensitive to the adaptive changes that have already taken place. The programming must recognize and build upon the advancements made, rather than assuming a uniform approach.
3. *Advanced training:* Beyond the intermediate level, advanced training related to exercise programming must be implemented. This phase is critical, as it prepares the athlete for the elite level, where minor adjustments can make a significant difference.
4. *Elite training progression:* Here, a 1 to 2 percent change can mean the difference between a gold medal and 25th place. The emphasis on specificity and individualization reaches its peak, with multidimensional capabilities being the focus.

Monitoring and Analytics

Finally, the analytical aspect of training comes into play. This stage requires common sense and context because without these, the monitoring of workouts and programming can become irrational, deviating from the fundamental need for strength, power, and the improvement of tissue density to prevent injury. Missteps here could lead to sawtooth progress in developing the athlete composite, disrupted by inadequate understanding of exercise stimuli and impact.

Day-to-Day Evaluation

As we will delve into in Chapter 5, the complexity and individuality of each athlete's development demand consistent monitoring and evaluation. Skill sets within the player development team must be advanced and aligned to fully comprehend and respond to the unique needs and context of the time for each athlete.

By recognizing the distinct phases and intricacies involved in athlete development, professionals can foster a more comprehensive, logical, and effective approach. By keeping these principles in mind, we can better ensure success at every level of competition and help athletes reach their fullest potential, both on and off the field.

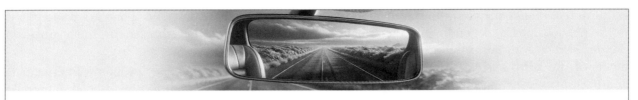

LOOKING IN THE REARVIEW MIRROR
- The big three for optimal training adaptation are (1) training program, (2) nutrition and hydration, and (3) sleep and recovery. All are equally important for maximizing athletic performance.
- The training program mediates the response-adaptation cycle. Proper manipulation of the acute program variables is the key to long-term progression for any fitness component.
- Recovery is a critical component for athletic development. The performance development team needs to invest in optimal recovery strategies and technologies to maximize athletic performance, deal with disruptors, and reduce the risk of overtraining and injury.
- Training workouts elicit acute physiological responses that help lead to chronic adaptations over time. The performance development team needs to understand the underlying physiological mechanisms that contribute to long-term player development.

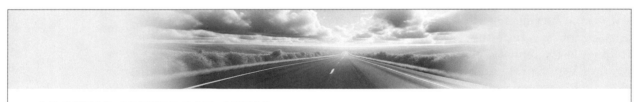

LOOKING AT THE ROAD AHEAD
As we look at the road ahead, one of the most important aspects of player development programming involves the assessments related to workouts and the different factors that contribute to the athlete composite. Proper accounting and monitoring of workouts are vital to making real-time assessments and changes in the program and provide insight into the different units of the player development team, which helps one understand whether the program is progressing as anticipated. Optimizing the technology used in the process is also vital to the individualization of each athlete's program.

Monitoring and Accounting in Player Development

A common question is "What is athlete monitoring?" Modern sport performance programs view athlete monitoring as a cornerstone of athlete injury prevention and improved performance. Often, technologies are applied globally and locally to collect a wide range of metrics, sensor information, and measurements. These multilegged approaches often result in the need for an *athlete management system*, more commonly known as an *AMS system* or simply *AMS*, which is used to disseminate information throughout the organization. However, before developing an AMS, practitioners should pause and look back to the origin and etymology of the word "monitor." Monitor is derived from the Latin root of *monere*, meaning

"To remind, recollect, or advise."

Since its inception, this word implied competence and a responsibility to intervene and ensure a desired outcome. It was not until 1924 that the word was used as a verb meaning to check for quality (originally of radio signals in particular). This context is relevant to today's practitioner because monitoring implies responsibility, competence, and an obligation to ensure successful outcomes. Programs must carefully select measurements and assessments that most directly improve the likelihood of preventing failure and that give ample warning for recommended interventions to the specific task at hand. Regardless of the situation, context, or sport, the first concern in designing an AMS is having precisely desired outcomes and coordinated interventions by the involved shareholders. Sending mass amounts of data and metrics to a team of isolated scientists without the context of the athlete's annual calendar, training program, or current emotional buy-in is counterproductive. Effective monitoring systems not only produce charts, facts, and figures but, more importantly, also give the day-to-day practitioners the greatest amount of situational awareness of each individual and directly improve their ability to make decisions about the proper training stimulus for that given moment.

The Importance of Proper Monitoring

When evaluating the installation of a new athlete AMS or reviewing a current system, all involved shareholders must be able to answer the following questions:

- Are the data being reported scientifically accurate?
- Are the data being reported in a feedback loop that allows time for an intervention?
- Does the staff have the expertise, competency, or capacity to implement the intervention required to make a change?
- Do all shareholders understand their required commitment to making sure the implementation can be maintained for the prescribed period of time?

If these four questions cannot be fully agreed upon and emphatically supported by all parties involved, then the player development team must go back and reevaluate. This process of synthesis and recollaboration takes time and is often cyclical because iterations are tweaked and revisited quarterly and thoroughly assessed once a year. Many administrators not directly involved with the day-to-day operations of the high-performance team need to better understand the raw amount of staffing and hours of review it takes to operate an optimal or moderately effective program. The sheer volume of data produced daily with today's technology, even for one athlete, is exponential compared to just a few years ago. As organizations improve this refinement process and establish key parameters known to lead to sport-specific outcomes, the process will become less about global assessment and more about greater individualization.

Importance of Accounting

For contemporary practitioners, the most essential data set is an accurately maintained athlete's training log during a workout or training session. However, the training log, as described here, transcends being merely a record of an athlete's workouts. It is, in fact, a comprehensive account capturing not just what was prescribed but also the actual execution, the methodology, and the subsequent feedback from the athlete. Although the term "vital historical exercise medical record" might sound like an exaggeration, it emphasizes the importance of this record. Ignoring such a critical document could lead to poor oversight that may contribute to athlete injuries or even graver situations. Given the numerous ways of monitoring workout logs today, any institution supervising an athlete must be prepared to address relevant questions about their training.

- Who was in charge of writing the program?
- Who administered the program?
- What stimulus was prescribed for the individual and why?
- What was the actual dosage of the exercise stimulus that was administered?
- What was the athlete's feedback regarding notes?

The player development team should be able to produce answers to all of these questions within hours rather than days or weeks. Too often, papers go missing, details need to be completed, and many programs struggle to clearly and accurately answer these questions with any level of detail if even at all. In a time of greater push for increased earnings and athlete safety in every program, this level of documentation is the minimum standard for safely administering any player development plan. A culture of documentation and detail is the bedrock of a great program. When injury or death occurs in a program, a lack of documentation and too much stimulus often turn out to be the causes of the biological failure. Modern athletes typically gravitate to digital platforms and appreciate it when coaches use the information they log to provide greater individualization to their plans. This attention to detail further drives commitment and faith in the program and the training culture.

Proper monitoring is only possible through a precise and detailed accounting of the individual training stimulus either by the athlete themselves or the training staff administering the plan. As stated earlier, monitoring in the active sense is crucial in providing an appropriate response or intervention that ensures success and prevents failure. One must make sure that the proper competence is in place so that the staff can make the appropriate decisions; for example, additional hours of manual therapy for soft tissue treatment by a certified athletic trainer may be needed. Conversations about training room availability should be had ahead of time in anticipation of this need. Especially in the university setting, many athletic training staff members are only 10-month employees. Before the training block begins, it should be well planned out what human capital and financial support will be needed and what will actually be available.

An evidence-based critical analysis of resource requirements should be completed before the start of every off-season. An annual plan and resource inventory are vital to ensuring that all training teams can adequately anticipate what to expect from each of the different shareholders in the form of time, money, and services for the given year. Too often, the support staff is stretched thin, and athletes face limited access. Very often support staff are asked to "go above and beyond" their job description, without any additional resource or financial compensation. Since its inception, this unspoken disparity between workload and compensation has plagued the industry, greatly contributing to burnout across the profession. However, with proper annual planning, departments can expect to have a tremendous impact on the quality of care for their employees by creating a working document and plan. The hallmark of any great program is the pride with which the entire team speaks about the organization's clear progression in career trajectories. Conversely, high attrition in support staff roles may indicate that the senior leadership is unable to maintain the three Cs.

Lastly, the athletics industry is in a fluid state that is constantly changing due to revenues, scholarships, and coaching staff. Striking a balance between rigidly adhering to standards of excellence and being agile and responsive enough to get the job done can be challenging. Nobody likes surprises, so the best course of action is to clearly outline to everyone involved with the athletes what they can and cannot expect. This way, even if support is limited for some time, the staff will at least be aware of it. It is up to leadership to respond to requests and provide additional resources, but without a good inventory and optimized monitoring and successful interventions, there will never be any documentation to roadmap these experiences and what is commonly referred to as institutional knowledge will be lost for future generations of staff.

Accounting: What Has Been Done?

Accounting is different from monitoring because it does not require analysis or intervention. It is merely the practice of producing repeatable and reliable data sets for shareholders to analyze and discuss in the decision-making process. Accounting must be accurate, timely, and without bias: As with financial accounting, individuals who produce numbers must provide accurate data and not omit or manipulate information to fit a narrative. If data sets are seen as incorrect or do not reflect an individual's progress, coaches will become distrustful. At a minimum, proper accounting should fall into the following categories (table 5.1) of documentation and feedback loop time cycles.

Responsibilities of the Player Development Team

Every member of the team matters, regardless of whether it is the senior coach or the newly minted undergraduate. Everyone on the team must be assigned roles and responsibilities appropriate to their career and certification levels (French and

TABLE 5.1 Key Data to Use During Accounting

Variable	Comment
Postworkout training load hours	The exact repetitions, sets, loads, and distances that were performed, with subjective athlete feedback and any technology sensor data.
Weekly training load stimulus	Prescription, actual performed, and biological adaptation are arguably the most important and overlooked parts of sport science. This is a radar to visualize where the disruptions occurred. This report will contain a treasure trove of vital information to facilitate conversations among the staff about training prescriptions in the following weeks.
Training block adaptations	The specific changes to the targeted biological system. This report should precisely answer the following questions: Did this training cycle achieve its objective? For whom did it work? For whom did it not work? What were the patterns, and who and what associations showed a clustered connection?
Annual review	The annual review provides the information required to update player profiles, discuss future resources needed to enhance outcomes, and determine what skills should be focused on for staff development. Tonnages and the intensities they occurred at should be analyzed with each of the major lifts in daily and weekly time frames. Intensities and velocities of the top and worst performers should be available for necessary exercises. A detailed participation timeline is not for record-keeping and punishment but for the coaching staff to create year-round buy-in. Creating a culture of consistency in training is the most effective way to prevent sawtooth player development in which players make progress when under direction of the coaching staff but detrain and regress to a baseline on their own.

Torres Ronda 2022). The vast majority of system failures occur when senior leaders need to formally address the other shareholders or members within their division about what is expected of them. Coaches often say, "you should have known better" or "you should communicate more," which may reflect a management style that itself fails to communicate effectively with the rest of the high-performance unit. We recommend using the "one throat to choke" model to define roles and responsibilities. This eliminates the tendency to blame others when objectives are uncompleted. Instead, no matter what happens, one person is responsible for monitoring the situation and ensuring its success. For example, at the start of a semester or year, the following conversation may be had in the team setting:

> Head coach: "Hey, [assistant coach's name] … You are in charge of room scheduling and equipment inventory. Nothing should be out of stock, and I would like a minimum of two weeks' inventory for all disposable items. Can you do this?"
>
> Assistant coach: "Yes" or "No"

There should be nothing said other than yes or no. This is important because accepting responsibilities often comes with hesitation or conditional caveats. Senior leadership must create a culture where individuals are encouraged to speak up and say no if they are not confident in their ability to execute the task that is being asked of them. The reason for saying no could range from "I don't have access to the purchasing department software," to "I've never done an inventory before." This is an excellent opportunity for senior leadership to provide the required training, resources, or support to get a solid yes.

Assigning roles for the programming of an athlete starts with a firm, confident, and excited "yes." When changing cultures, individuals may have the credentials and competence but may not want to implement the newly instructed commitment. These refusals will typically be in the form of "I don't have time," "we've never done it this way before," or "I don't get paid enough to do that." These types of "no's" are less about training and education and more about the cultural state of the group. This is where department and division heads need to take a closer look at the department and make necessary personnel changes. The assignment of duties, whether big or small, and their guaranteed execution is where the rubber meets the road between institutional rhetoric and athlete development. It is essential to constantly perform quality control reviews of what is being effectively implemented and what is being missed.

Importance of Tracking Metrics in Player Development

Technology integration has arguably been the bridge between science and the practice of resistance training (Haff and Triplett 2016; French and Torres Ronda 2022). The modern practitioner currently has access to an unimaginable number of resources and technology that practitioners 30 years ago would think sounded more like a science-fiction movie than a college weight room. The shutdowns associated with the COVID-19 pandemic forced individuals outside their comfort zone; training someone in a squat rack on the other side of the world using video conferencing became a weekly routine. Technology can come in hardware or software and can produce mountains of information. This information is either prepacked commercialized reporting or open-ended API tools that allow dissertation-level deep dives into the minutest aspects of the human machine. As the field continues to optimize the integration of barbells and web-based dashboards, one aspect

---

What to Look for in Incorporating Metrics

- Is this device or output validated?
- Can this information provide greater insight and enhance the development of mutable characteristics to maximize potential?
- Is this technology reliable or constantly inconsistent, and does it create gaps in the data?
- Can these data be produced by everyone on staff or only a selected individual?

should be noticed: The purpose of any of these technologies is to aid and assist in creating individualized programs that produce better on-field results. Seemingly limitless capital has been spent on technology, inviting questions about who will use it and what data it will generate. The corporate machines of the performance industry have long tried to capitalize on the psychology of the individual who is looking for an edge. This fear of loss is deeply hardwired into human psychology and is the focal point of every marketing department. Since the days of Eugen Sandow's Chest Expander to the modern "injury prevention" devices, the commercial market will try to fully leverage a technology or concept. This is where one must use the evidence-based practice model and develop a clear roadmap for player development that identifies the metrics that matter the most and have tremendous gain potential at any given time for any individual. Once this has been done, technology can be added; otherwise, the technology just creates distraction and dysfunction.

As research is integrated into the daily practitioner's construct, the data being produced must be accurate, reliable, and repeatable. Commercial companies are often forced to make choices between profit and precision, but sadly many often choose only to make the product just good enough. Good-enough manufacturing and measurement historically fails to pass peer-review validation studies protecting the field's knowledge base and preserving scientific integrity. Modern practitioners, unfortunately, must perform this quality control themselves before incorporating these metrics into their practices. The real-world consequences of wrong data or metrics without context can often lead to poor performance or ignorance that harm the athlete. The sidebar on page 128 depicts some core questions relating to the selection of monitoring metrics.

Understanding Disruptors to the Program

As previously explained, a *disruptor* may be defined as something that interferes with or alters the function of human physiology. Disruption of a consistent training plan is the most significant risk factor for underperformance and injury. Many practitioners may focus on outcome metrics such as the 1RM for an exercise, sprint speed, or the highest vertical jump. However, what many practitioners must realize is that after the initial normative training range of 6 to 8 weeks, the most significant factor in success is not what is done in the 4 to 6 hours a week of training but rather in the other 168 hours of the week. This is where elite departments separate themselves from other programs. When shareholders from a wide range of departments successfully address ongoing issues that arise, the stage is set for the most significant era of athlete development. Historically, a single strength and conditioning professional would have to deal with a vast array of topics, including nutrition, sleep, psychology, academics, and rehabilitation. Now, entire departments are dedicated to becoming masters of their domain and practice. History can

---

Examples of Disruptor Comments from Athlete Workout Logs

- "The dining hall closes at 7 p.m., but we don't finish training until 7:30 and I can't afford to eat out."
- "I slept 2 hours last night so that I could submit my paper on time."
- "I didn't sleep well because I went to my best friend's funeral this weekend."
- "I'm lactose intolerant and can't drink our protein shakes."
- "I can't do my sprints because we are in an active war zone when I go home, and I'm only allowed to work out on my rooftop with security."
- "Coach intended us to do leisurely tempo runs after practice. After checking GPS data, coach ended up doubling the distance—all at top speed."
- "My country doesn't allow us to go outside due to COVID, and if I leave my apartment my GPS tracker will notify the authorities. I need an in-home workout."

be made when egos are put aside and alignment is unshakeable. Disruption is the detectable deviation from positive trait development, which is why accounting and record-keeping are so vital. There is no point in only detecting disruptions at the end of the year. What is most important is for the player development team to identify interventions and address staffing requirements based on the current state of the program and its subsequent direction. The sidebar on page 129 presents some examples of both expected and unexpected disruptors that have been tracked through the years.

Skill Sets Needed

The player development team needs a multitude of skills and proficiencies to optimize the level of instruction for the athletes. These are discussed throughout this book. Figure 5.1 depicts a general list of several proficiencies and content knowledge expertise areas needed by competent members of the player development team (Ratamess 2022). In this section, we focus on other skills needed, such as computer competencies, staff training and software education, basic statistics, graphing, and data management.

Computer Competencies

The arrival of computer technology in the weight room and sport performance has come. Love it or hate it, the staff needs to interact with it. The modern practitioner must have a baseline understanding of each domain's capabilities and applications. This is not to say one must possess an elite level of competence, but one should have a general understanding of the context of the capabilities of the computer platforms and how they may help or hinder the current training infrastructure. Ideally, those who can instruct and inform those around them about areas of proper application can have a tremendous effect on the athlete's developmental outcomes and the quality of life for the support staff.

Introducing computers and related technology to staff is about integration. Athletics has followed a similar path of data and technology integration that was seen in the finance industry since the early 1990s, and cybersecurity since the 2000s in regard to the "data gold rush," data overload, and trying to derive a competitive advantage with meaningful data insight. Some practitioners will refuse to learn and adapt to the new role of technology in

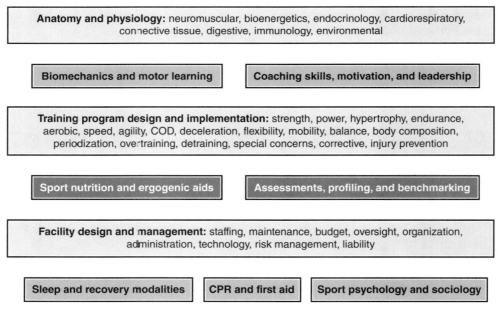

FIGURE 5.1 Proficiencies and content knowledge expertise areas.

the weight room and will quickly be left behind. Young talent will make promises about technology solving all of the problems of previous generations, but those promises will not materialize. What will most likely emerge in the coming generations of human performance are savvy practitioners who understand their strengths and weaknesses and how to use technology as a force multiplier for saving time, quality control, and thus creating better training outcomes.

In today's industry, each staff usually has someone in charge of the data. This role is typically given to one of the most junior staff members who lacks experience but is enthusiastic about learning and working in a digital environment. What is most important is to not fall into the trap of siloing responsibility but instead to use this individual or group of individuals to build scalable applications and platforms to be used by all practitioners. To the best of their abilities, modern practitioners must find a way to optimize their current practice by integrating the digital environment into their programs. Regardless of experience or track record, staff members are often limited by redundancy and inefficiency, which limits their ability to do what they love, which is to work with people. The failure to successfully integrate into a digital environment is usually due to the egos and insecurities of those who do not want to seem foolish or obsolete. Truly elite practitioners are always searching for ways to iterate, refine, and improve their craft because their true motivation is to serve their athletes in the best possible way they can.

Staff Training and Software Education

Training and education in the digital environment are no different than in the physical environment. Since software is not tangible, it is often overlooked during instruction, compared to the back squat, for example. With any digital platform, it is essential to follow these guidelines for proper instruction, application, and proficiency before using the product in the day-to-day workflow.

- It takes roughly 90 days of hands-on interaction, training, and application before staff members can gain an intuitive feel for any piece of software they use in their practice.
- The leadership staff should hold an all-hands meeting to discuss any ongoing problem before rolling out the new platform (see the sidebar on page 132 for an example). The problem should be broken down into great detail concerning how it has negatively affected the athletes, the full-time staff, and any other shareholders. Leaders often provide some new and "exciting" or "game-changing" application to streamline daily processes, but adding any application, be it hardware or software, for no other reason than novelty creates a technology bottleneck problem and eventually technology creep. *Technology creep* occurs when an organization rapidly accumulates technology without any formalized plan. The management, upkeep, and integration of new technology should be thoroughly thought through because it will ultimately become a full-time job for an individual on staff and take time away from their day-to-day responsibilities. This phenomenon may result in resistance and sometimes the refusal of the staff to comply, and they may become so frustrated that the technology gets shelved and forgotten about.
- When adding any technology platform, there should be an enthusiastic or at least understanding acceptance of how it is the best decision for the program. A good litmus test for any practitioner is to ask the staff to verbally articulate the platform's importance and give their honest take on how it makes a positive impact.
- Training should be broken into the following phases:
  - Overview and history of the product and its capabilities
  - Validation
  - Reliability
  - Accuracy

> ## The Rollout
>
> The planned rollout should be broken into phases. Here is an example of the process:
>
> ### The Problem
> Athletes need to improve linear speed. The department has decided to use a laser timing gate system that integrates with the university's data science department.
>
> ### The Phases
> - Phase 1: Start on a small scale with a population that is highly committed and diligent and will give honest feedback about its application.
>   - Action: Laser-test one specific group of athletes on the 10-yard dash.
> - Phase 2: Target the specific rollout to the entire population.
>   - Action: Laser-test all athletes on the 10-yard dash.
> - Phase 3: Use laser testing for a broad-spectrum battery set of field tests to measure agility and athletic profile for the entire department.
>   - Action: Share data with data science staff for cluster analysis.

Software Training

There are countless software platforms that the modern practitioner must interact with. The most important thing is that the individual directly responsible for an application demonstrates sufficient competency and expertise. If the individual does not directly interact with a particular software platform, it is still important to know about it and, more specifically, to know who the point of contact is if a question arises. Typically, in athletics, a firewall protects an organization's electronic medical records. These medical files may contain restricted or private information protected by an individual's medical rights. Practitioners should thoroughly understand what is possible and whom to speak with to request information. For example, if an operations assistant was instructed to purchase food for a road trip for an upcoming tournament, it would be reasonable and perfectly legal to reach out to the sports medicine staff and ask if anyone on the trip has any allergies or any medical condition that would require specific nutritional needs outside of what is normally provided. Knowing that this information is available allows the departments to align and work in synergy to properly care for the nutritional needs of all players and avoid an allergic reaction.

Data Entry

Raw data without context can be useless. Data entry ultimately falls into two categories: *timeliness* and *integrity*. Data streams from sensors and tablets come in predictable waves and require automated database integration, such as CSV files that can be formatted at a later time. Other data streams may come straight from an athlete or coaching feedback. Sample size, completion percentage, and compliance become extremely important in the later stages of interpretation and analysis. As a general rule of thumb, any subjective data should reside in a 24-hour feedback loop, which will ensure that days and weeks do not pass where information is being missed or ignored.

Data Quality Demands

In every instance of data capture, quality control is the best safeguard against analyzing insufficient data. Data are useless if they come from a sensor that has not been correctly calibrated. Workout cards on which athletes report load lifted in kilograms one week and then pounds the next week can lead to false conclusions about program efficacy. As a rule, quality control procedures should follow these guidelines:

- Quality control is performed by someone objective who is not directly associated with the information collected. For example, body composition tests are performed by the institution's medical staff on a DEXA scanner instead of with hand calipers by the strength and conditioning staff that wrote the training plan for improved body composition and increased muscle mass.

- A brief program defense should be performed and presented to the staff at the end of every training block. This is an excellent opportunity to exchange experiences, insights, and obstacles faced during training. Additionally, this is where the blend of experience and technology becomes synergistically beneficial. These sessions often provide growth opportunities for young coaches and advancements in the department's institutional knowledge that help guide future policy initiatives.

See the following sidebar for an example.

Data Quality Example

The coach discusses the speed training plan to address linear speed improvement. The coach states that there was a significant increase in speed and the program worked better than expected. During the defense, the coach is asked what the average 10-yard dash time was and states that it was 1.45 seconds. The senior coaches respond that this number seems inaccurate because it would make the high school tennis team faster than every NFL DBs of the past year's combine. With any testing, technology needs to be set up correctly, and the testing procedures need to be followed exactly. Still, if the data provided during the defense seems incorrect, it should not be validated until after an investigation into what happened. Using this data set for future testing benchmarks would be an example of poor data integrity and setting unrealistic training benchmarks for future training groups.

Basic Statistics

Statistics is the science of collecting, classifying, analyzing, and interpreting data (McGuigan 2017). Data obtained from athlete assessment may be used for intra-athlete comparison (e.g., comparing the individual athlete's data over time), comparing different athletes or groups, comparing an athlete relative to the group, or comparison to norms. Coaches may compare data over time and calculate a difference score or percentage difference. These data help quantify the efficacy of the program but are limited in their capacity to determine higher levels of meaningfulness. Further analysis could provide the team with solid evidence-based changes that may be used for various purposes throughout the organization (e.g., the level of precision seen in a scientific study). Thus, further statistical evaluations may provide added benefit to the program.

A basic understanding of descriptive, inferential, and magnitude-based statistics is helpful for today's practitioners. *Descriptive statistics* include calculating the mean, median, mode, variability (variance, range, standard deviation, and standard error of measurement), percentile ranks, t-scores, and z-scores. Relationships may be investigated by calculating correlation coefficients or using regression analysis. *Inferential statistics* are used to draw conclusions about the population from a sample. Statistical significance may be tested ($p \leq 0.05$) with normal data distributions (figure 5.2) or nonparametric statistics may be used for unequally distributed data. Some examples of inferential tests include *t*-tests, analysis of variance (ANOVA) and covariance (ANCOVA) with subsequent post hoc tests (e.g., tests used to denote specific areas of statistical significance). Here, significance can be determined by comparing one group of athletes to another group. Comparing effect sizes, or the magnitude of difference between groups, could

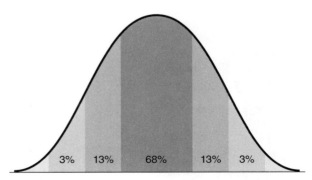

FIGURE 5.2 Normal data distribution.

Reprinted by permission from M. McGuigan, "Administration, Scoring, and Interpretation of Selected Tests," in *Essentials of Strength Training and Conditioning*, 4th ed., edited by G.G. Haff and N.T. Triplett (Champaign, IL: Human Kinetics, 2016).

provide meaningful data as well. Although mandatory for scientific inquiry, statistical analysis of group data is optional, but it could be useful for critical program analysis. The team should use high-quality statistics software (e.g., SPSS or another statistics package) because these software programs allow for easy data input and the use of many statistical procedures. For example, if a sport science member of the player development team presents data to higher shareholders in an organization, determining statistical significance could strengthen the argument for the program's efficacy. This could lead to other benefits stemming from program evaluation success. While many strength and conditioning professionals have a limited background in mathematics, the new generation of data scientists will frequently speak in this statistical jargon in everyday conversation. Thus, it is essential for the practitioner to facilitate meetings to discuss the findings and research and thoroughly understand the statistical parameters they choose to implement during a given phase.

Graphing Capabilities and Data Storage

After data are collected, members of the player development team may organize, clean, store, analyze, and present the data in understandable and meaningful ways. This is a critical part of the athlete monitoring process because visual data assists in the inspection of progress or tracking over time. Graphs play an important role in modeling and understanding data. Many types of graphs are commonly used to depict athlete data, including scatterplots, line graphs, bar and column graphs, spider (radar) graphs, pie charts, area graphs, box plots, violin plots, histograms, and a combination of column and scatterplot graphs. Figure 5.3 depicts an example of a spider (radar) graph simultaneously showing six metrics. Some

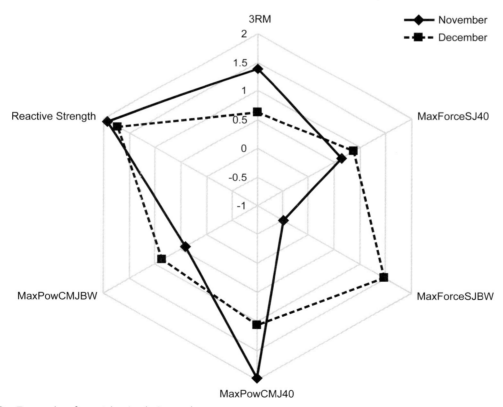

FIGURE 5.3 Example of a spider (radar) graph.
Courtesy of Dr Robert U. Newton, Exercise Medicine Research Institute, Edith Cowan University, Perth, Australia.

equipment software such as force plates allows for a graphical representation of the data as well as storage of large files of individual data points. Others may require one to input the data into spreadsheet software, such as Excel, or into AMS software. Spreadsheets are good for relatively small data sets, but a database management system such as the AMS is needed for managing large amounts of data. AMS software is a web-based application designed to store, organize, analyze, and present graphic visuals of data sets. These programs allow users to choose metrics and KPIs, customize data collection forms, dashboards, apps, questionnaires, and analytic features, and integrate data from other technology while maintaining integrity standards.

Creating Data Visualizations

Visualizations format data and information in a way that is easy to understand and visually appealing for the athlete. Data visuals can easily and quickly show coaches or athletes how performance changes and how it relates or compares to other performances. Figure 5.4 shows a system we used previously, titled the *4 Pillars of Visualization* created by Noah Illinsky. The directives were intended for staff to optimize visualizations for data presentation.

Responsibilities of the Athlete

Every athlete should be able to articulate the purpose of what they are doing in their training plan. While some athletes enjoy following the plan as prescribed, understanding what they are doing and why it is important to their player development contributes to the level of buy-in from the athletes. Great programs acknowledge that buying into the process starts with driving intent into every aspect and detail of preparation. Intent drives habits, and habits drive culture. Great team cultures can often be limited or reduced to their smallest component by a lack of buy-in from the athletes.

Understanding the Exercises

Regardless of the modality, every intervention combines kinematic coordination with some load demand. These demands range from maximal motor unit recruitment to strategy assessments under fatigue and duress. The modern athlete should have a thorough understanding of how to safely perform any exercises or drill, not merely to the point of getting it right—but until they cannot get it wrong. Exercise movement can be broken down into four levels of competence:

- *Level 3:* The movement mechanics are near exemplary, and the athlete can articulate and coach fellow teammates in the fundamental coaching cues and progressions.
- *Level 2:* The athlete demonstrates sufficient technical capacity under low RPE or low fatigue status. This is where the 80/20 rule applies: The athlete may never achieve Olympic world record outputs but can safely perform the exercise to the point that there is ample motor transferability to the sport of choice.
- *Level 1:* The athlete displays limited proficiency in the mechanics of the exercise, and any form of loading would most likely be detrimental and not result in sport transferability. This level of motor control would be best used as an opportunity for technical improvement. The coach must dig into their toolbox and use experiential progression and regression drills from their years of practical coaching experience.
- *Level 0:* The movement pattern looks terrible and sometimes unrecognizable as to what the original intent of the exercise was. Any attempt to load these pathways would result in injury or catastrophic failure. This can often be the case during early player development when the training age is young or when the athlete is coming back from an injury.

Players and coaches must develop similar coaching eyes so that staff and players can agree on proper movement mechanics. This not only helps develop a better training culture; it can also be a source of pride for the older athletes who act as proxy coaches to the younger teammates. These grading assessments can easily be woven into the training program with little disruption to the actual training sessions.

The 4 Pillars of Visualization

1. PURPOSE: The Who and Why
   - The purpose must be specific to the audience being addressed
   - Think about who the audience is and why they need to know this information
   - What will they now be able to do with the data that they couldn't do before
2. CONTENT: The What
   - Identify what data set matters
   - Identify what data will be excluded
   - Eliminate the data that does not contribute specifically to the particular point you are making. Ask yourself these questions:
     1. What data matter the most?
     2. Do the data change over time?
     3. What relationships might the data have?
   - People are good at noticing patterns and differences; therefore, the visualization should use those patterns and differences to highlight the most important information
3. STRUCTURE: The How To
   - Decide how the data will be displayed
   - The graph type depends on your purpose and what you are trying to show
     1. Bar graphs: comparison between data sets
     2. Line graphs: changes in data over time
     3. Scatterplot: correlation between data sets
4. FORMAT: The Appeal and Focus
   - Know how your data will be consumed (digital vs paper)
   - Understand the impact that proper encoding can play in correctly conveying your findings

FIGURE 5.4 The 4 Pillars of Visualization.
Courtesy of Thomas Newman and Noah Illinsky.

Understanding the Program

The following scenario is a dialogue among a coach and three athletes about understanding their training programs:

> Coach: "What does your training plan look like today?"
>
> Athlete A: "I don't know, I just do what I'm told."
>
> Athlete B: "I'm in a strength phase for the next two weeks."
>
> Athlete C: "I'm trying to up my 1RM strength so I can be on track to start the power program before I go home for winter break."

All three of these answers are correct, but which is best? One of the most significant barometers of program buy-in is when athletes can articulate the "why" of their program. The days of merely following instruction without question are gone. The "what" of a program is easy to read off a card, but the "why" and how it matters both short-term and long-term are critically important in driving intentionality and commitment to details. Taking the time to answer any athlete's questions regarding their program is a critical opportunity for the modern coach to reinforce buy in. Athletes should be able to articulate confidently not only what is occurring in the plan but also why it is best for them and what success looks like. Athletes by nature are hardwired to win, so why should a

Visual Encoding Properties and Best Uses

Visual encoding		Properties		Best uses			
Example	Encoding	Ordered	Useful values	Quantitative	Ordinal	Categorical	Relational
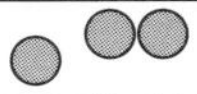 ○ ○○	Position, placement	Yes	Infinite	Good	Good	Good	Good
1, 2, 3; A, B, C	Text labels	Optional (alphabetical or numbered)	Infinite	Good	Good	Good	Good
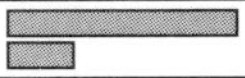	Length	Yes	Many	Good	Good		
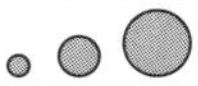 ∘ ○ ◯	Size, area	Yes	Many	Good	Good		
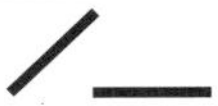 / ⁄ _	Angle	Yes	Medium/few	Good	Good		
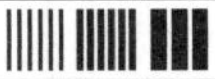	Pattern density	Yes	Few	Good	Good		
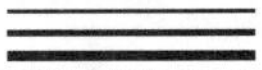	Weight, boldness	Yes	Few		Good		
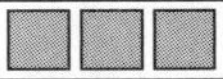	Saturation, brightness	Yes	Few		Good		
	Color	No	Few (<20)			Good	
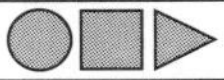 ● ■ ▶	Shape, icon	No	Medium			Good	
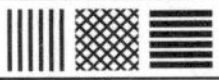	Pattern texture	No	Medium			Good	
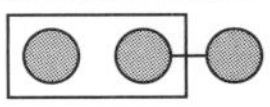 ○─○─○	Enclosure, connection	No	Infinite			Good	Good
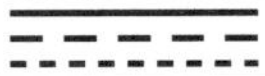 - - - - - -	Line pattern	No	Few				Good
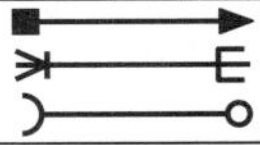 ▬─▶ ⇥─E ↳─○	Line endings	No	Few				Good
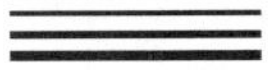	Line weight	Yes	Few		Good		

FIGURE 5.4 The 4 Pillars of Visualization.

workout be any different? The workout environment is a great opportunity for driving consistent, year-round commitment to development.

Recording the Workout

Recording workouts has become easier given the improvements in technology. Recording and tracking workouts helps monitor progression and provides accountability since changes can be made based on past workout data. Workout logging allows the athlete to record not only training data (e.g., sets, repetitions, and weight) but also other observations or feelings that affect overall performance. Apps and software programs have made it easier to record elements of the workout. Figure 5.5 depicts an instructional document to educate athletes on the standards of workout logging. The document consists of background information to educate athletes on proper logging, athlete and coaching standards for both entities, and an evaluation rubric coaches can use to score the workout cards. It is important for athletes to be shown how to log workouts and provide good detail so that coaches can accurately review the day's workout and develop program modifications when necessary.

Sport Coach's Responsibilities and Roles

Sport coaches will always be involved in the athlete development process. At the collegiate level especially, there is often tremendous overlap

STANDARDS OF WORKOUT CARD LOGGING

The use of the workout card log is one of the most important practices in resistance training. The training log establishes a high standard of work for the athlete to fulfill. The strength coach should maintain and update the card constantly based on observed task completion. It serves as the benchmark for improvement in the scope of long-term athletic development.

ATHLETE STANDARDS

1. Record body weight.
2. Adhere to exercises, programmed percentages, sets, and repetitions prescribed by the coach. If an athlete is unable to complete any exercise or load, the coach should be conferred with before any alterations to the prescription. Record modifications on card.
3. Athlete is responsible for recording:
- Weight moved
- Fatigue rating, sleep, or other questionnaire prompts.
- Notes that provide insight about training sessions (perceived effort, pain, soreness, reps in reserve).

COACH STANDARDS

1. Assign player prescriptions at the beginning of the daily, weekly, or monthly block based on season and injury.
2. Review cards at the end of the day for completion of objective measures such as exercises, 1RM percentages, and set and repetition adherence. Review subjective measures and address statistics with athletes.
3. Prescribe progression and regression adjustments to the program based on short-term and long-term review.
4. Coaches will score workout cards.

WORKOUT CARD EVALUATION AND SCORING RUBRIC

0 - Standards Not Met:	1 - Below Average:	2 - Average:	4 - Above Average:
Workout card or weight/rep prompts are empty. Exact values have not been recorded. Card is not filled out on the day of lift. Card does not reflect modifications.	Surveys, weight entry, or rep prompts are entered. Some modifications are accounted for. There are no notes to provide insight regarding training to progress the next workout.	Surveys, weight entry, or rep prompts are entered. Modifications are accounted for. There are notes on main lifts to progress for the next week, but not on other accessory exercises.	All surveys, weight entry, rep prompts are entered. All modifications are accounted for. There are notes on all exercises to provide insight into the training session and guide progression.

FIGURE 5.5 Example of the standards of workout logging.
Courtesy of Thomas Newman.

between the sport coach and the support staff in guiding athletes through their journey. Coaches typically fall into several archetypes, and some slide along the spectrum throughout their careers. Regardless of title, coach involvement slides on two axis: involvement and detail. It is up to the modern performance coach to effectively identify and package their messaging and services for the needs of the team. Sport coaches, when left with no alternative, attempt to maintain total control of the program, making interdepartmental collaboration cumbersome.

Decisions on What Data Need to Be Entered

Once the shareholders agree about their roles and responsibilities, it is time to surgically select from the sea of possible metrics commercially available a list of metrics to establish an ironclad chain of command and assign responsibility for interventions. Referring back to the three Cs, the assigned shareholders must demonstrate competence in and commitment to their responsibilities. Regardless of bureaucracy, red tape, or other impediments to success, they are responsible for getting things done. Too often, perfectly qualified individuals lack real-world competence or the patience to fight through unpredictable adversity of athletics and get the job done. Especially under the modern paradigm of collaborating performance, team individuals should not be judged by the nature of their responsibilities but rather by how often they successfully complete their assigned tasks. This is particularly important when developing younger coaches. The capacity and commitment in a younger coach to execute a task regardless of barriers is a priceless trait that cannot be taught. The people who make positive and decisive interventions based in common sense complemented with analytics are typically the backbone of any great performance program.

Types of Data

Data comes in many forms, but in general it is classified into two categories: acute and chronic. In the early implementation stages of a program, it is imperative to focus on acute variables that have an immediate effect in order to bring about the largest possible change and help participants buy into the program. However, it cannot be overstated that long-term data structures must be collected and monitored during the initial implementation of any development program. The law of large numbers is often overlooked in the athletic industry and when there is a change in the coaching staff, the data previously collected are ignored or discarded. This hard reset of institutional knowledge has a devastating effect on programs. Data are disregarded for many reasons, but as today's sensors become more universal, the failure point tends to be at the point of human collection. Did the jump occur with an arm swing or with hands on hips? Was the bar loaded in kilograms or pounds? Was there a spotter or no spotter? These metadata points are crucial when establishing confidence in the meaning of potential interventions that may be required.

Great care must be taken with chronic data collection, and other complementary sets should cross-reference any assumptions. Academic researchers tend to obsess about establishing large-scale studies of athletic programs. These researchers will be quick to state that any true data analysis requires large volumes to make any real scientifically valid recommendations, sometimes even one year of collection. The modern sport coach is not focused on these long-range studies; they are trying to win games and keep their job. This misalignment of priorities can cause friction with the researchers, especially if the in-season record of the team is poor. Erroneous conclusions can be drawn from chronic data if collected with tunnel vision because the output of the data is seen as a sign of the times and not vice versa. Some examples of complementary data sets that have worked well in the past for chronic collection include the following:

- DEXA scans for muscle mass
- Force plate power output
- 1RM back squat totals
- Participation in fuel station shakes/nutrition interventions
- Academic year
- Workout card completion percentage

Identification of Disruptors in the Program

The most important and overlooked metric in modern sports is the level of disruption to the athlete. A disruptive event or stressor negatively affects an individual and causes a suboptimal training state. This will be the focal point of the performance industry and will largely be dealt with in individualized recovery programs that resemble current training programs. Staff members who have a thorough understanding of the physiological and psychosocial underpinnings of high performance and can detect, identify, and intervene will bring great success.

Historically, emphasis has been placed on the positive social reinforcement of praising those who consistently increase their output. This was typically done with leaderboards, medals, and trophies for off-season accomplishments—all to gamify off-season development in the hopes of increasing in-season performance. However, for many reasons, especially the lack of technology at the field's inception, focusing on disruptors was not possible in daily practice. With the emergence of commercially available technology, it has become easy to extract data from workout cards, especially weekly or monthly training block trends, and identify anomalies during a specific exercise, set, or repetition.

A common theme throughout this book is the idea that exercise is modern medicine. Even at its earliest inception, Selye's concept of stress adaptation and the subsequent planned supercompensation is the foundation of the performance industry (Selye 1976). Elite practitioners are already beginning to see a substantial effect from studying these disruptors. With tremendous success, they have already begun more commonly administered recovery modalities such as float, chiropractic, massage, and sleep hygiene. However, a great emphasis is being placed on prescribing a good overload and tailored rebound stimulus to help catapult individuals out of the deeper alarm states. Tracking disruptors helps staff understand other factors that could have affected an athlete's performance at a given time and develop enhanced mitigation strategies for the future.

Workouts and Load Monitoring

Data collected from workouts are the most critical data set for any individual or sport coach. Given the field's current financial and economic structure, one practitioner may be in charge of many athletes and not have the time to successfully collect and analyze sizeable data sets from daily training at scale. In 2023 and beyond, serious programs must implement a digital collection platform for workouts. Plenty of commercial products exist, ranging from free to several thousand dollars per year, to solve this problem. These pay for themselves in a matter of weeks considering the number of hours sport coaches spend formatting and transposing paper to Excel. Following the NCAA's catastrophic event planning guidelines, departments should be legally able to produce workout cards and medical training history with the same efficiency and accuracy with which a doctor produces records for a liability case from an electronic medical records system. In addition, markers of internal and external load should be easily tracked and monitored over time. In chapter 6 we discuss these variables in more detail. Here, we present a brief overview of some of them to see how tracking is important for the development of the athlete.

Variables

A researcher would say, before performing any analysis, that one must limit confounding variables, account for the placebo effect, and have a solid control group. Unfortunately, as science and technology are integrated into modern athletics, one cannot control everything. Confounding variables play a role in sport performance and can be tracked, but often the entire athlete training program can be influenced by sport coaches who are neither part of the sport performance team nor care about research. The sole focus of these coaches is to win championships, and deviation from that goal is considered a distraction. This is typically where practitioners who fail to establish relationships with the sport coach will see programs shy away from participating in performance programs that focus heavily on individualization and metric-based program decisions.

Competition variables are commentaries on the team's current recruiting, development, and strategic proficiency. Great caution must be taken in drawing conclusions about game data other than a win or loss. Game data and on-field success are often the greatest points of friction in any program and at the center of many bad decisions in the off-season development program. An assistant coach comments, "We need to be faster!" and the strength and conditioning professional may then question the level of running volume. Data science may point to an imbalance in ground strikes. The athletic trainer identifies issues with neuromuscular synchronicity. The subsequent cascade occurs after nearly every game around the world, especially if a team has underperformed for the season. Success is often a multivariate problem, and knee-jerk reactions often fail to address the more significant issues at hand. At the same time, there may be some truth in every shareholder's view on how to fix the problem. The elephant in the room, however, may be that the recruited players lacked the required genetic endowment to reach the desired velocity outcomes, even with the most comprehensive program. Every athlete is governed by genetic endowment, so great emphasis should be placed early on in the composite profile to select largely nonmutable traits that will limit their final potential gain.

Recovery

Recovery is the new frontier of performance. What was once considered taking a day off has developed into a calculated, choreographed effort to help reinforce and aid the recovery of the body's underlying biological substructures. This strategy of implementing recovery acts as a biological trampoline to launch individuals out of the alarm state and into supercompensation. Recovery methods should be tracked as part of the athlete monitoring program.

Sleep and Heart Rate Variability

Sleep is the most widely misunderstood variable under the performance paradigm. Sleep is a process of the physical hardware of human existence, yet modern technology mostly disrupts this aspect of human life. Research is just beginning to understand not only the positive effects of sleep on the daily performance of athletes but also its effect on longevity in the second half of life. Not sleeping has culturally been perceived as a sign of toughness and positively reinforced by coaches for decades. We can now measure and monitor the effects of sleep with commercial products. *Heart rate variability* (HRV) is a measure of the variation in the time interval between heartbeats and is considered an indirect, noninvasive measure of cardiac autonomic activity. Sleep and HRV technologies are used to track and collect qualitative and quantitative information on the body. As technology and research continue to discover sleep's impact on performance, it can be expected that in the future, coaches will need to program and periodize recovery and sleep hygiene as part of the resistance training programming.

Behavior

The psychological and psychosocial effects of team culture can be quantified by measuring either adherence to instruction or collective buy-in to a cause greater than the individual. There has been considerable research on the relationship between team cohesion and elite output. Some researchers suggest that team cohesion may be linked to pathological structures in the brain that predispose individuals to buy into a greater cause. Self-selection further confirms this in high-performance athletics and the military. Upon reaching full genetic potential, there are specific untrainable attributes that nearly all elite performers possess. Coaches prophesied that "heart," which may refer to the willingness to compete regardless of outcome, cannot be measured. There are specific untrainable attributes that nearly all elite performers possess, and have a keen sense in detecting in others, that can't be explained but must not be ignored.

Nutrition

Tracking macronutrient and micronutrient intake is part of the athlete monitoring process. Nutrition must keep up with advancements in research and technology. Gone are the days of protein, fats, and carbohydrates. The simplification of "calories in" and "calories out" underestimates the problem. If an athlete eats 2,500 kilocalories of donuts and another athlete eats 2,500 kilocalories of grass-fed beef, there would be a drastic difference in their training performance. The future of nutrition will be individualized for not only the task-specific demands of the sport but also the athlete's genetic predisposition. Nutrition should be measured in the sense of classical dietetics as well as with regard to the social and cultural norms of the group. Strategies that promote consistency and community often provide immediate transformation in both body composition and performance. Simply creating metrics on time, frequency, and consistency may provide the most immediate change in a program.

Perceived Exertion and Session RPE

Perceptual feedback from athletes comes in many forms. With digital surveys, coaches can quickly gain insight into an athlete's perceived difficulty or physiological state. This type of data is essential when trying to turn around a program or individualize training programs. Initially, individuals begin to learn the range of psychological and physiological soreness encountered in the program. Interestingly, the perceived difficulty decreases over time with consistent training density. This down-regulation of prescribed stress is vital to preparing athletes for competition. While competition is unpredictable and sudden, long-term tracking of training load can give incredible insight into the time needed to get an athlete ready and the acute training loads required to perform at a high level. Ideally, the training sessions should require more than potential competition demands, thus driving psychological confidence to accomplish the task. The *session RPE* takes into consideration the athlete's perception of exercise intensity and workout duration (Foster et al. 2001) and is useful for tracking over time (discussed in more detail in chapter 6).

Injury

While injuries are often perceived as a setback in an athlete's career, it is a data goldmine for the program. Through the review of six months of the initial training load, the performance staff can begin to develop a program and a position-specific risk analysis matrix. These roadmaps typically contain fairly consistent developmental milestones across several predictable monthly and weekly time intervals. These matrices are the crown jewel of any program because coaches are inherently chasing loss prevention or injury reduction with the hope that viable bodies give them the greatest chance of winning. Attention should also be paid to the training load and the requirement to rehabilitate.

Health Biomarkers

Health is a universally contentious topic in athletics. However, health can be considered a biological subsystem that may not provide a 1:1 correlation to performance. Evaluating health can come in the form of assessing individuals for sleep apnea via a sleep study if they have a neck circumference greater than size 18. It could also include comprehensive eye exams, which are often overlooked in childhood. Evaluating HBA1C or administering a glucose tolerance test with individuals that have immediate family members with diabetes all provide practitioners with a long-term perspective. Especially for athletes who possess physical traits on the fringe of the human spectrum that allow them to excel at the tasks of their sport, these same traits may not be conducive for their long-term life span or health span (e.g., a 330 pound [150 kg] lineman allows them to compete in a Super Bowl, may not be a great trait at 60). Health biomarkers are becoming increasingly easier to administer, and the long-term consideration for the athlete's well-being is virtually always received with tremendous support from family members.

Biomechanics

Biomechanics is a field of study unique to performance development and is one of the original cornerstones of performance. Its history is rooted in the medical community's search for better ways to rehabilitate after surgery and therapeutic treatments for various musculoskeletal disorders. Unfortunately, over the past century, time and money have been two of the greatest limits on integrating biomechanics into modern athletics. However, with advances in strain gauges, transistors, and wireless technology, biomechanics is in the midst of a renaissance of practical application. Currently, there are ways to measure not only the output of an individual compared to their peers in the classical sense but also the strategies through which that output was accomplished. With further research, it can be expected that high-speed biomechanical analysis and subsequent training suggestions will become standard for high performance.

Data Input and Quality Entry

With so many shareholders involved in current athlete development programs, data input and quality are more important than ever. Not only are the values important; the frequency of the sampling rate and feedback loop cycles is also critical. Any technology used to collect data must be reliable and valid, which means everything from ensuring proper calibration and maintenance to holding user-specific training seminars. Fragmented data or inherently flawed data provides practitioners with misinformation and sows doubt in the sport coaches who invest time in the program. As a matter of good housekeeping, any data set should always pass common sense analysis. Additionally, great caution should be used whenever adding a data stream. Too often, departments are bogged down in technology creep, and collected data turn out to be useless or simply a vanity metric providing no actionable value. Also, repeatedly assessing the same biological marker in various ways does not confirm findings but only decreases confidence. Anything collected should have a purpose and an individual or department with a subsequent plan of action to increase the athletes' performance development.

Checks and Rechecks

As the collection and use of data move away from research and into a more practical setting, great care must be taken to install consistent quality control procedures before announcing a finding or suggesting an intervention. If sensitive data are being used while being shielded from certain shareholders, the data must be correct. As a matter of practical experience, there is always an error in the data field, although many go unnoticed. The error could be an incorrect weigh-in, the weights on the bar having been recorded initially in kilograms and then later in pounds (this is more common than people would like to admit, especially with international technology companies). Regularly scheduled quality control checkpoints are standard practice at the highest levels of the industry. Independent staff members often perform them to ensure data integrity and that the practitioners have not manipulated the data to seek praise from the sport coaches or athletes themselves. Not only does corrupted data create short-term problems but it also damages any long-term value by corrupting the data pool.

Documentation of Who Entered the Data

The best way to express the core of programmed resistance and performance training is through the idea that exercise is medicine. To put this theoretical concept into practice requires tight control of the data chain of command and ownership. Just as a doctor must provide detailed post-surgical notes, modern practitioners must consistently be able to answer the following questions, as well as why it is significant, when discussing any data set.

- Who: Who collected the data? Coaches, athletes, the sport information department, or medical staff?
- What: What was collected and what procedure was used (countermovement arm swing versus hands on hips)?
- When: When were these data collected? Team setting, individual training, morning versus afternoon, or scattered across a week?
- Where: Was the data collection carried out on turf field A or turf field B?
- Why: Were the data collected from an impromptu test by the coach or a planned training session or test?
- How: Were the data collected with a laser timer or stopwatch?

Accountability

During the quality control assessment and review process, it must be made clear that the individual and the employing program are responsible for data integrity. If there is a technical problem with a piece of hardware, it must be fixed or removed from daily operations. Individuals who have struggled to administer tests correctly should receive training. If repeated training sessions fail to remedy the situation, the individual should be removed from the process.

Auditing

The *audit* is a central component of any athlete development program. An audit of a workout is a formal collection and analysis of the post-workout stimulus (figure 5.6). This accounting style of tracking and evaluating individual stimuli provides the single most significant opportunity for a sport franchise to improve on-field results while at the same time outlining the value of a practitioner in comparison to the industry average. The coordinated application of science and the art of coaching is often difficult to quantify; however, we fully expect that the future economics of the industry will be based on objective data-driven changes that a coach can produce over a career. The audit in its most granular form is the key to the development of optimal training plans across a wide range of modalities and training paradigms.

How to Audit

Auditing is a critical component of any player development program. The following sections provide details on how to conduct preworkout and postworkout audits, mesocycle analysis, and annual audits.

Preworkout In the preworkout audit, the coach must first assess the expected load for the session, exercise, and each individual set (figure 5.7). There must be an intended target that can be used as a reference for each workout. Other than during initial exposures at the start of a career, at each transition of a microcycle, mesocycle, or macrocycle there should be a seamless transition between expected maximal and load prescriptions. All of this information is contained in the workout card. The workout has several vital components, regardless of the formatting:

- *Maximal weight or corresponding percentage.* This informs the practitioner of the neurological demands expected from the exercise, including the tissue recruited for the event and the demand placed on the soft tissue substructures. Practitioners must fully understand the concepts of the size principle and the repetition continuum.

- *Total repetition load.* How many repetitions are expected in relation to the continuum for intensity and the entire repetition load of the session? Guidelines can be established to not over- or under-prescribe repetition load.

- *Tonnage as it relates to pounds per repetition.* Tonnage receives criticism for its inability to distinguish a thousand pounds lifted once from one pound lifted a thousand times. However, it provides tremendous insight into tissue growth related

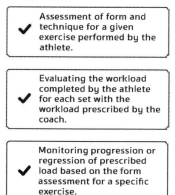

FIGURE 5.6 Auditing on TeamBuildr.
Courtesy of TeamBuildr.

AUDITING WORKOUT REPORT & VIDEO JOURNAL

This workout and video journal report should contain 1. updated maxes (or metric that is used to track the programmed exercises), 2. sets, repetitions, and tempos corresponding to intensity prescribed by the coach, and 3. load and repetition the athlete completed for each specific exercise.

1. Compare the actual weight used, reps completed, and tempo followed by the athlete to the prescribed intensity, rep, range, and tempo.

2. Record any deviations from prescription and review notes from athlete on subjective evaluation of their performance and effort.

3. If video journal was uploaded, review for safety, form/technique, and adherence to program.

SAFETY CONSIDERATIONS

- Spotters, if necessary
- Squat crash guards
- Appropriate attire (footwear, clothing that does note pose a safety issue or sacrifices technique)
- Environmental/equipment hazards (no plyos on concrete)

TECHNIQUE CONSIDERATIONS

- posture
- hand/foot placement
- bar speed/bar path
- joint angles
- grip

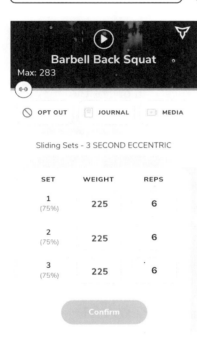

FIGURE 5.7 Auditing a workout report.
Courtesy of TeamBuildr.

to hypertrophy and repeated muscular endurance, which is why tonnage relating to pounds (or kilograms) per repetition is critical. Tonnage is useful in planning future training sessions and forecasting *anticipated biological* adaptations heading into the next testing cycle.

- *Documented qualitative feedback.* Diligent notetaking by athletes and staff is critical and often overlooked in the audit. A number without context is limited in value, but an exercise with subjective feedback is incredibly effective for planning subsequent workouts. As athletes reach the ceiling of their genetic endowment, producing manufactured outputs can be quickly affected by disruptors and may require unplanned default workouts.

As commercial external sensors are added to the sport paradigm, practitioners must resist the temptation to collect data for the sake of collecting more data. Too much data collection can cause great confusion and doubt when making programming decisions. For each athlete, it is recommended that there be a clear mesocycle focus and daily training goal. For example, on a high force day, the focus may be on achieving 3% more intensity than in the previous training session. Velocity profiling, video feedback, and other sensors may provide valid information but can distract from the goal of the day, which is to move weight at a greater intensity. This cluttering of the workout occurs largely unintentionally when one of the performance shareholders is attempting to collect team- or position-wide data for comprehensive spectrum data collection, overlooking the fact that, for the specific individual in question, the ancillary data collection detracts from their individual training plan for the day.

After establishing a clear and focused target for the workout, practitioners should encourage the athlete and the staff to solely focus on achieving the tasks of their workout. While the athlete focuses on completing the task, the practitioner should monitor the following items:

- How did the warm-up sets look? Was there a breakdown in the form? Was it very easy?
- What is the athlete's emotional state? Is the athlete nervous or excited to attempt the workout?
- The last warm-up set should be a final checkpoint to either green-light the working sets, back off and default, or shut it down.
  - This type of autoregulation can use many formulas, but the Epley formula is a good starting point either as a true effort or true effort + repetitions in reserve to the ballpark estimate if the intensity is appropriate. [(Reps + RIR / 30) + 1] × weight lifted = 1RM. Repetitions in reserve is discussed in more detail in Chapter 7.
  - Evaluate if the max is within 5% of preworkout projections. Given the athlete's state of readiness and this difference in perceived max, evaluate whether the current training plan needs to be modified or the athlete should default entirely.
- After each set, the athlete should document the weight lifted, how it felt, and any additional comments. This prevents the scenario of an athlete reporting they did 4 × 15 = at 95% of their 1RM. These situations of impractical volume/load entries happen quite often. It is well understood that it is impossible to do 15 repetitions with 95% of 1RM. However, the athlete may have actually lifted the weight 15 times, and a closer inspection of the expected max needs to be evaluated or it's just an error in filling out the workout log. This is also an excellent teaching opportunity for interns to practice the perceived exertion of the theoretical training loads used for the workout.

Postworkout Postworkout, the coach should be able to answer the following questions within an hour of the workout's conclusion:

- Did the individual hit the prescribed intensity?
- Did the individual hit the prescribed repetition scheme for that intensity?
- Did the individual hit the prescribed tonnage and pounds (or kilograms) per repetition?

Postworkout, the individuals are placed in one of three groups:

- Achieved in one of the three areas
- Achieved targeted weights within 5% intensity, 3% of the tonnage, and corresponding pounds (or kilograms) per repetition
- Underachieved by more than 5% intensity, 3% of the tonnage, and corresponding pounds (or kilograms) per repetition

In any biological system there is a natural fluctuation, but three consistent days of underperformance should initiate a modification to the training plan and more than five days of underperformance should trigger a conversation with the relevant shareholders of the high-performance staff to identify and develop a mitigation strategy to the main cause of the disruptor. As athletes develop in training age and adaptation takes multiple coordinated days of training stimulus, it should be expected that proper monitoring of these "bad days" becomes especially important.

Despite seemingly endless marketing of the best training method or training philosophy, every workout will include individuals who default from what was originally planned for training due to biological readiness. The ability to quickly and safely pivot training to address this default and create rapid responses will separate the industry elites in the future. With more data accessible to practitioners, this has become increasingly important. Other key questions of interest include the following: Are the athletes completing the intended workout? Was this the correct workout for the athlete, based on the quantitative and qualitative feedback loops? Meticulous auditing in the quality control process drastically increases the likelihood the athlete will achieve the goal of the mesocycle.

Mesocycle Analysis Regardless of the programming style or philosophy, every program has a fixed duration of time, usually a 4-to-6-week window, to implement a new training cycle to build on the success of the previous block's adaptation. In an ideal programming situation, every program of an athlete's career is systematically coordinated to establish preparatory movement patterns, underlying physiology, and technical lifting acumen. The longer an individual is engaged in a development plan, the further from the initial genetic baseline that individual should be. Regardless of the sport composite or technical requirements, every individual should display greater biological and physiological traits for improved game performance the longer they are involved in the program. Even a simple trend line of traits over time can quickly assess whether the programs have an overall efficacy. These macro assessments can drive commitment and buy-in and serve as a reality check for the coach in charge of the development program.

Upon completing any training cycle, the coach should perform the following assessment:

- Was the training objective accomplished?
  - If yes, what were the objective training outcome numbers? *Example:* Muscle (individual muscle gain in 4 weeks was 3.7 pounds [1.7 kg])
  - If not, what were the objective training outcome numbers? *Example:* Muscle (individual muscle gain was only 1.2 pounds [0.5 kg] of muscle in 4 weeks)
- After assessing the training outcome, all proxy measurements are analyzed within the workout to assess the effectiveness of the application.
- What was the corresponding tonnage and pounds (or kilograms) per repetition for each individual?
  - How many defaults occurred within the training block? *Example:* This cycle contained 40 defaults as a group.
  - How many defaults were there compared to previous cycles and the same time the year prior? *Example:* Last year there were only five defaults.
  - What was the nature of the default?
    - Coach practice loads
    - Social interface
    - Team commitment level
    - An honest assessment of what worked and what did not work from a subjective coaching staff evaluation. Ask questions such as the following:
  - Was the technique good enough for this cycle?
  - Did we have an optimal equipment layout to administer the plan?
  - Did the athletes have an effective recovery strategy for the new stimulus?
  - Did the coaching staff as a whole hold everyone to standard for every workout?

The mesocycle audit combines subjective and objective data points to determine whether the strategy and stimulus plan fit perfectly and effectively. In reality, any plan that is effective above the 80th percentile should be saved for future use. These programs may have been very effective for a select few but only a good fit for some. Outlining the prerequisite characteristics of those who are exceptionally successful is imperative for future implementation. A great example of this would be an aggressive Olympic lifting plan that required both strength and solid lifting technique. For those who meet this prerequisite, the effect could be profound, while those who are not strong enough may consistently miss the catch. It was not that the program was wrong, but the prerequisite athlete training composite needed to be revised to reap the desired training effect. Additionally, plans that demonstrate consistent, predictable, and repeatable results across multiple populations should be achieved and saved and further developed and optimized for future training cycles. Normative teaching programs emphasizing motor unit coordination and foundational strength are especially valuable to deploy and set solid foundations for any program in the early months of training. Especially as they relate to sport-specific annual intricacies, great programs should be treasured. Great programs (1) produce repeatable and reliable results across multiple staff members, (2) produce objective training outputs greater than previously recorded, and (3) offer enough consistent stimuli to drive change without creating cultural complacency.

Annual Audit The annual audit is a culmination of objective and subjective assessments of the program's effectiveness. *Effectiveness* means here the successful increase of biological traits within one's genetic endowment to aid the athlete's ability to demonstrate improved in-game production. Traditionally this audit has been limited to pre- and post-data, typically reflected in annual average increases across the team. This primordial assessment fails to capture meaningful change and is often biased toward effective or ineffective recruiting and the analysis of single metrics, usually an output metric, in isolation (i.e., vertical jump height). With today's modern technology, the annual audit can become much more detailed and provide tremendous insight into the effectiveness or ineffectiveness of the training plan. Every team's annual audit may be customized, but the final result should be succinct in answering the following questions:

- Did our training plan identify the biological and physiological traits resulting in increased individual or team performance?
- How much objective change was accomplished due to the biological and physiological traits we as a staff chose to develop?
- How many training defaults occurred this year, and what is the per-cycle breakdown?
  - What can we learn about scheduling the sport staff?
  - What can we learn about the athlete's technique level?
- Did our blocks sequentially link together to create a synergistic effect or a training interference effect?
- Did the athletes who demonstrate development above the team average composite see additional playing time or acknowledgment from the coaching staff for their efforts?
- What plans were ineffective or less effective?
  - Why were they ineffective?
  - What could be done to fix them?
  - Should this style be thrown out altogether?

While many early practitioners attempted to evaluate program effectiveness, sense of self-worth, and competence by administering a max-out day or testing days throughout the year, with today's technology the actual test of a program is the training itself. By consistently and carefully analyzing training logs throughout the entire training year, coaches can quickly address areas that need to be adjusted long before they become failure points. Additionally, coaches should be able to forecast what components of the athlete composite are critical to on-field production. They should be able to identify the required trait and how long it will take to train someone up to that level. Traits that must be recruited during early assessment will become well-known and shared with the coaching staff. Attributes such as height, wrist girth, and tibial plateau combine to give a relatively effective prediction of the ability of an individual to gain muscle mass. Other elements such as tendon length and relative muscle fiber power output capacity also aid in calculating the likelihood that someone will be able to achieve the required traits to become a top performer in a sport.

Reports to Coaches and Athletes

When designing reports, the modern practitioner must follow the basic rules of successful visualization design. The four pillars, as described by visualization icon Noah Illiskny, are as follows:

- *Purpose (the why):* Why are you making this report? Is there currently a problem? If there is a problem, do you have a solution? Is this problem independent of the individual or interdependent among the other athlete development shareholders? Defining the problem with clarity is often overlooked. Especially in today's era of athlete monitoring, practitioners can sometimes find themselves immersed in a sea of data with no clear purpose.

This can lead to what is commonly referred to as *vanity metrics*. Vanity metrics are data sets that present no real sense and are only displayed to show what is being collected.

- *Content (the what)*: The data streams that support your specific purpose should be the focal point of the visualization, and data that do not contribute should be removed. The emphasis of content is to specifically highlight and target the data that matters most to answer the specific question that is being asked. The report can provide the viewer with greater insight and contextual relevance. The report's content can come from single-source or multi-source inputs.

- *Structure (the how)*: The data collected dictate how it will be displayed. Whether the information is fixed or constantly flowing will have a tremendous effect on what type of structure will most effectively help convey your message. When dealing with data over time, an X or Y axis could be used to show trend lines, while a postseason evaluation of injuries may be better displayed with a pie chart.

- *Formatting (everything else)*: Formatting is where the final, personal touches can be added to help the end-user process your findings. Where many sports scientists fail is when they produce product in the format that they personally enjoy, and not the optimal format for the end consumer. Busy charts shown to sport coaches leave them feeling overwhelmed or, worse, insults their hard-earned experience as a coach. A good rule of thumb is that you should not have to explain what anything means when presenting a report. Just as no one has ever read the manual to use their iPad because it is so immediately intuitive, your reports should be equally intuitive. If the coach does not understand the report, you need to go back and rework it. Attempting to demonstrate your intelligence by painstakingly reviewing each graphic does not represent your expertise or value. It will instead most likely be a friction point in future conversations.

Coaches

Ideally, proper reporting should provide to the end-user context, insight, and clarity on what steps must be taken next. As outlined in the first section, genuinely understanding the report you are developing and the purpose for which it will be used is crucial. Creating a report that offers no constructive feedback does not help the relationship between the shareholders and creates cultural resistance toward future collaborations.

Athletes

When designing reports for athletes, the practitioner must remember that what every athlete wants to get out of a report is clear feedback if they are going to see improvement in their sport. The most prominent mistake coaches make when presenting information to athletes is to use the same data set and display shown to the coaches. This mistake is often a significant problem in underperforming teams. Historically, coaches have shown players weightroom leaderboards, team rankings by tests, and averages, only to have the athletes reply that those weightroom numbers don't mean anything since they are still going to start every game. The motivation to participate in the weight room and offseason training, with a few exceptions, is usually to become better at a sport, not to lift weights. Coaches need to show their athletes how their efforts in the weight room positively affect their playing time and on-field performance.

When creating reports for athletes, it is essential to keep the focus on specific goals and how the data relates to performance. Instead of displaying team averages or leaderboards, focus on the individual athlete's progress and how it relates to the specific sport. Use data visualization techniques that are easy to understand and explain how the athlete's progress is directly affecting performance on the field.

When creating reports, it is essential to have a clear purpose, content, structure, and formatting that is easy to understand and relates to the end-user's specific goals. Whether the report is for coaches or athletes, it should provide context and insight and help guide the next steps. By following these guidelines, practitioners can ensure that their reports will be well-received and have a positive impact on the athlete development process.

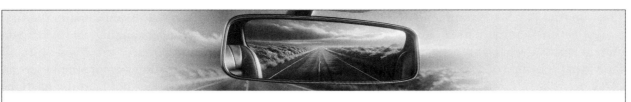

LOOKING IN THE REARVIEW MIRROR
- Athletic monitoring is imperative for a player development team, and an AMS must be carefully constructed for implementation. The three Cs matter for every member of the player development team.
- Effective accounting of an athlete's performance, with valid and reliable metrics that can be acted upon immediately, is crucial.
- Evidence-based critical analysis of resource requirements should be completed before the start of every off-season.
- The performance development team must understand and anticipate the program disruptors and use evidence-based practices to obviate adverse effects if a disruptor occurs.
- The program development team must receive computer and software training to use technologies optimally.
- Data quality and data entry are paramount to an AMS, and data checks must be routine.
- The player development team needs to understand basic statistics and the intentions of the different programs for each athlete.
- Proper reports for coaches and athletes must be carefully constructed to provide optimal messaging to the target audience.

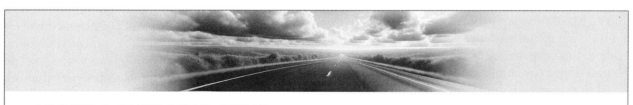

LOOKING AT THE ROAD AHEAD
Looking ahead, it is crucial to evaluate and interpret the different metrics from testing that define a specific athlete composite. Understanding how each intervention program was designed to address a specific targeted goal for an individual is essential for the player development team. Evidence-based practices are vital for optimizing the interpretation and context of the findings from testing protocols. Organizing the databases and using individual and team data is important for evaluating the next steps in an athlete's workout or training cycle. Analyzing data and interpreting the individual athlete's data and its role in the team's progress help predict the individual's trajectory for future performance. Understanding testing metrics and their context for each athlete's exercise prescription within a specific training cycle is vital to optimal athlete development.

6

Interpreting and Evaluating Testing Results of the Athlete Composite

After the player development team has collected data related to the athlete composite, it is time to evaluate and interpret the results. At this point in the evolution of player development, many organizations do not have a proper player development team. At best, they may have an ad hoc group that reflects the necessary components discussed in chapter 1. Typically, responsibility for the whole process falls on one or two members of what is supposed to be the player development team. Usually, the evaluation and interpretation processes are the purview of strength and conditioning professionals. However, this can create blind spots in decision-making due to a lack of expertise in certain testing areas. The testing area should be able to draw on the entire player development team along with its multiple backgrounds and information resources to help in player testing evaluations. This can allow for a more global perspective. As discussed in chapters 1 and 3, a successful player development team needs professionals, each having the appropriate credentials, competence, and commitment (the three Cs) required to optimize the athlete composite.

Roles of Player Development Team

As noted in chapters 1 and 2, many of the player development team components are well-known in the field yet still need to be connected with one another or better defined. Some components, such as sport science and sport performance, have evolved only within the field of athletics. The keys to the player development team are related to the chain of command and the organization and communication structures that have been developed to integrate all available expertise to work with the athletes. Currently, most organizations are centered around head coaches who make decisions based on personal relationships and structures within the athletic organization. The influence of sports medicine has led the way due to the obvious importance of injury, surgery, and rehabilitation. This has been closely followed by athletic training, physical therapy, and rehabilitation sciences. Strength and conditioning professionals continue to have an impact on every sport due to their high exposure to athletes year-round and their roles in enhancing factors related to sport performance. As sport coaches have accepted more science and technology, sport science and sport performance professionals have become the newest types of athlete performance professionals. They have been further complemented by sport psychologists and sociologists in the augmentation of other aspects of the athlete composite.

It has been noted in previous chapters that each of the team's professionals needs to acknowledge and appreciate the different areas of expertise. Doing so promotes respect and limits authoritarian drift into other areas of expertise. This is accomplished by clearly understanding each area's professional task analysis and by each team member presenting their background and credentials. These presentations must be considered when expanding the player development team. Everything comes back to the three Cs, and this is vital for respect and communication. Each area should have professionals in the player development team structure. The biggest issue outside of communication is expertise drifting from one discipline to another due to the lack of understanding or respect for that area's expertise.

The role played by each individual on the player development team has to be carefully examined. The strength of this model resides in integration and communication among the areas that make up the team. However, many day-to-day activities depend on the expertise and competence of individuals within each area. For example, sports medicine professionals work within their area of expertise and then coordinate with other areas as handoff points for the rehabilitation. The most common example of this is the injured athlete who has surgery, proceeds to physical therapy and athletic training, and then to strength and conditioning and sport performance to complete the return to play. Along this path, any disruptors that reduce the efficiency of the athlete's movement along this pathway must be carefully documented. For each of the handoffs from one area to another, communication must be carefully crafted so that each area is confident of the next step in the path from rehabilitation to performance. The handoffs to other areas must be formalized to avoid conflicts with the team. There are many examples of area handoffs, including a handoff from strength and conditioning to nutrition, from sport performance to sport psychology, or from sport science to scientific faculty advisers. For larger questions, evidence-based practices should be used to seek answers. Individual areas should also use evidence-based practices when the questions are discipline-specific, but even here input from other units and areas is helpful for gaining other perspectives. Regular meetings of the whole player development team are vital for this process, despite the almost suffocating schedules that each professional works within.

Sources of Knowledge

There are many different sources of knowledge used in the day-to-day practices of our different professions. No source of knowledge is devoid of criticism or the need for careful examination. This includes scientific studies that need to be carefully evaluated for efficacy regarding the question at hand. All kinds of perspectives can be brought to the table for discussion and examination. In the world of big headlines in the media, social media hype, websites, and blogs, there can be a natural tendency to act before carefully examining the information. Someone once said, "Be careful when you jump on the bandwagon, to make sure the bandwagon is not a manure spreader." In another presentation early in the evolution of the National Strength and Conditioning Association, I (WJK) stated, "Be careful: what you don't know can hurt you." This was a plea for coaches to get back into the books and study. All knowledge is tentative and in need of evaluation to determine its context for any use in practice. Typically, knowledge arises from unscientific methods, after which the scientific method can be used to validate or invalidate it. Again, all knowledge can have flaws and therefore must be carefully studied when looking for answers.

Types of Knowledge

In everyday life, everyone uses unscientific methods to evaluate the world. This also occurs when there is a need for rapid answers in player development programs. Such methods might yield correct answers but can lead to a disconnect between perception and reality if the answer is wrong. All sources of information should be put through the process of evaluation using evidence-based practices. At some point in time, the best available information can be used to frame practices and answer questions that relate to player development, with the proviso that when new information arises, reevaluation of the practice should occur.

Typical unscientific sources of knowledge:

- *Intuition:* This means knowing something without any reasoning or evidence to substantiate it. The answer to the question is just sensed or felt to be right, often independent of any previous experience or empirical knowledge.
- *Tradition:* This is the idea that something has always been done a certain way and has been successful.

- *Bias:* This is typically thought to be negative because it is nothing more than a preference or inclination based on personal reasons. If, however, the bias is based on scientific facts, it may be effective. Thus, the use of evidence-based practice may be a bias that is worth having among all the professionals of a player development team.

- *Myths:* In many sports, myths are widely held. These are often unfounded beliefs and often they are part of the cultural history of a sport. Differentiating myth from facts is an important factor in optimizing decision-making and problem-solving processes.

- *The rationalistic method:* This approach uses reason to produce facts. Its efficacy is based on the veracity of the assumptions made and their factual basis. Reasoning is a solid method for making decisions, but producing knowledge based on reasoning alone is not a valid approach in science.

- *The empirical method:* This method is based on one's own observations and experience. It is part of the scientific method and involves collecting data. However, conclusions reached with this method are affected to the extent that our observations and experiences are based on personal context. What works for one person may not work for another. Therefore, depending on the background qualifications and factual basis of the individual's experience, the empirical method may or may not provide correct conclusions.

- *Trial-and-error:* This method is commonly used to find an answer but is a hit-or-miss technique. This approach is to try some practice and see if it elicits the desired outcome. In many ways, it is a miniature scientific experiment and can prove effective. However, caution must always be used with this approach because random trials are not true experiments and can result in incorrect answers to the questions being asked due to a lack of control of conditions and context.

There are many sources of knowledge that arise from unscientific methods yet are part of the evidence-based practice pool of knowledge and are considered for their efficacy when solving problems in a player development program.

Scientific Method

The scientific method involves some basic steps, which include observation, asking a question, gathering information, forming a hypothesis, testing the hypothesis, making conclusions, reporting, and evaluating.

In the book *An Introduction to the Study of Experimental Medicine*, Claude Bernard, the renowned French physiologist, makes some important points relative to the scientific method. "Experimental ideas are by no means innate, to have our first idea of things, we must see those things; to have an idea about a natural phenomenon, we must, first of all, observe it. The mind of man cannot conceive an effect without a cause, so that the sight of a phenomenon always awakens an idea of causation. All human knowledge is limited to working back from observed effects to their cause. Following an observation, an idea connected with the cause of the observed phenomenon presents itself to the mind. We then inject this anticipative idea into a train of reasoning, by virtue of which we make experiments to control it."

The scientific method of answering a question is based on a series of steps needed to provide a very specific and contextual answer to the hypothesis being tested. To understand knowledge, one must understand the hierarchy and stability of facts, theories, principles, and laws.

- *Facts:* Facts are observational data confirmed repeatedly by many independent and competent observers. However, important to this observation is the context, which stipulates the conditions surrounding the observation. Therefore, facts must be interpreted within the context of observation.

- *Theory:* A theory is typically a conceptual framework of ideas or speculations regarding a certain topic, and hopefully it is based on facts. Here again, theories have a great deal of context for their meaning and applications. Thus, there can be different theories on the same topic due to the fact that the context of interpretation is different. In science we often say that theories are never really proven, only disproved. Therefore, it is important to understand that we can think about things differently due to the context in which they are represented. Furthermore, the stability of a theory is based on the available facts that go into its composition.

- *Principles:* We use facts and theories to derive guiding principles in our approach to a problem or question that arises. A principle describes how something should be done, the rules that explain a phenomenon, or guidelines to adhere to for the optimal performance of a task, such as developing a resistance training workout.
- *Scientific laws:* The description of an observed phenomenon supported by a large body of scientific evidence. A scientific law does not explain why the phenomenon exists or what causes it. An explanation for a phenomenon is called a scientific theory. It is a misconception that theories turn into laws with enough research.

All of these concepts are mutable and can be discarded, modified, or operationally expanded as new discoveries come about in the world of science.

The Scientific Process

In a player development program, questions can arise from the local level of a particular unit or the global level of the entire program. The scientific process is one of discovery in which one tries to figure out what the possible answers are to a question or what solutions there may be to a problem. This has been written about extensively insofar as it relates to the scientific research process (Armstrong and Kraemer 2016). The first step is to look into the body of knowledge, primarily the peer-reviewed literature, which will consist of many components. Through a process of evidence-based practice, one combines these findings with anecdotal evidence and Internet results from members of the team (Amonette, English, and Kraemer 2016). The quality of these answers and their possible solutions are then vetted for efficacy and validity. The process of understanding how these solutions can be implemented practically can then begin.

For the scientist, if the answers are not available in the scientific body of knowledge, then there is a need for further studies to be conducted. The question and the possible answer then serve as the hypothesis that should be tested under controlled conditions with independent and dependent variables. These variables will dictate how the generalized data can be used in specific practical applications. This is where a study that already exists in the scientific literature may not completely align with your specific situation due to differences in variables such as age, sex, training level, sport, and level of competition. Thus, the player development team and its units, including, more specifically, the academic adviser's unit, may be able to conduct a collaborative study that more directly answers the specific question for your program.

In science, which is the core of any player development program, scientists use the scientific method to determine facts, each of which has a very specific context for its use and interpretation. In looking for answers to questions, the first step is to look to the body of knowledge to see if the answers exist. This is what the use of evidence-based practice starts with. From this process of seeing what we know both in the scientific literature and from the practical world, we decide what we think we know. We then decide on what in fact we think will happen based on our assessment of the body of knowledge. If the answer is not there, scientists will go one step further and use the scientific method to develop a study that will test the guess or hypothesis. An experimental design will be created for the study. The experiment will have different conditions or contexts related to the question at hand for a particular sport in the player development program. This has to do with experimental design, which is also very important when reading other scientific studies. Experimental design involves what we call independent variables—anything from age, sex, environmental conditions, the type of program being used, and training level. Each of these will determine an important context for what we find in the study. The dependent variables are the measurements that we want to determine. The scientists will then collect data and evaluate it to see if the hypothesis is correct.

The investigative process that uses the scientific method has been laid out in a stepwise fashion in a research book that takes one through the entire process, from the question to the final application of the findings (Armstrong and Kraemer 2016). While beyond the scope of this book, it is important that each of the player development team members understand this particular process and how it relates to research procedures (Kraemer,

Fleck, and Deschenes 2021). Furthermore, it is important for the sport coaches to also understand how research works and how it can be beneficial for their own athletes and coaches. Player development programs are now taking on many sport analytics, yet many of the studies that need to be done are tracking and training studies readily available from the testing and monitoring analytics used in the program. These have been discussed in detail in chapter 5. Ultimately, such research that is completed at the sport- and program-specific levels will yield direct evidence for answering questions that may exist in a number of areas, such as training programs, recovery technologies, nutritional interventions, and sleep.

Use of Evidence-Based Practice Approaches

A book that should act as a training guide for evidence-based practice has been published with extensive examples of how professionals can use this practice to their advantage (Amonette, English, and Kraemer 2016). A common question is whether a program is evidence-based or whether a professional uses evidence-based methods. Unless the programs are completely random or the decisions made are based on nothing, the program is evidence-based. However, the fundamental question is how current and sound is the evidence from which one is developing decisions. In other words, are you committed to being an evidence-based professional in finding, evaluating, and incorporating the best evidence to steer programs for the benefit of the athletes?

The six steps in the evidence-based process have been outlined in chapter 2. For over 25 years, the introduction of evidence-based practice in medicine and other fields, such as nursing, dentistry, and physical therapy, has also made its way into the U.S. military and is now emerging in the field of athletic performance. Science and knowledge are very dynamic and shaped every day by new discoveries. Often, new research adds to the knowledge base but only prompts minor adjustments in daily practice. However, at times there are new discoveries that are so disruptive and unexpected that they necessitate major practical changes. This is often called a *paradigm shift*. The evidence-based practice draws heavily on empiricism but recognizes the dynamic and continuous flux in knowledge resulting from new clinical, practical, and scientific discoveries.

The intent of the process is to provide a standardized methodology for integrating scientific and practical knowledge. Three basic terms have been presented to describe the knowledge source on which practice is based. It has been called *experience-based practice*, *science-based practice*, and *evidence-based practice*. Implicit in each of these terms is the recognition that the information that is obtained from multiple sources, experiences, and observational opportunities is used to help gain a global perspective on the question and practice being examined.

There have been criticisms of this practice, but its strength outweighs any limitations. These different criticisms and rebuttals have been extensively reviewed. The major concern is often one of communication and competence of the individual or group to address the question at hand. Lack of experience in the field, lack of scientific training to interpret experimental studies in the literature, and insufficient training in the area of the experimental study being interpreted can each result in a mistake in interpretation. This is why the player development team approach is needed to respectfully challenge individuals to see if further outside assessments are needed. This is why it is important for both individuals and team to be evaluated each year for their competence and the role they play on the team. An overview of an evaluation method for scientific studies is shown in the sidebar on page 156.

Understanding Context of Training Steps and Target Goals

In the field of player development, each team has target goals for success. The head sport coach must carefully look at the total landscape of the team for its weaknesses and strengths. The level of competition that the team faces is an important factor. Athletes should be evaluated for their potential to contribute to the team's success. The potential for improvement in each of the team's athlete composites is related to the starting points that each athlete brings to the table. Proper placement of each athlete into an optimal position

> ### Evaluating a Scientific Study
>
> In evidence-based practice, one of the biggest challenges is evaluating studies that are found in the scientific literature. Here is where trained scientists come into play. Understanding what has not been said in a scientific study as well as any deception for the purpose of being published is what the experience and knowledge of scientists bring to the process. Critical analysis of the scientific study is essential for the evidence-based practice process. There are many "junk studies," which cause a great deal of confusion when trying to make decisions on questions related to player development. Each area of science has this problem because of the prolific number of studies that come from a variety of published outlets. Authors are becoming very effective at writing studies so as to minimize their weaknesses, distort context, or, worse yet, not describe competing theories or studies that contradict their conclusions. Therefore, internal or external members of the team who know the literature in that particular area must weigh in on the study's efficacy and its influence on answers to practical questions and decisions. Furthermore, the player development team, including scientists involved in the program, should take special care to study and train in the evaluation of scientific studies.

based on athlete composite is a vital part of the decision-making process. The player development team can dramatically assist in determining the athlete composite through testing. Additionally, the player development team can develop recruitment profiles for each position on the team. This will be addressed later in this chapter. Mistakes in position placements or unrealistic expectations for improvements in the athlete composite will result in losses. Therefore, the athlete composites play a very specific role within the team structure, which depends on the sport, the position, and the game strategies. Whether for an individual sport or a team sport, the athlete composite, and its potential to develop over time to meet competitive demands, will determine success or failure.

While the team will have specific goals related to wins and losses in competition, each athlete will have very specific target goals for the development of their athlete composite. This process involves a broader team perspective as well as the perspective of the individual athlete. Each of the units plays a very specific role in contributing to success and has specific interfaces to take the athlete composite from the current level to the next. Integrating the different target goals from each unit over a particular training phase or cycle is vital for training, monitoring, and testing programs and protocols. Communication and fluidity concerning these target goal challenges for each athlete is important.

The program should ensure a seamless transition over time so as not to create confusion and complexity in the athlete's demanding schedule. The process begins with educating and communicating with the athletes so that they understand the what and why of their programs and how they relate to improving their potential to meet competitive demands.

Organizing the Database

Decisions about the types of databases and software systems that will be used in the program need to be carefully assessed and determined by the player development team. Each team member is responsible for proper data entry using the appropriate software system. A database or sport analytical professional can also be used to make sure that the data are properly formatted for use by members of the team.

Concerns for the development of a database include the following:

- Choice of software applications to be used
- Database security measures
- Proper entry of variables with significant digits
- Verification and notation of units associated with the variables

- Double-checking database for proper entry and partial support by software limits
- Electronic translation from testing instruments
- Translation from one database to another (e.g., tracking to statistics software)

Looking to Analyze the Data

In a player development program, data analytics can range from simple to complex. Extensive statistical methodologies have been presented in detail and knowing them is an important skill for members of the player development team (French and Torres Ronda 2022; Armstrong and Kraemer 2016). However, the key factor is to understand how data will be used. As we have pointed out several times in this book, the primary goal of a player development program is to improve the individual athlete composite. Therefore, the data that is collected with testing and training become the primary databases that require careful scrutiny, interpretation, and evaluation. The development of target testing goals for each athlete's composite determines what units become the inputs for the athlete's program. As will be discussed later in this chapter, graphics such as spider graphs can help athletes visualize where they are and their progression over time.

Statistics

Statistics is a tool for the evaluation of data. The first thing it does is to look at the specific measurement value. In a player development program, the primary data that is important for the athlete composite is the individual data point. Statistics begins with the accuracy of this data point and then proceeds to interpret it with normative comparisons appropriate to the level of competition.

After prior research on testing protocols and measurements, one may ask whether the value for a measurement makes sense. If the individuals involved with the initial evaluation of the data point are not clear about the expected range of values, then one has to go back to the original testing protocol and normative data for the variable. Mistakes in this area typically are related to test data from technology that individual members of the player development team (e.g., the sport coach) may not be familiar with. For example, power output in watts (W) may not be particularly well known if one has not worked with force plate technology (French and Torres Ronda 2022). While this term has become more familiar in sport communities, it is important to differentiate values that are generated with different force plate technologies on the market because the values can differ from one company to the next. This is very important when studying normative values for different sports. The first step is to validate the individual measure as accurate and within the realm of reality. Rapid determination of accurate values during testing, data input, and analysis is necessary. Otherwise, the athlete needs to be retested, which can result in logistical problems. One would quickly see that a 3.8-second 40-yard dash time is a measurement error, but it may not be as obvious when looking at a force plate power output of 15,000 W. The accuracy of the measure is the first step in evaluating a data point.

Measurement Error Considerations

One of the most important aspects of data analytics in a player development program is the reliability of testing methods. Here is where the basic statistical procedures for calculating different correlation coefficients for testing are part of an important statistical skill set that members of the player development team need to have (see chapter 3) (French and Torres Ronda 2022; Armstrong and Kraemer 2016). Even more important is the collection of data for such reliability calculations. When a value is determined from a testing protocol, it must be put in context with the error factor in the reliability of that measure (chapter 3). For example, in performing skinfold measurements and calculations of lean body mass and percent fat, generated from standardized regression formulas, one has to consider the error factors for such measurements. Many times, there is at best a 4.0% error factor associated with the values, not including the error that might exist locally with your team's testing. Therefore, a body fat measure of 12.0% could be as high as 16.0% or as low as 8.0%; therefore, evaluation of such a data point needs to be done in a range that would be considered acceptable for the athlete's position and sport. If the error factor is not taken into account, dramatically negative program interventions (e.g., dietary restrictions that are not needed) may be implemented due to the data not being evaluated correctly. Each measurement arising from the testing protocols must be interpreted with error factors taken into consideration.

Other types of statistical analyses of athletes or teams can be performed and used for a variety of reasons, including for reporting to the coaching staff, athletic and academic administration, external funding, and comparison of team statistics to other normative studies in the literature. Such statistical analysis of group data can also be used by the different units in the player development team for scientific publications; therefore, proper informed consent and institutional review board approval are necessary. Methods for data analysis and presentation have already been published and are beyond the scope of this particular book on player development program organization (Armstrong and Kraemer 2016; French and Torres Ronda 2022; Fukuda 2019).

It should again be emphasized that the context of a measurement depends on how a test is conducted, what instrument is used, the exact settings of the instrument, and the homogeneity of external factors such as time of day, hydration status, and arousal levels.

Interpreting the Results

In chapter 3 we discussed several ways in which athletes are tested for mutable health- and skill-related fitness components. We also listed a few examples of sport-specific tests. The player development team must determine which tests are needed for their athletes and design an appropriate testing schedule. Some tests may be performed frequently as a form of player monitoring or load management, while other tests are best used periodically following a specific training phase (e.g., off-season or preseason). Regardless of the test or its frequency, the player development team must not only test and collect data on athletes but must also be able to understand the results and apply them in a meaningful way for comparisons or *intraplayer analysis*. Player test results may be obtained, stored, analyzed, and plotted over time during a career with the team as a form of progression analysis. In addition, it is a value to the player development team to know how its players rank or compare to other players either on their own team, from opposing teams, or from teams at higher levels of competition. For example, we previously discussed the dichotomy in which athletes playing at higher levels of competition show test results of health- and skill-related fitness components that are higher in magnitude (which may help explain why some of these athletes are able to compete at higher levels). Measures of maximal strength, speed, power, agility, endurance, and aerobic fitness tend to be higher at higher levels of athletic competition. These data provide levels, or *norms*, which can be used as goals for the athletes to target in training. Thus, it is imperative for the player development team to understand the context of testing data on the team (for team-sport athletes), in a specific position within the sport, and at higher levels of competition so that the data can be used as progression targets.

Norms may be acquired from different sources. For example, player development teams are highly encouraged to develop and use their own data from years of testing athletes. Norms can be developed from years of collecting player data in a database. The testing team should input data results into a spreadsheet or similar software program and be able to access these data when needed. Subsequent testing sessions allow the player development team to make comparisons between athletes or to compare athletes over time to other players in similar positions. Detailed information should be included to describe the testing environment, including the testers, equipment used, clothing worn, ergogenic gear used (e.g., a lifting belt, wraps, and sleeves), and temperature experienced. This information should be noted because testing on the field should mimic testing in the laboratory and use the most stringent procedures possible. Little is gained from comparing a 40-yard dash time obtained using infrared sensors (speed trap) to one obtained the year before using hand timing by a coach. The error associated with hand timing is much greater, so any difference noted could be due to error or differences in the testing environment (equipment) rather than reflect a training adaptation. For meaningful norms to be established for a sport team, highly stringent and identical testing procedures should be used; furthermore, any change or difference must be included in the spreadsheet so future comparisons will accurately reflect it. In the research laboratory, it is common practice to keep a lab notebook to log any observations or relevant information that can be used to properly interpret results. The same analogy can be made here: The testing files should contain relevant information so that future comparisons can be accurately made.

Another excellent source of data norms is a literature search using *evidence-based practice*—that is, a process used to review, analyze, and translate the latest scientific information available. Here, the player development team can compare the performance of their athletes to other athletes in similar positions and levels of competition documented in published literature. Excellent resources for published norms include scientific textbooks, coaching efficacy textbooks, peer-reviewed narrative and systematic reviews, and original research (descriptive and experimental) studies. Reviews and meta-analyses are examples of *analytic research* where critical thinking skills are applied to evaluate a research question in the literature. *Descriptive research* is a type of research that describes a population being evaluated—that is, a cross-sectional group of athletes is tested on several performance measures and the results are published. Different types of descriptive approaches may be used and be of value to the player development team, but observational and normative studies specifically provide valuable data on athletes intended to be used for comparison. *Experimental research* involves designing a study treatment, manipulating independent variables, and measuring the results in the dependent variables. As such, data from athletes may be determined as descriptive data from pre-study measures or extrapolated from the results of fitness tests. Textbooks review the literature and may compile useful normative data for athletes. The player development team may use these valuable resources to compile norms that can be used for comparison to their athletes. Here, we provide some examples of norms or descriptive data from studies that coaches may use in order to evaluate athletes. For a more detailed discussion, the reader is referred to (Hoffman 2006; Fukuda 2019; Ratamess 2022).

Evaluating Body Composition and Anthropometric Testing Data

Body composition testing can give the player development team valuable information on percent body fat, fat distribution, lean body mass (LBM), BMD (if DEXA is used), limb and segment lengths and ratios, somatotypes, and circumferences gained through body composition assessment. In chapter 3 we reviewed several methods of body composition testing. It is important to note once again that each method has different levels of accuracy. Accurate comparisons can only be made when the same test is conducted by the same person over time. Body composition assessment is noninvasive, nonfatiguing, and may be used frequently throughout a training period (with the exception of DEXA, which involves low-level radiation exposure) or used as a monitoring tool. Several anthropometric tests measure largely nonmutable characteristics (height, limb, and segment lengths). We discussed the importance of collecting anthropometric data and common athlete profiles in chapter 2. We also discussed how these anthropometric measures affect sport performance and how they are used for talent identification, recruiting, and sport selection. A full anthropometric testing battery may occur early in the process as part of recruiting or during initial testing when an athlete is new to the sport or team. Unless one is working with youth athletes, some anthropometric measures (e.g., limb, segment lengths, and height) are tested infrequently since they change only marginally. Other measures, such as girth assessments, can be tested routinely as a measure of body segment mass changes or as an indirect measure of muscle size.

Interpretation of body fat percentages is complicated because there are no accepted universal standards for percent body fat and all methods are indirect and involve error. Body fat percent data should be presented and interpreted with the understanding that the standard error of estimate can be high, and errors could be 3% to 5% in some cases. Levels of percent body fat in athletes may vary greatly (table 6.1). In general, several male athletes show values of approximately 5% to 13%, while female athletes show values of approximately 12% to 20%.

TABLE 6.1 Select Body Fat Range Data from Athletes

Sport	Percent Body Fat
Baseball	12%-20% (men)
Basketball	6%-21% (men); 18%-33% (women)
Bodybuilding	5%-8% (men); 10%-15% (women)
Boxing	5%-19% (men); 10%-30% (women)
Cycling	5%-15% (men); 15%-20% (women)
American Football (positional)	9%-30% (men)
Gymnastics	5%-12% (men); 10%-16% (women)
Handball	8%-20% (men)
High and long jump (track)	7%-14% (men); 10%-20% (women)
Hockey (ice and field)	8%-17% (men); 12%-20% (women)
Marathon running	5%-11% (men); 10%-18% (women)
MMA (elite)	5%-18% (men); 12%-28% (women)
Soccer	6%-18% (men); 13%-24% (women)
Softball	16%-35% (women)
Sprinting	6%-12% (men); 12%-20% (women)
Strongman (elite)	6%-28% (men)
Swimming	7%-18% (men); 15%-28% (women)
Tennis	8%-18% (men); 16%-25% (women)
Triathlon	5%-12% (men); 10%-15% (women)
Volleyball	9%-17% (men); 16%-28% (women)
Weightlifting	7%-25% (men); 12%-35% (women)
Wrestling	5%-26% (men); 12%-30% (women)

Human body fat may be categorized as essential or nonessential. *Essential body fat* has important functions in the body and is found in the heart, lungs, liver, spleen, kidneys, intestines, muscles, bone, and central nervous system. It ranges from 4% to 5% in males and 10% to 12% in females. Percent fat should not fall below these minimal levels. *Nonessential fat* includes subcutaneous and visceral fat tissue. This type should be kept low for health and athletic purposes. Often, a lower percent fat is desirable in many groups of athletes. Athletes competing in weight classes require low percent fat to maximize LBM and compete in a desired weight class. Athletes involved in endurance sports or sports where one competes against gravity (gymnastics and some track-and-field events) benefit from a low percent body fat. Physique athletes require low body fat as well. Body composition measurement is useful for athletes in sports such as gymnastics, wrestling, and bodybuilding where weight cutting may be used and there is potential for malnutrition. Regular body composition assessment can be used as a monitoring tool to benefit these athletes. Athletes involved in inertial sports or who compete in heavyweight or super heavyweight classes can afford a higher percent body fat, although it should not be excessive. Lowering body fat requires a multicomponent approach involving proper diet, aerobic training, and anaerobic training. Lastly, percent fat data should be viewed within the context of the testing period or season (i.e., the off-season period versus the preseason or precompetition periods). For example, strength and power athletes can benefit from a slight increase in percent fat during the off-season when the main goals are to increase muscle size, strength, and power; however, they will lower percent fat preseason while trying to maintain their performance gain. The player development team should view the percent fat data of athletes in the context of the training phase.

Percent fat measures, as well as girth measures with skinfolds, can be used to estimate changes in LBM. Ultimately, DEXA provides a gold standard for LBM assessment, but other technologies can be used, provided that proper testing procedures are followed. The sport may dictate how much LBM is required or targeted in training. For example, some strength and power athletes who require large body size are better served by maximizing LBM. American football players (e.g., linemen), weightlifters, bodybuilders, strength competitors, powerlifters, and track-and-field throwers benefit from having high LBM (relative to weight class, when applicable). In fact, we have shown that NFL linemen, and some of the strongest men in the world, have very high levels of LBM (118 kilograms ± 11.7 kilograms for strongmen [Kraemer et al. 2005; Kraemer et al. 2020]). These athletes have high mesomorphic physiques that contribute to the strength and power needed for the sports or to aesthetic qualities in the case of bodybuilding. Athletes in hybrid sports (e.g., boxing, MMA, wrestling and grappling sports, and basketball) benefit from having higher LBM as well. Given the hybrid of strength and endurance components in these sports, increased LBM is good, but endurance must also be emphasized. The magnitude may depend on the weight class and interaction with performance since, in some cases, too much muscle mass may compromise some elements of endurance. Many other groups of athletes benefit from hypertrophy as well. The size of athletes in many sports has increased in recent generations because, in part, of improvements in strength and conditioning programs as well as genetic modifications that affect subsequent generations. In baseball it was thought that increased LBM would compromise performance, but MLB player size increased significantly from the 1980s to the present day and performance was not compromised. Rather, we are in an era when pitchers attain record high velocities and hitters are hitting the ball harder than ever. In fact, some of the most successful MLB players in recent history have had high levels of LBM. Thus, increased LBM is a necessity for some anaerobic sports and a benefit for others. Given the relationships between muscle size (and LBM) and strength, power, and other specific sport performance characteristics, the player development team should routinely monitor LBM as a function of training efficacy. The level of desired increase depends on the sport. Athletes who compete against gravity (e.g., pole vault and high jump) require high speeds (e.g., sprinters), or are endurance athletes who may benefit from getting stronger but may need to limit changes in body mass since body mass is a major determinant of sport success. These athletes can focus on increased strength-to-mass ratio to balance potential LBM gains with performance.

BMD data can be acquired if the player development team uses DEXA technology. As discussed in chapter 4, BMD changes are slow, and responses are based mostly on the magnitude and rates of loading. Higher BMD values are seen in anaerobic athletes, especially those who participate in collision sports, have explosive running and jumping ground reaction forces (plyometrics, sprint, and agility), or do heavy lifting (figure 6.1). For example, we have shown high total-body BMD values in some of the world's strongest men (1.80 g/cm^2) (Kraemer et al. 2020). A study by Antonio et al. in 2018 compared BMD values of male and female collegiate (DII) athletes (Antonio et al. 2018). The highest values were seen in American football players (1.60 g/cm^2) and MMA athletes (1.57 g/cm^2), followed by resistance-trained men (1.44 g/cm^2) and women (1.24 g/cm^2). Values of 1.27 to 1.34 g/cm^2 were seen in track athletes and distance runners. Lower values were seen in male (1.27 g/cm^2) and female (1.18 g/cm^2) swimmers. We showed mean BMD values of 1.42 g/cm^2 in Division III American football players (Ratamess et al. 2007). Mean values of 1.32 g/cm^2 (basketball), 1.26 g/cm^2 (soccer), 1.29 g/cm^2 (track-and-field sprinters and jumpers), 1.30 g/cm^2 (volleyball), and 1.14 g/cm^2 (swimmers) were shown in Division I female athletes (Stanforth et al. 2016). Swimming is less effective because the buoyancy of the water decreases stress on the skeletal system; thus, it is important for the player development team to target BMD increases via land-based training in swimmers. The player development team can target increased BMD in athletes who score lower by using explosive training (plyometric, speed, agility), heavy resistance exercise, ballistic resistance and high-velocity movements, as well as ensuring proper diet (kilocalorie, macronutrient,

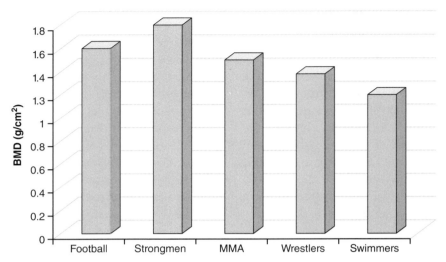

FIGURE 6.1 Bone mineral density (BMD) data from select male athletes.

Data from Antonio et al., "Bone Mineral Density in Competitive Athletes," *Journal of Exercise and Nutrition* 1, no. 2 (2018): 1-11. Kraemer et al., "Body Composition in Elite Strongman Competitors," *Journal of Strength and Conditioning Research* 34 (2020): 3326-30. Sagayama et al., "Bone Mineral Density in Male Weight-Classified Athletes is Higher Than That in Male Endurance-Athletes and Non-Athletes," *Clinical Nutrition ESPEN* 36 (2020): 106-110.

and micronutrient intake), rest (and sleep), and recovery in between workouts.

Male athletes have shown higher BMD than female athletes because of several factors, including differences in hormones, muscle size, and strength. Female athletes are more likely to be affected by *relative energy deficiency in sport* (RED-S), formerly known as the *female triad*. The relationship among low energy availability, menstrual function and dysfunction, health risks, and reduced BMD has been noted for some time. Female athletes who consume less than or equal to 30 kcal/kg LBM/day are more susceptible to RED-S. Factors such as moderate-to-severe energy restriction in order to make a weight or for appearance, eating disorders (e.g., anorexia nervosa, bulimia nervosa, and binge-eating disorder) or abnormal behaviors (e.g., use of laxatives or diuretics), poor dietary choices or limited types of foods consumed, and excessive energy expenditure from exercise to further reduce body weight can all result in energy deficiency. Screening and diagnosis of RED-S in susceptible athletes should be undertaken as part of a routine assessment by the player development team. Screening may include patient history profiles, physical exams, and laboratory testing. Treatment recommendations include a multicomponent approach involving increased energy intake and reduced energy expenditure, nutrition counseling, and psychological counseling for eating disorders (Mountjoy et al. 2014).

Evaluating Muscular Strength Testing Data

Muscular strength is a critical component in many sports. Maximal strength testing should be implemented periodically to assess the efficacy of the training program and to use as a basis if the player development team assigns loading based on a percent of the 1RM for certain structural exercises. It may also be used in the regular monitoring of athletes via loading during training (e.g., tracking the weights and repetitions lifted per exercise) or as a measure of force and velocity if special technology is specifically used (e.g., during jumps, cycling, striking, running, and VBT). Maximal strength testing may assess different types of strength (e.g., dynamic CON, ECC, and ISOM and isokinetic) in an exercise-specific manner. Strength is velocity-specific, so maximal dynamic and ISOM strength testing involves strength produced at unintentionally slow velocities or without movement. Sport-specific strength and peak and average force can be measured using force plates, transducers, or specialized equipment with load cells or force-measuring devices. The player development team should assess the exercises that are most critical to the program and sport. There is no need to test the maximal strength of every exercise because training load data can also provide the player development team with valuable information. Strength results depend on many factors, including body weight, gender, exercise, training experience and technique, type of test, the testing environment, and several other factors (see chapter 3), so results must be properly interpreted in the context of the athlete's sport and position and the athlete's progression over time. In addition, the athlete's anthropometrics absolutely must be taken into consideration to properly interpret strength test results (see chapter 2). For example, an athlete with a very long wingspan would not be expected to bench press as much weight, given the mechanical disadvantage this athlete has for this particular exercise. Strength data must be viewed in the context of the entire athlete composite. In this section, some data norms for several exercises and strength ratios are discussed.

Dynamic Maximal Strength

Maximal strength is a key component for many athletes and has been shown to relate to many factors, including rate of force development, jumping ability and power, upper-body power, sprint speed, change-of-direction ability, and sport-specific movements such as bat speed, punching power, and track-and-field throws (Suchomel, Nimphius, and Stone 2016). Testing maximal strength is important for the assessment of athletes. The exercises may vary depending on the athletes in question, although core structural multijoint exercises, such as the squat, bench press, deadlift, power clean (or other OL derivatives), leg press, and rows, may be commonly used. For example, the barbell squat is a key exercise in the training of athletes. Figure 6.2 depicts a figure modified from (Suchomel, Nimphius, and Stone 2016) depicting the importance of relative squat strength and athletic performance. They present three basic phases:

1. Strength deficit: novice athletes are beginning to get stronger but are not yet capable of having enough strength to maximize performance
2. Strength association: increases in strength often directly translate to an improved performance
3. Strength reserve: athletes continue to gain relative strength but make less significant performance gains or hit a point of diminished returns

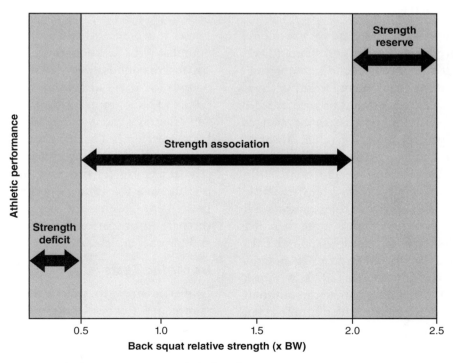

FIGURE 6.2 Importance of relative squat strength and performance.
Adapted from Suchomel, Nimphius, and Stone (2016).

The figure also notes that a relative back squat strength of 2.0 × body weight is desirable in adolescent-to-adult male athletes.

Dynamic maximal strength norms have been presented in absolute and relative terms. Relative norms are based on body weight, and absolute norms are used in reference to specific body weight classes. Both depend on gender and age. In addition, relative strength measures tend to favor small- to medium-sized athletes, so results must be interpreted with this in mind when evaluating large athletes. Below are some published relative norms for young adults that would place the athlete in the top 10% (Hoffman 2006; Ratamess 2022; Fukuda 2019):

- Bench press: (M) = 1.5 × BW; (F) = 0.5 to 0.75 × BW
- Leg press: (M) = 2.3 × BW; (F) = 2.0 × BW
- Deadlift: (M) = 2.0 to 2.75 × BW; (F) = 1.5 to 2.0 × BW
- Back squat: (M) = 2.0 to 2.5 × BW; (F) = 1.3 to 1.8 × BW
- Power clean: (M) = 1.0 to 1.8 × BW; (F) = 0.7 to 1.2 × BW
- Lat pulldown: (M) = 1.15 to 1.20 × BW; (F) = 0.80 to 0.85 × BW

Absolute strength increases are easy to monitor and track over time. Precise and standardized measurement techniques (e.g., hand and foot position, posture, ROM, equipment, warm-up, and ergogenics) for each exercise must be used in order for data to be meaningful because slight changes can significantly affect the 1RM value. Absolute strength norms and percentiles and descriptive data have been published (see Hoffman 2006 for review). For example, the top ten percentile of strength for a Division III American football player is the ability to bench press more than 365 pounds (166 kilograms) and squat 470 pounds (213 kilograms), whereas the values are 370 pounds (168 kilograms) and 500 pounds (227 kilograms), respectively, for Division I American football players. For Division I female athletes, the top ten percentile 1RMs are 124 pounds (56 kilograms) for the bench press and 178 pounds (81 kilograms) for the squat in basketball, 117 pounds (53 kilograms) and 184 pounds (83 kilograms) in softball, 116 pounds (53 kilograms) and 145 pounds (66 kilograms) in swimming, and 113 pounds (51 kilograms) and 185 pounds (84 kilograms) in volleyball (Hoffman 2006). In addition, a 1RM power clean of at least 130 pounds (59 kilograms) and 122 pounds (55 kilograms) was seen in female basketball and softball players, respectively. For male Division I baseball players, the bench press, squat, and power clean top ten percentile 1RMs were more than 273 pounds (124 kilograms), 365 pounds (166 kilograms), and 265 pounds (120 kilograms), respectively, while for basketball players they were more than 269 pounds (122 kilograms), 315 pounds (143 kilograms), and 250 pounds (113 kilograms), respectively. The strength and conditioning professional Mark Rippetoe has published extensive strength standards for the bench press, overhead press, back squat, deadlift, and power clean based on five training status classifications from novice to elite (Rippetoe 2011). For example, for elite male athletes weighing 181 to 275 pounds (82 to 125 kilograms), elite thresholds are 343 to 407 pounds (156 to 185 kilograms), 218 to 272 pounds (99 to 123 kilograms), 479 to 567 pounds (217 to 257 kilograms), 548 to 602 pounds (249 to 273 kilograms), and 310 to 367 pounds (141 to 166 kilograms) for the bench press, shoulder press, back squat, deadlift, and power clean, respectively. For elite women athletes weighing 132 to 181 pounds (60 to 82 kilograms), elite thresholds are 150 to 192 pounds (68 to 87 kilograms), 110 to 140 pounds (50 to 64 kilograms), 211 to 268 pounds (96 to 122 kilograms), 273 to 329 pounds (124 to 149 kilograms), and 152 to 193 pounds (69 to 88 kilograms) for the bench press, shoulder press, back squat, deadlift, and power clean, respectively. The critical element for the player development team is to increase the athlete's strength in all exercises prescribed. Coaches can track strength data and compare athlete performance to their previous tests and to other athletes of similar caliber.

Isometric Tests

Isometric strength tests measure static performance, and the results depend on the evaluation angle, standardization between athletes, feedback (visual and from coaches), and level of motivation. The best comparisons for a single athlete are made using the same equipment, testing standards, and environment. Comparisons to published norms must factor in the potential differences due to variance of testing. Isometric grip strength is commonly assessed. General norms (classified from good to excellent) for maximal grip strength of the dominant arm are more than 51 to 54 kilograms (112 to 119 pounds) in adult men and more than 33 to 36 kilograms (73 to 79 pounds) in adult women between 20 and 39 years of age (Hoffman 2006). We reported mean values of 53 to 63 kilograms (117 to 139 pounds) in Division III wrestlers (Ratamess et al. 2013). In fact, starters had greater total (i.e., both hands combined) relative grip strength to body mass than nonstarters (approximately 0.82 compared to 0.72). Elite Division I wrestlers (from The Ohio State University) showed similar levels of dominant hand grip strength combining the different weight classes at a mean of about 59 kilograms (130 pounds) with values lower or higher depending on body mass in the different weight classes. Grip strength is only sensitive to body mass changes or changes over a tournament or season due to weight loss or hydration status but is not sensitive as a measure to differentiate sport success.

Two common ISOM tests used in athletes are the ISOM squat and ISOM mid-thigh pull (leg press and bench press have also been used). These exercises are performed on a force plate against an immovable resistance and peak force (with or without body weight included), mean force, and rate of force development (RFD) are commonly assessed. In some cases, they may be a preferred test mode because they are applied easily, have high test–retest reliability, and pose a low risk for injury (Brady, Harrison, and Comyns 2020). Standardization of joint angles is critical, and variability may be seen among studies since different force plates yield different numbers. For example, knee angles of 120° to 150° and hip angles of 124° to 175° have been used to assess the mid-thigh pull, while knee angles of 90° to 150° and hip angles of 110° to 140° have been used for the ISOM squat (Brady, Harrison, and Comyns 2020). Changes in joint angle affect force production; thus, athletes have shown a wide variety of force values, making it difficult to establish norms. Figure 6.3 depicts a force–time curve from the ISOM mid-thigh pull. Baseline force represents the athlete's body weight. Peak GRF (total) or peak minus BW can be used as the delta force. RFD is calculated in different ways (see the sidebar on page 166).

For the mid-thigh pull, averaged peak force values have ranged from 1,500 N to nearly 6,000 N (Brady, Harrison, and Comyns 2020). Higher values were seen in male weightlifters and powerlifters (5,000 N to 6,000 N) and female weightlifters (3,500 N to 3,740 N), while athletes from other sports ranged from 2,100 N to 3,800 N. Relative force ranged from 28.0 N/kg to 64.0 N/kg in weightlifters. Peak RFD values ranged from 6,500 N/sec to 29,693 N/sec. For the ISOM squat, averaged peak force values have ranged from 1,318

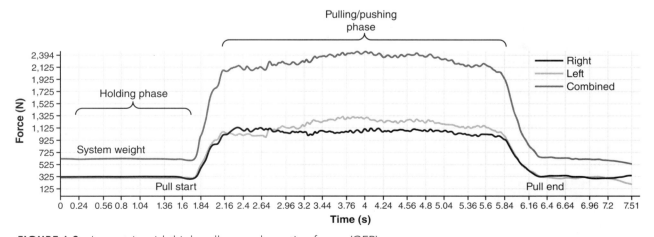

FIGURE 6.3 Isometric mid-thigh pull ground reaction forces (GFR).

ISOM Test F-T Variables

- Peak force (N): highest force attained
- Absolute peak force (N): peak force – body weight (BW)
- Relative peak force (N/kg): absolute peak force and body mass (kilograms)
- Force at specific time point (N): any F measure at 50, 100, 150, 200 milliseconds, etc.
- Left and right peak force, absolute peak force (N): values for left and right limbs
- Rate of force development (RFD) (N/s): change in force / change in time
- Peak RFD (N/s): highest RFD during time window
- Impulse (N × S): average force × time
- Impulse (N × S) per time: impulse per specific time window

N to 3,522 N, with peak RFD ranging from 6,100 N/sec to more than 14,000 N/sec (Brady, Harrison, and Comyns 2020). These values can provide the player development team with a framework, but each coach should develop their own norms given the high variability of testing differences seen in these studies.

Direct Dynamic Force Measures

In chapter 3 we discussed the use of force plates, transducers, and IMUs for measurement of force, velocity, and power. Force transducers may be strategically placed in sport-specific training equipment to measure force and power. Collecting force data allows the player development team to get direct measures of force in sport-specific movements such as jumping, running, and striking. Increasing 1RM strength is a major goal for many strength and conditioning programs, but transferring strength gained from heavy training to sport-specific movements is also of the utmost importance for athletes. The key is to increase strength across a spectrum of velocities and not just slow or moderate velocities. Although some athletes may be very strong as defined by their 1RMs, they may not always be strong at faster velocities to the same magnitude. Monitoring force and velocity during sport-specific movements allows the player development team to assess the connection between strength gained in the weight room and sport-specific force development. Field tests have been developed for coaches to estimate average force when expensive technology is not available. For example, (Samozino et al. 2008; Samozino et al. 2016) have developed methods for calculating force, power, and velocity during squat jumps with progressive loading and running sprints.

Norms for force measures are sparse since there is great variability in the technology used to measure force. In addition, several metrics may be used to gauge performance (see chapter 3). The higher the force (per velocity) during propulsion or striking, the better the outcome. For example, peak propulsive forces observed during jumping have ranged from 1,000 N to 5,000 N (at elite levels) and during running from 200 N to 1,100 N (French and Torres Ronda 2022). We reported averaged peak force values during the CMJ (with hands on hips) of approximately 1,900 N to 2,500 N (with peak values of approximately 3,000 N seen at higher weight classes) in Division III wrestlers (Ratamess et al., 2013). We profiled force at four time points and monitored force decrements that occurred during the preseason and in-season periods. The peak force values were higher in starters than in nonstarters per weight class, showing how important high force characteristics are to sport performance.

The Nordic hamstring curl (or reverse leg curl), which emphasizes the ECC component, has been shown to help reduce injury risk when incorporated into strength and conditioning programs. A device (NordBord) has been developed as a more specific alternative to isokinetic testing to measure ECC force of each leg via uniaxial load cells built into the leg support unit. In the initial studies, averaged peak knee flexion ECC force per leg values of approximately 340 N to 410 N (3.65 to 3.85 N/

kg) were reported in Rugby Union players (Bourne et al. 2015) and 250 N to 330 N (3.04 to 3.81 N/kg) in Australian footballers (with peak values of approximately 500 N) (Opar et al. 2015). Ranges of relative ECC strength of 2.5 N/kg to 6.5 N/kg body mass per leg have been shown for athletes in other sports, including American football, soccer, basketball, and track-and-field (Wille et al. 2022). These initial studies showed that low levels of ECC hamstring strength were related to the risk of injury but not limb imbalance between right and left sides. However, subsequent studies in similar and other groups of athletes did not find a relationship between increased injury risk and lower ECC strength levels (Opar et al. 2015). These conflicting results notwithstanding, monitoring of peak ECC hamstring strength may still be a useful testing and monitoring tool to assess progression in running-based athletes.

Technology has been adapted to measure force production during striking in boxers, martial artists, and MMA athletes via force transducers embedded in a target. Striking force depends on the type of punch, speed and technique of the punch, size and muscle mass, gender, and profile of the athlete. Elite athletes tend to develop more force during punching than less elite or non-elite athletes, possibly due in part to greater contributions of force and power from the lower body. Due to differences in technology used, a broad range of values for maximal punching force have been shown in various studies. In a review of the literature, Chaabene and colleagues reported absolute peak punch force data ranging from 1,600 N to 5,400 N (relative force ranges of 25 to 45 N/kg body mass) across several studies, with higher force seen during crosses, uppercuts, and hooks with the rear hand (with more rotational elements) versus lead-arm jabs (Chaabene et al. 2015). Lab-tested punching force values tend to be higher than those seen during live action. Newer technologies may display different measures of impact, so the team should develop its own norms for comparative purposes.

Strength Ratios

Strength testing data also serve as a guide for examining balance in strength improvements across the entire body during training. Muscular balance is critical because imbalances (or large strength differences between antagonistic muscle groups or right and left sides of the body) are known to increase the risk for injury. Although athletes have a dominant side, the strength differential between the two sides should not exceed 15% to 20% in most cases, and training should keep this percentage as low as possible. In addition, low peak hamstring and quadriceps strength ratios are related to higher injury risk in the lower body. Having knee flexion strength that is at least 70% to 75% as high as maximal knee extension strength (for a ratio between 0.70 and 0.75) is highly recommended for athletes, especially those in sports with large sprint and agility components. It has been recommended that athletes have a hip adduction and abduction strength ratio greater than or equal to 80% to prevent groin injuries (Dallinga, Benjaminse, and Lemmink 2012). Among throwing athletes, balance is needed between external and internal shoulder rotation strength. An isokinetic external and internal rotation strength ratio of 66% or an isometric strength ratio of 75% to 100% (depending on the testing position) has been recommended (Berckmans et al. 2017). The strength and conditioning program should target total-body strength development. Although some focus may be given to strengthening weaknesses, the goal is to increase maximal strength throughout the body so that the athlete will be well rounded in strength development. In addition, every exercise is unique and requires a specific level of neuromuscular activation; thus, maximal strength differs per exercise. Given that not all exercises are tested, coaches over the years have used ratios that could provide a framework for examining the strength (or weight lifted) for exercises that are not tested. The renowned Canadian strength and conditioning professional Charles Poliquin has suggested structural balance strength ratios for strength-trained athletes, shown in the sidebar on page 168 (Poliquin 1999; Thibaudeau, 2018).

Evaluating Muscular Endurance Testing Data

Tests of muscular endurance involve the athlete performing body weight exercises for a maximal number of repetitions or a maximal number in a specified time, repetitions for a resistance training

1RM Strength Ratios Compared to Other 1RMs

Percent of the 1RM back squat:
- Front squat: 85%
- Clean deadlift: 100%
- Snatch deadlift: 90%
- Deadlift: 120%
- Bench press: 75%
- Close-grip bench press: 67.5%
- Push press: 63.75%
- Incline bench press: 60%
- Military (shoulder) press (standing, strict): 45%
- Weighted dip: 78.75% (body weight included)
- Supinated chin-up: 67.5% (body weight included)
- Chest-supported barbell row (torso parallel): 52.5%
- Preacher curl: 30%
- Standing reverse curl: 26.25%
- Clean and jerk: 80%
- Snatch: 66%
- Clean: 81.6%
- Jerk: 84%
- Power clean: 68%
- Power jerk: 72%
- Power snatch: 54%
- Front squat: 85%

Percent of the 1RM clean and jerk:
- Snatch: 82.5%
- Clean: 102.5%
- Jerk: 105%
- Power clean: 85%
- Power jerk: 90%
- Power snatch: 67.5%
- Front squat: 110%
- Back squat: 125%

Percent of the 1RM Bench Press:
- Close-grip bench press: 90%
- Push press: 85%
- Incline bench press: 80%
- Military (shoulder) press (standing, strict): 60% (75% of the 1RM push press)
- Weighted dip: 105% (body weight included)
- Supinated chin-up: 90% (body weight included)
- Chest-supported barbell row (torso parallel): 70%
- Preacher curl: 40%
- Standing reverse curl: 35%

exercise at an absolute percentage of the 1RM and sustained maximal duration tests. In chapter 3 we discussed several local muscular endurance tests. Here, we present some norms that represent the top ten percentile for young adults, athletes, or a blend of values from multiple sources (Hoffman 2006; Haff and Triplett 2016; Ratamess 2022):

- Sit-up (1 minute): (M) = >57; (F) = >47
- Curl-up: (M) = >75-82; (F) = >60-70
- Push-up: (M) = >57; (F *modified*) = >42
- Pull-up: (M) = >12-15; (F) = >1-2
- Squat (depending on body weight): (M) = >120-215; (F) = >82-165
- Flexed arm hang: (M) = >56 sec; (F) = >29 sec
- Biering-Sorensen test: (M) = >157 sec; (F) = >167 sec
- Prone ISOM chest raise: (M) = >187 sec; (F) = >173 sec
- Prone double straight-leg raise: (M) = >130 sec; (F) = >126 sec
- Trunk flexor test: (M) = >144 sec; (F) = >140 sec
- Plank: (M) = >126 sec; (F) = >80 sec
- Side plank: (M) = >94 sec; (F) = >72 sec

The aforementioned norms were developed from a variety of sources for athletes between the ages of 18 and 30. Some studies have shown that collegiate, national, and professional athletes (in football, basketball, baseball, judo, and canoe and kayaking) may perform, on average, approximately 45 to 83 sit-ups, 8 to 44 pull-ups, 32 to 73 push-ups, and 23 to 32 dips (Hoffman 2006). Thus, great variability exists among different groups of athletes. The core stability test duration values were generated from only a few studies that examined athletes and non-athletes, so more research is needed in athletic populations for these norms to gain further acceptance. The player development team should select a few endurance tests and assess at various time points depending on the season. Clearly, the higher the value, the more muscular endurance the athlete will have. It is important to stress the need once again for highly standardized procedures because, just as with strength testing, any improper deviation in technique or methodology could result in a large difference in duration or repetition number. Coaches are highly encouraged to establish and use their own norms for comparison purposes. Although these values can give some important information to coaches, the key is to chart the progress each athlete makes for each of the desired tests. Lastly, the 225-pound bench press test is used mostly to assess American football players at the NFL combines. Norms are presented in table 6.2. The higher the number of repetitions completed, the better the score and the higher the predicted maximal bench press. Higher scores are just one of many factors that can help improve a player's draft status.

Evaluating Aerobic Endurance Testing Data

Aerobic capacity assessments involve the direct measurement or estimate of $\dot{V}O_2max$ or $\dot{V}O_2peak$. Endurance sports require high $\dot{V}O_2max$. For example, elite athletes such as Bjorn Daehlie (retired Olympic champion cross-country skier) and Greg LeMond (retired multi–Tour de France winner) had $\dot{V}O_2max$ values of approximately 96 and 92 mL/kg/min, respectively. Aerobic endurance athlete performance is ultimately determined to a large extent by the big three: $\dot{V}O_2max$, lactate threshold, and exercise economy. The higher the $\dot{V}O_2max$, the larger the aerobic capacity of the athlete, which, coupled with the aforementioned factors, leads to optimal endurance performance. Other sports may benefit to some extent, but $\dot{V}O_2max$ improvements need to be viewed in the context of the sport. For example, ATP-PC athletes do not require a high $\dot{V}O_2max$; however, improved $\dot{V}O_2max$ may help with metabolic recovery, so there is still a benefit to an increase. Figure 6.4 depicts $\dot{V}O_2max$ values from various groups of male athletes. Note that aerobic endurance athletes have the highest values, followed by hybrid aerobic and anaerobic athletes and ATP-PC athletes. In general, top ten percentile norms for $\dot{V}O_2max$ are greater than 51.4 mL/kg/min in men and greater than 44.2 mL/kg/min in women (Hoffman 2006). However, aerobic endurance athletes have shown very high values (greater than 70 mL/kg/min in men, 60 mL/kg/min in women); hybrid athletes in sports such as soccer, basketball, wrestling, tennis, judo, and hockey have shown above average to high values (approximately 48 to 62 mL/kg/min in men, approximately 44 to 53 mL/kg/min in women); and ATP-PC athletes in sports such as baseball, softball, powerlifting, weightlifting, and American football have shown average values (approximately 44 to 51 mL/kg/min in men and approximately 35 to 43 mL/kg/min in women) (Hoffman 2006; Haff and Triplett 2016). It is important to note that these are relative $\dot{V}O_2max$ values. Thus, a large athlete will not have a high relative value, although large athletes may have large absolute $\dot{V}O_2max$ values. Relative $\dot{V}O_2max$ is a better predictor of endurance performance. If $\dot{V}O_2max$ is estimated from a running field test, then following norms may also be used to demonstrate the top ten percentile (Haff and Triplett 2016; Hoffman 2006):

- 1.5 mile (2.4 kilometer) run (min:sec): (M) = <9:34; (F) = <11:10
- 12-minute run: (M) = >1.74 miles; (F) = >1.54 miles

Descriptive data have been reported for the Yo-Yo intermittent recovery (YY1R1, YY1R2) and beep tests. Figure 6.5 depicts data modified from Bangsbo and colleagues (Bangsbo, Iaia, and Krustrup 2008). Male elite, moderate-elite, and sub-elite soccer players covered 2,420 meters (2,647 yards), 2,190 meters (2,395 yards), and

TABLE 6.2 Percentiles for the Bench Press and the Predicted 1RM for Players in the NFL Combine

	DB			DL			LB		
		PRED 1RM			PRED 1RM			PRED 1RM	
% rank	Reps	lb	kg	Reps	lb	kg	Reps	lb	kg
90	18.0	345	157	28.1	416	189	29.3	423	192
80	17.0	340	155	26.0	400	182	27.0	405	184
70	15.0	325	148	25.0	395	180	26.0	400	182
60	14.0	320	145	24.0	385	175	25.2	396	180
50	13.0	315	143	23.0	380	173	22.5	378	172
40	12.0	305	139	21.6	371	169	21.6	372	169
30	10.0	295	134	20.0	360	164	19.1	356	162
20	10.0	295	134	18.8	353	160	15.4	329	150
10	8.0	280	127	17.0	340	155	13.7	319	145
X	13.2	315	143	22.8	378	172	22.2	375	170
SD	4.1	28	13	4.4	29	13	5.7	38	17
n	62			68			26		

	OL			RB			TE		
		PRED 1RM			PRED 1RM			PRED 1RM	
% rank	Reps	lb	kg	Reps	lb	kg	Reps	lb	kg
90	30.0	430	195	23.0	380	173	27.4	411	187
80	27.0	405	184	20.0	360	164	24.2	389	177
70	25.6	398	181	19.0	355	161	22.4	377	171
60	24.0	385	175	18.0	345	157	20.4	363	165
50	23.0	380	173	18.0	345	157	19.0	355	161
40	22.0	375	170	17.0	340	155	18.0	345	157
30	21.0	365	166	16.0	335	152	18.0	345	157
20	20.0	360	164	15.0	325	148	17.4	342	155
10	17.0	340	155	14.0	320	145	13.8	320	145
X	23.3	382	174	17.9	346	157	20.1	361	164
SD	5.1	35	16	3.3	22	10	4.2	28	13
n	97			67			11		

Pred 1RM = predicted 1RM; DB = defensive back; DL = defensive line; LB = linebacker; OL = offensive line; RB = running back; TE = tight end.

Reprinted by permission from J. Hoffman, *Norms for Fitness, Performance, and Health* (Champaign, IL: Human Kinetics, 2006).

2,030 meters (2,220 yards), respectively, during the YY1R1, while female soccer players covered 1,600 meters (1,750 yards), 1,360 meters (1,487 yards), and 1,160 meters (1,269 yards), respectively. Data from other athletes are also included. Distances covered of at least 1,760 meters (1,925 yards) were seen in male athletes with $\dot{V}O_2$max data of greater than or equal to 51.3 mL/kg/min.

For the beep test, data show that men ($\dot{V}O_2$max of approximately 58 to 59 mL/kg/min) complete an average of 11.4 to 12.6 levels with 105 to 121 total shuttles (laps), and women ($\dot{V}O_2$max of approximately 47.4 mL/kg/min) complete an average of 9.6 levels with 85 total shuttles. Completing greater than or equal to 13 levels is considered excellent in men and greater than or equal to 12 is considered excellent in women.

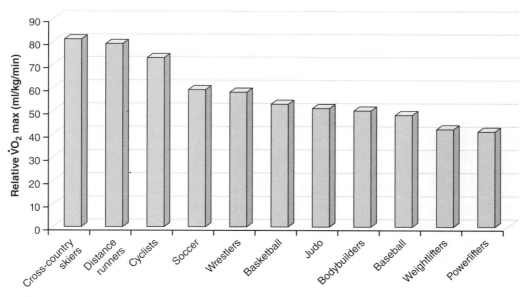

FIGURE 6.4 V̇O₂max data from various male athletic groups.

Data from Hoffman (2006); Haff and Triplett (2016).

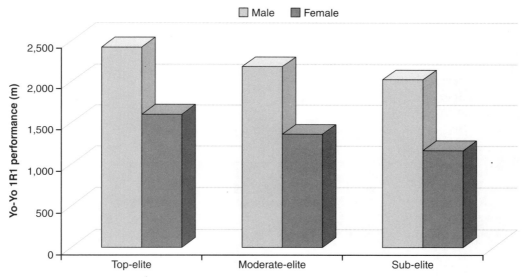

FIGURE 6.5 Performance of Yo-Yo test in different levels of athletes.

Data from J. Bangsbo, F.M. Iaia, and P. Krustrup, "The Yo-Yo Intermittent Recovery Test: A Useful Tool for Evaluation of Physical Performance in Intermittent Sports," *Sports Medicine* 38 (2008): 37-51.

Cardiovascular Monitoring of Athletes

It has become customary for the player development team to monitor internal load and fatigue in athletes. Given the rise and popularity of wearable technologies, such as HR monitors and positional systems (GPS, IMUs), it has become easy for the coaching staff to monitor the athlete in real time during practice or competition. Two cardiovascular measures commonly used to monitor athletes are heart rate (HR) and HR variability. *Heart rate variability* (HRV) is a measure of the variation in the time interval between heartbeats (e.g., R-wave to R-wave intervals) and is considered an indirect, noninvasive measure of cardiac autonomic activity, specifically the balance between sympathetic (SNS) and parasympathetic (PNS) branches. Following data collection and artifact correction, HRV can be determined in multiple ways, including with time- or frequency-domain measures.

Time-domain measures are more common and are computed by taking the standard deviation of the R-R intervals (SDRR) and the root mean square (RMSSD) or standard deviation of successive differences in R-R intervals. Decreased PNS activity (and increased SNS activation) is characterized by decreased HRV and vice versa. Increased SNS activity represents a stressor, so HRV can be used to monitor stress levels in athletes. Exercise elicits a curvilinear dose–response reduction in HRV until a threshold point is reached (figure 6.6). HRV demonstrates a time-dependent recovery and a return to preexercise levels after the exercise. Rapid recovery takes place within minutes, but full recovery could take 48 hours or longer if exercise intensity is very high. Chronically, aerobic training can increase HRV at rest, which may occur alongside a reduction in resting HR. The increase in HRV reflects greater cardiac parasympathetic tone at rest (e.g., reduced cardiac stress). Athletes in different sports display an overall increase in HRV at rest and a moderate increase in postexercise HRV (compared to untrained individuals), indicating an increase in postexercise parasympathetic HR modulation (Bellenger et al. 2016). The best data are obtained when the time of day of measurement, nutritional intake, temperature, and body position are standardized.

In chapter 4 we discussed acute and chronic changes in exercise and resting HR. HR can also be used to monitor the training load of athletes. HR can be monitored for long periods of time with wearable technology and can be used to calculate training load. First proposed by Banister et al. (1991), HR data can be used to calculate *training impulse* (or *TRIMP*). $TRIMP_{Banister}$ is calculated from training duration and maximal, resting, and average HR during exercise. It recognizes training intensity as a function of the HR reserve (%HRR) multiplied by a nonlinear factor (based on the intensity–blood lactate relationship) multiplied by workout duration where:

$$TRIMP = \text{wkt duration (min)} \times \Delta HR \times 0.64 \times e^{1.92} \text{ (for men)}$$

$$TRIMP = \text{wkt duration (min)} \times \Delta HR \times 0.86 \times e^{1.67} \text{ (for women)}$$

where $\Delta HR = (Avg\ HR_{exercise} - RHR) / (HR_{max} - RHR)$; e = natural logarithm

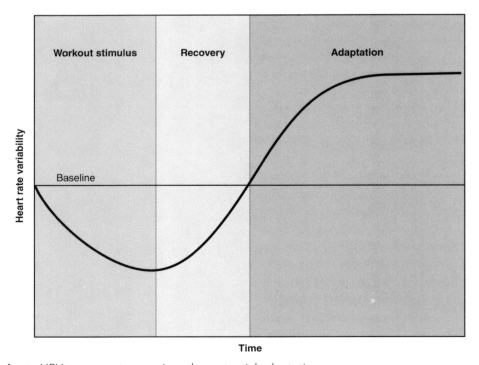

FIGURE 6.6 Acute HRV response to exercise, plus potential adaptation.

A limitation of this TRIMP calculation was that it relied on mean HR measures (mostly steady-state) and did not consider the intermittent nature of some activities, especially interval training. For these reasons, TRIMP was modified to account for HR zones. The use of HR zones enables the player development team to quantify the time spent during the workout between 50% and 100% of maximal HR in five approximately 10% increment zones. In 1993 Edwards extended Banister's TRIMP by calculating the product of the cumulated training duration in minutes for each of five HR zones, multiplied by a corresponding coefficient denoting higher values at higher HRs, where:

50%-60% HRmax = 1
60%-70% HRmax = 2
70%-80% HRmax = 3
80%-90% HRmax = 4
90%-100% HRmax = 5

$TRIMP_{Edwards}$ = duration in zone 1 × 1 + duration in zone 2 × 2 + duration in zone 3 × 3 + duration in zone 4 × 4 + duration in zone 5 × 5

Both methods have been validated (as well as other TRIMP methods and the session-RPE discussed later in this chapter) and used with athletes. Other TRIMP calculations have been introduced; for example, Lucia's TRIMP model uses three HR zones based on the athlete's lactate threshold and onset of blood lactate accumulation (Halson 2014). Other models have been developed using HR, blood lactate, or both (e.g., iTRIMP, team TRIMP, LacTRIMP) (French 2017). There are a number of limitations to regular lactate monitoring of athletes during training and competition. Regardless of the methods used, the higher the value, the greater the internal load on the athlete. Although each method has limitations, they do provide the player development team with another measure to quantify internal load during various training and competition phases.

Evaluating Flexibility Testing Data

Flexibility testing is simple and does not require expensive equipment. Certain groups of athletes require high levels of flexibility in parts of the body while others require good-to-moderate flexibility depending on the sport or position. Often, the shoulder, spine, and hip regions may be targeted with routine flexibility assessment of athletes. A direct relationship between flexibility and injury potential has not been established, but it appears that a lack of flexibility may contribute in part to certain types of injuries and not others. Nevertheless, the sport or position may dictate the level of flexibility needed. Average joint ROMs are presented in table 6.3. Some tests described in chapter 3 are pass-fail, so a failed test would prompt focus on strength and conditioning. Other tests yield quantitative data that are easier to use for comparison. In general, top ten percentile norms for the modified sit-and-reach are more than 17.2 inches (43.7 centimeters) in men and more than 17.9 inches (45.5 centimeters) in women (Hoffman 2006). For the trunk rotation test, more than 20 centimeters (7.9 inches) is excellent; 15 to 20 centimeters (5.9 to 7.9 inches) is very good; 10 to 15 centimeters (3.9 to 5.9 inches) is good; 5 to 10 centimeters (2 to 3.9 inches) is fair; and 0 to 5 centimeters (0 to 2 inches), or a negative score, is poor. For the shoulder elevation test, a score of less than 6 inches (15.2 centimeters) in men and less than 5.5 inches (14 centimeters) in women is considered excellent; 6 to 8.24 inches (15.2 to 20.9 centimeters) and 5.5 to 7.49 inches (14 to 19 centimeters), respectively, is good; 8.25 to 11.49 inches (21 to 29.2 centimeters) and 7.5 to 10.74 inches (19 to 27.3 centimeters), respectively, is average; 11.5 to 12.5 inches (29.2 to 31.8 centimeters) and 10.75 to 11.75 inches (27.3 to 29.8 centimeters), respectively, is fair; and more than 12.5 inches (31.8 centimeters) and 11.75 inches (29.8 centimeters), respectively, is considered poor (Johnson and Nelson 1986).

Evaluating Power Testing Data

Jump testing provides a simple method for assessing lower- and total-body power. Standing long jump (broad jump) performance (top ten percentile) in elite male and female athletes is more than 134 to 148 inches (340 to 376 centimeters) in males and more than 116 to 124 inches (295 to 315 centimeters) in females (Hoffman 2006). Top ten percentile performance from the NFL Combines indicate jumps (depending on the position) of more than 108 to 127 inches (274 to 323 centimeters).

TABLE 6.3 Average Joint Ranges of Motion

Joint	Joint motion	ROM (degrees)
Hip	Flexion	90-125
	Hyperextension	10-30
	Abduction	40-45
	Adduction	10-30
	Internal rotation	35-45
	External rotation	45-50
Knee	Flexion	120-150
	Rotation (when flexed)	40-50
Ankle	Plantar flexion	20-45
	Dorsiflexion	15-30
Shoulder	Flexion	130-180
	Hyperextension	30-80
	Abduction	170-180
	Adduction	50
	Internal rotation	60-90
	External rotation	70-90
	Horizontal flexion	135
	Horizontal extension	45
Elbow	Flexion	140-160
Radioulnar	Forearm pronation (from midposition)	80-90
	Forearm supination (from midposition)	80-90
Cervical spine	Flexion	40-60
	Hyperextension	40-75
	Lateral flexion	40-45
	Rotation	50-80
Thoracolumbar spine	Flexion	45-75
	Hyperextension	20-35
	Lateral flexion	25-35
	Rotation	30-45

Reprinted by permission from Hoffman *Norms for Fitness, Performance, and Health*. (Champaign, IL: Human Kinetics, 2006).

Studies have shown mean values of 78 to 102 inches (198 to 259 centimeters) in various groups of male athletes and 58 to 85 inches (147 to 216 centimeters) in female athletes (Haff and Triplett 2016). Vertical jump norms (top ten percentile) for athletes are more than 34 inches (86 centimeters) in men and more than 30 inches (76 centimeters) in women. Male players of American football at the NFL Combine have shown top ten percentile vertical jumps of more than 33 to 40 inches (84 to 102 centimeters) (depending on position). Studies have shown mean values of 15 to 25 inches (38 to 64 centimeters) in various groups of male athletes and 10 to 21 inches (25 to 53 centimeters) in female athletes (Haff and Triplett 2016). As discussed in chapter 3, jump heights and lengths only give a measure of a kinematic displacement and do not actually denote power output, unless a power prediction equation is used to estimate power, or unless the athlete jumps on a force plate (or uses a linear position transducer). A wide range of power outputs have been reported in the literature due to different populations tested, testing techniques, loaded and unloaded, and equipment.

For example, McMaster and colleagues reported ranges of peak concentric power values of 3,000 W to 9,000 W during jumps of body weight only, ballistic jump squat with up to 60% of the 1RM squat, and mean concentric power values of 1,500 W to 4,000 W (McMaster et al. 2014). In addition, chapter 3 discussed other measures that force plates can provide the coach using countermovement jumps, squat jumps, or depth jumps. Some norms include approximately 0.5% to 6.8% (peak power) and approximately 12.5% to 25% (peak jump height) for the prestretch augmentation percent; approximately 1.12 to 1.25 (peak jump height) and approximately 1.01 to 1.06 (peak power) for the eccentric utilization ratio; and top ten percentile values of greater than or equal to 0.547 in male DI athletes; greater than or equal to 0.434 in female athletes for the RSI (Sole, Suchomel, and Stone 2018).

Peak upper-body power has been assessed using ballistic bench press and the plyo push-up on a force plate. Athletes were shown to produce peak power outputs during the ballistic bench press between 450 W and 1,500 W and mean concentric power outputs between 300 W and 800 W using 20% to 60% of the 1RM bench press (McMaster et al. 2014). For the ballistic bench press, values of 477.7 ± 115.2 W and 185.4 ± 55.7 W in male and female athletes, respectively, have been reported (Bartolomei et al. 2021). For the plyo push-up, peak power of 939 ± 257 W, mean power of 516 ± 150 W, peak RFD values of 4,751 ± 1,862 N/sec, and mean RFD values of 2,342 ± 872 N/sec in male recreational athletes have been documented (Wang et al. 2017). Figure 6.7 shows the force curves obtained during the plyo push-up in a female athlete. In addition, medicine ball chest throws have been used to test upper-body power. Data vary considerably depending on the size of the medicine ball (usually 3 to 5 kilograms), but some descriptive distance data for athletes have ranged from 2.5 to 6 meters (2.7 to 6.6 yards) (Hoffman, 2006; Ratamess 2022).

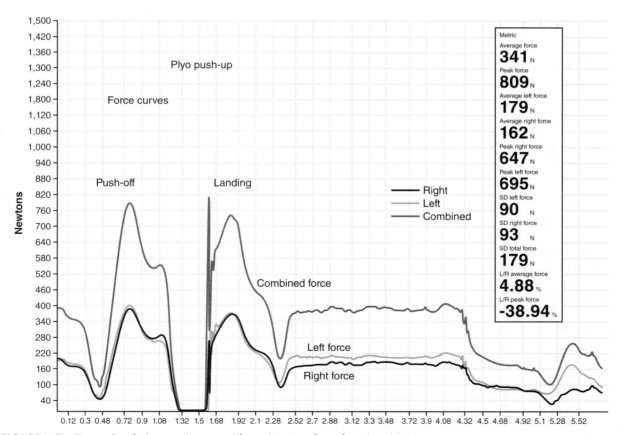

FIGURE 6.7 Example of plyo-push ground force kinetics for a female athlete.

Force Plate Monitoring During Training

Force plates may be used for load–response monitoring. Coaches may use force plate tests (usually with a jump variation) to monitor fatigue, fatigue resistance, and recovery from previous workouts or competitions. Monitoring may be used prior to a workout or competition, and 24, 48, and 72 hours postworkout to monitor fatigue and the athlete's recovery ability. These data can also help the staff in measuring performance while an athlete is recovering from an injury. For example, bilateral, unilateral, and asymmetry data (and potential deficits) can be used to assist in the decision-making process of the athlete's return-to-play training program. In addition, force plates may be used to help coaches determine the type of workout used during training. For example, in flexible nonlinear periodized training programs, the workout may be prescribed based on athlete preparedness for the day. A benchmark profile may be created so that the athlete's workout matches the force, velocity, and power data generated via preworkout testing. Given the advances in force plate technology, the large array of measured variables, and the ease of use in conjunction with a device such as a phone or iPad, athlete monitoring has become much more efficient and provides pertinent data that can help the training and competition paradigm. In addition to plates, other force and power measuring devices, as discussed in chapter 3, can be used for athlete monitoring. For example, we mentioned that boxers have been shown to produce various levels of peak and mean punching force (depending on weight class, gender, type of punch, skill level, and technology used to measure or estimate force) from approximately 1,600 N to approximately 5,400 N (Chaabene et al. 2015). The coaching staff can collect real-time force data and use that information to monitor the athletes and set benchmarks that may be targeted per workout.

Evaluating Anaerobic Capacity Testing Data

Anaerobic capacity tests measure power endurance and typically last 15 to 90 seconds. The Wingate anaerobic power test is an all-out maximal cycle ergometry test lasting 30 seconds. For lower-body maximal testing, top ten percentile data indicate peak power values of more than 822 W (10.89 W/kg relative peak power) and 560 W (9.02 W/kg relative peak power) in men and women, respectively, and mean power values of more than 662 W (8.2 W/kg relative mean power) and 470 W (7.3 W/kg relative mean power) in men and women, respectively (Ratamess 2022). Averaged peak power values of 842 W to 1,900 W and 406 W to 785 W were shown in male and female athletes, respectively (Hoffman 2006). Elite athletic performances are peak power more than 1,163 W and more than 730 W and mean power more than 823 W and more than 541 W in men and women, respectively (Peterson, 2012). For upper-body Wingate performance, data in nonathletic populations show peak power more than 658 W and mean power more than 477 W in men (Hoffman 2006).

The 300-yard shuttle run and line drill were discussed in chapter 3. Top ten percentile performances for the 300-yard shuttle run (determined from Division I male baseball and basketball players and female basketball and softball players) are 54 to 57 seconds in men and 58 to 63 seconds in women (Hoffman 2006). For the line drill (determined predominately in basketball players), mean times of approximately 28 to 29 seconds in men and 30 to 32 seconds in women were noted.

Evaluating Speed Testing Data

Assessments of speed involve maximal linear movement. Short sprint tests assess maximal speed and acceleration ability, while long sprint tests assess speed endurance. Mean 10-meter (11-yard) sprint data reported for various groups showed mean times of 1.69 to 2.27 seconds in male athletes and 1.67 to 2.31 seconds in female athletes (Haff and Triplett 2016). Ten-yard sprint times of 1.52 to 1.59 seconds and 1.99 seconds were shown in male and female athletes, respectively. Mean 20-meter (22-yard) sprint data reported for various groups showed mean times of 2.91 to 3.38 seconds in male athletes and 3.17 to 3.38 seconds in female athletes (Haff and Triplett 2016). Top ten percentile 40-yard (37-meter) dash times in American football players measured at the NFL Combines range from 4.41 to 4.44 seconds in defensive backs, running backs and wide receivers to 4.72 to 5.07 seconds in defensive and offensive linemen (Hoffman 2006). Mean times of 4.68 to

5.34 seconds have been shown in other groups of male athletes (e.g., soccer, basketball, and rugby players). Mean times of 5.34 to 6.45 seconds have been shown in groups of female athletes. Periodic testing of speed is critical to assessing the efficacy of the strength and conditioning program as well as the nature of practice for athletes who require fast linear speed.

Kinematic External Load Monitoring in Athletes

The tracking of athletes using GPS technology began in the mid-1990s. GPS technology enabled reliable measures of speed, distance, and distance covered during different speed zones. The use of GPS and other wearable microsensor technology has made it easier for the player development team to track and monitor speed, player load, and contact. Inertial Measurement Units (IMUs) allow tracking in three motion planes and consist of *accelerometers* (triaxial, measure movement), *gyroscopes* (measure rotation), and *magnetometers* (measure orientation), all of which complement each other to provide accurate kinematic data. This technology is easily used and worn between the scapulae of the athletes and has shown good validity and reliability. Collectively, these technologies are very useful for tracking player speed, distance, acceleration and deceleration, change of direction, impact and collisions, jumps, speed thresholds, metabolic power, and quantification of player load. These wearable technologies have made it possible for coaches to quantify training and practice load, manage fatigue, develop player databases, and use the data to manage the athlete's training and playing time. Manufacturers may use their own metrics obtained from accelerometers, but often the Catapult PlayerLoad is calculated by quantifying the sum of the individual accelerometer vectors using the following equation:

$$PlayerLoad = \sqrt{\frac{(a_{y1} - a_{y-1})^2 + (a_{x1} - a_{x-1})^2 + (a_{z1} - a_{z-1})^2}{100}}$$

where

a_y = Forward accelerometer
a_x = Sideways accelerometer
a_z = Vertical accelerometer

The player development team can use player load data to monitor athletes throughout a competitive season. A study tracked Division I female basketball players over a 4-year period (Ransdell et al. 2020). They were able to track four metrics over a 4-year period and compare the data between positions (guards and post players) and in games that were won versus lost. The metrics monitored were average PlayerLoad (in arbitrary units), PlayerLoad per minute, average high inertial movement analysis (combines acceleration, deceleration, COD, and free running above an acceleration threshold), and average jumps. These data provide coaches with valuable information used for tactical decision-making, practice, and training.

GPS data have made it possible for coaches to determine an athlete's speed zones or windows during training, practice, or competition. This information is helpful for determining the number of sprints and moderate- to high-intensity runs or sprints incurred during the workout and the amount of time spent in each speed zone. The key element is to individualize the speed zones for each athlete. This may be done by assessing maximal speed and then developing intensity thresholds or bands to determine the speed windows or modifying zones from published studies. Typically, six speed zones are identified, with zone one being the lowest and zone six being the highest, ranging from 0 to 36 km/hr with each zone linked with a description (e.g., walking through to sprinting) (Cummins et al. 2013). Each zone differs depending on the athlete monitored and subsequent speed capacity. There is disparity in the literature, which is why it is important for coaches to develop their own speed zones or at least modify the zones for the abilities of their own athletes. Cummins and colleagues reviewed the literature and showed the ranges of speeds per zone were as follows (Cummins et al. 2013):

- Zone 1 = 0 to 1-6 km/hr; 0 to 0.6-3.7 mph (standing, walking)
- Zone 2 = 1 to 12-14 km/hr; 0.6 to 7.5-8.7 mph (walking, jogging, cruising)
- Zone 3 = 7 to 18 km/hr; 4.3 to 11.1 mph (jogging, cruising, striding)
- Zone 4 = 12 to 21 km/hr; 7.5 to 13.0 mph (running, striding)
- Zone 5 = 18 to 24 km/hr; 11.2 to 14.9 mph (high-speed running, sprinting)
- Zone 6 = >18-25 km/hr; >11.2 to 15.5 mph (maximum intensity sprinting)

Microsensor technology can also determine body load and provide impact or collision data for athletes from sports such as American football and rugby. The intensity of the collision is typically measured in g-force. Impact intensity is graded into six zones as well. This allows coaches to quantify the number or percent of collisions per zone or body load. As reviewed by (Cummins et al. 2013), these zones are as follows:

- Zone 1 = 5-6 g-forces (light)
- Zone 2 = 6-6.5 g-forces (moderate)
- Zone 3 = 6.5-7.0 g-forces (moderately heavy)
- Zone 4 = 7-8 g-forces (heavy)
- Zone 5 = 8-10 g-forces (very heavy)
- Zone 6 = >10 g-forces (severe)

Evaluating Agility and Change-of-Direction Testing Data

Agility tests assess the athlete's ability to rapidly accelerate, decelerate, and change direction in a controlled manner using forward, backward, and side-shuffling movements. They are made up of change-of-direction ability and reactive ability. Completing each test in the shortest time possible is indicative of better acceleration, deceleration, and COD ability. For change of direction and the 505 COD test, mean values of 2.30 to 2.51 seconds were shown in male rugby players and 2.66 to 2.69 seconds in female basketball and softball players (Haff and Triplett 2016) using the traditional version starting with a 10-meter (11 yard) sprint. In a review, Ryan and colleagues reported mean times of 2.49 seconds in male athletes and 2.65 seconds in female athletes, a 6% difference (Ryan et al. 2022). Elite male athletes had mean times of 2.37 seconds, while sub-elite and novice male athletes had mean times of 2.47 to 2.57 seconds (Ryan et al. 2022). Modified versions of the test (where there is no 10-meter (11 yard) sprint preceding the timing) have been used, yielding mean times of 2.78 seconds in male athletes (2.75 seconds in elite athletes, 2.80 seconds in novice athletes). In addition, times may slightly differ depending on which leg (dominant versus nondominant) the athlete performs the 180° turn with. If *change-of-direction deficit* is calculated (i.e., the difference between 505 time and 10-meter [11 yard] sprint), mean times of 0.62 to 0.67 seconds have been shown in male athletes (Nimphius et al. 2016) and 0.52 to 0.59 seconds in female athletes (Dos'Santos et al. 2019).

t-test times of less than 9.5 seconds and 10.5 seconds in men and women athletes, respectively, are excellent; 9.5 to 10.5 seconds in men and 10.5 to 11.5 seconds in women are good; and 10.5 to 11.5 seconds in men and 11.5 to 12.5 seconds in women are average. Top ten percentile performance in Division III male American football players is 8.17 to 8.51 seconds for QBs, WRs, RBs, DBs, and TEs and 8.36 to 9.24 seconds for LBs, OLs, and DLs (Hoffman 2006). Groups of female athletes have shown mean values of 9.94 to 12.52 seconds (Haff and Triplett 2016). Top ten percentile pro agility times in Division I female athletes (in volleyball, softball, and basketball) is 4.65 seconds to 4.88 seconds and 4.21 seconds to 4.25 seconds in male athletes (in baseball, American football, and basketball) (Hoffman 2006). Top ten percentile performances from NFL Combines show times of 3.89 to 4.02 seconds for RB, WR, DB, 4.07 seconds to 4.18 seconds for QB, LB, and TE, and 4.22 seconds to 4.45 seconds for DL and OL (Hoffman 2006). Analysis of NFL Combine data from 2002 to 2016 showed a range of times of 6.42 to 9.12 seconds with a mean of 7.28 ± 0.42 seconds for the three-cone drill (Hedlund 2018). Top ten percentile performance shows values of 6.85 to 7.66 seconds for all positions (Hoffman 2006). For the hexagon test, values of approximately 12.3 seconds in male athletes and 12.9 to 13.2 seconds in female athletes were shown (Ratamess 2022).

Evaluating Balance Testing Data

Balance tests include timed static standing tests, dynamic unilateral standing tests that involve a measurable movement with opposite limb or upper extremities, tests using unstable surfaces, standing tests on force plates, and tests using specialized balance testing equipment. Some tests may be evaluated through visual inspection of technique (e.g., single-leg squat). For the balance error scoring system test, better balance is indicated by a lower score (the worst possible score is 60). Mean scores shown in men (ages 20 to 29) is 10.4 ± 4.4 and 11.9 ± 5.1 in women (Haff and Triplett 2016). For the Y balance test, composite scores of 85% to 108% have been shown in male and female athletes, with an anterior reach of 57% to 106%, a posteromedial reach of 93 to 123%, and a posterolateral reach of 86% to 108% (Plisky et al. 2021). Comparisons showed across all studies that differences were noted in the posteromedial (109% versus 102%) and posterolateral (107% versus 102%) directions where male athletes had higher scores. No differences were noted in the anterior direction (72% versus 71%) or composite scores (95%) (Plisky et al. 2021). A higher score indicates greater balance and strength. For the landing error scoring system, a lower score denotes better landing technique. The highest score possible is 17, so athletes should strive for the lowest score possible. Padua and colleagues reported mean scores of 4.43 ± 1.71 in uninjured male and female athletes and 6.24 ± 1.75 in athletes who were injured (e.g., had a prior ACL injury) (Padua et al. 2015).

Subjective Measures of Monitoring Training Load

Our previous discussions of calculating and monitoring training load involved some form of technology to track athletic performances, such as HR, speed, and acceleration. A subjective and inexpensive method to monitor training load is to use the session rating of perceived exertion or the *session-RPE*. Developed by Foster in 2001, the session-RPE takes into consideration the athlete's perception of exercise intensity and workout duration (Foster et al. 2001). It is calculated by multiplying the workout duration in minutes by an RPE rating on a 10-point scale. The Foster RPE scale indicates that 0 = rest; 1 = very, very easy; 2 = easy; 3 = moderate; 4 = somewhat hard; 5-6 = hard; 7-9 = very hard; and 10 = maximal.

One can see that the scale is nonlinear: The somewhat hard workout anchor begins at 4 and there are more values within the harder range of 4 to 10 than there are within the easy to moderate range of 2 to 3. The athlete is asked to rate a workout or practice session on the 10-point scale (as a measure of the mean intensity throughout the workout) and this value is multiplied by the time in minutes to calculate session-RPE in arbitrary units. The session-RPE value can be added during a specific time frame, whether short-term, such as for a day or week, or for a longer mesocycle. From these data *monotony* and *strain indices* can be calculated. Monotony is a measure of daily training variability (e.g., weekly mean training load divided by the SD), and strain is the weekly training load multiplied by the monotony (on off days, use a zero for both measures). Higher values for monotony represent less variability, and strain represents a composite of both variables. Research has shown that the session-RPE is a valid and reliable tool for quantifying training intensity and correlates to other monitoring measures such as TRIMP, $\dot{V}O_2$, ventilation, respiratory rate, lactate concentrations, and heart rate (Haddad et al. 2017).

Training load monitoring has implications not only for optimizing performance but also for reducing the risk of injury in athletes. Gabbett proposed modeling the athlete's acute workload to a chronic workload ratio in order to provide an index of the athlete's preparedness and to derive the athlete's susceptibility to injury (Gabbett 2016). Acute workload is defined as the current week's workload, and chronic workload refers to the average load of the previous 4 weeks as a measure of developed fitness. Gabbett also proposed that a ratio of less than 0.8 may indicate under training (and a higher injury risk); a ratio of 0.8 to 1.3 indicates an optimal load (well prepared) and low-risk zone; and a ratio of more than 1.5 indicates excessive load and increased injury risk. Thus, excessive increases in training load should be avoided, when possible, to optimize performance and reduce injury risk.

Player Monitoring via Biomarkers

Biomarkers refer to analytes from human specimens, such as blood, skeletal muscle tissue, saliva, urine, sweat, or other tissues, that can be measured and quantified. Biomarker monitoring allows the player development team to track variables of interest over time. Given the expansion of the player development team in years, it is critically important that a team member understands the physiological significance of each biomarker and why its monitoring is important to the athlete's development, load management, and general health. Biomarker selection must fit into the monitoring program of the team and each analyte must provide critical information that basic testing and monitoring does not address. From a coaching education standpoint, the team should relay this information to athletes and explain why biomarker analysis is important to training and player development. This is important since the monitoring may be invasive, depending on the analytes of interest, and requires strict procedures for accurate measurement (e.g., proper rest, hydration, and a standardized diet, activity level, and time of day). These data help steer program design and training toward individualization. Likewise, the player development team should work in tandem with the exercise science or kinesiology department at the college or university to carry out specimen collection and biomarker analysis. As some testing may be invasive and costly, the player development team should identify only those biomarkers critical to program development. In some ways, the modern-day player development team mirrors a sport science research lab: What was customary for sport science research in the past is now used in the context of athlete monitoring. Advances in technology may make it possible to analyze some biomarkers noninvasively so that the process is less disruptive to the athlete. As this technology rises to the forefront, simpler and less costly means of physiological monitoring may become available to the player development team.

The basic rules of science apply to presampling instructions for the athlete, equipment, correct labeling of tubes, obtaining specimens, processing, storing, assays, assessing of samples, and interpretation of biomarker data. Often, several biomarkers may provide a better picture of the athlete scenario since one in isolation may not accurately reflect the demands and stress of training. Some biomarkers are measured to examine the acute response to the stress of exercise, practice, or competition, while others are measured to examine recovery elements 24 to 48 hours postexercise. Chronic training responses and adaptations may be examined by analyzing acute exercise or resting biomarker data over time. Thus, biomarkers are often time-sensitive, and a thorough understanding of diurnal patterns is essential to proper interpretation of results. Specific details about biomarkers have been published elsewhere (French and Torres Ronda 2022). Figure 6.8 provides an overview of some potential biomarkers of interest.

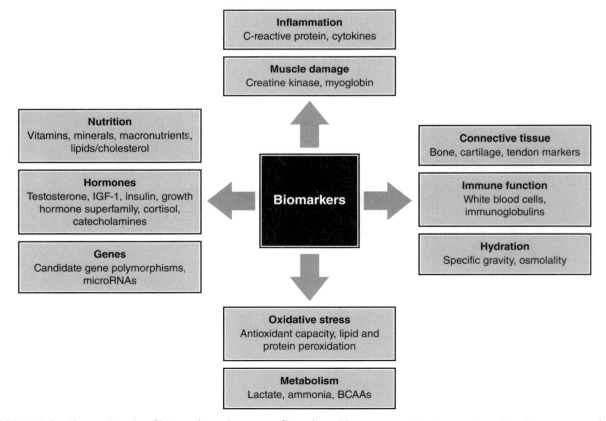

FIGURE 6.8 The multitude of biomarkers that can reflect the athlete composite at any given time in a macrocycle.

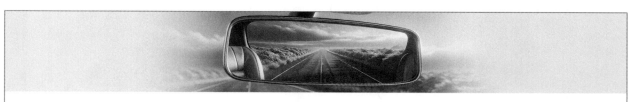

LOOKING IN THE REARVIEW MIRROR

- The player development team must not only test and collect data on athletes but must also be able to understand the results and apply them in a meaningful way for comparisons or for intraplayer analysis. This involves comparing data to established norms and previous player data.
- The player development team must have the three Cs of successful player development: appropriate credentials, competence, and commitment to optimize the athlete composite.
- The player development team must select appropriate sources of knowledge and use the scientific method in order to properly disseminate data and form conclusions.
- Periodic testing of selected health- and skill-related fitness components, as well as sport-specific performance, must occur on a regular basis to monitor performance and evaluate the efficacy of the training program. This includes subjective measures of training load and perhaps measures of biomarkers.

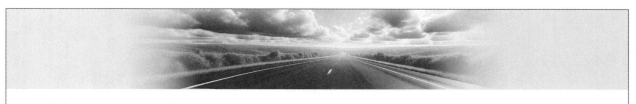

LOOKING AT THE ROAD AHEAD

The training of the individual athlete, as well as recovery capabilities, are vital to the success of not only improving the athlete composite but also getting the athlete composite ready for competition. Mistakes made in this area of player development can be detrimental to the athlete's progression toward genetic capability and the ability to recover optimally and reduce the potential for injury. The road ahead involves examining training principles and recovery technologies that affect the athlete composite.

Training and Recovery Approaches in Player Development

The training approach used in any player development program is essential. The training program is typically multidimensional and involves all of the different elements arising from the player development team. The physical exercise components related to sport-specific skills and strength and conditioning make up most of the demands, but nutritional, psychological, and behavioral programs (e.g., imagery, alcohol, and sleep) help move the needle for the player's mutable metrics.

There is a wealth of information on each of these elements. In this chapter, we go over some of the areas related to these concepts since decisions have to be made by the player development team about the direction of the player training approach. As previously discussed, an evidenced-based process should be used in making such decisions, along with the appropriate scientific principles and facts. The player development team's task is to take each athlete in the direction pointed to by the facts.

Importance of Individualization

Over the years, one of the most contentious issues in training programs has been the individualization of programs. Only when the popularity of personal training came into the fitness arena in the 1980s did this become an important topic of discussion. By the 1990s, some professional athletes hired personal trainers to help them get ready for a season. As the number of players managed by professionals increased, the issues with individualizing programs became about the limitations of technology in conducting rapid assessments. As noted in chapter 5, monitoring technologies and software have dramatically improved over the last five to ten years. It still takes much work to manage the workout data and other associated data (e.g., nutrition, sleep, fatigue, and injury) specific to each athlete, but individualizing training programs is the only way to optimize and enhance each player's athlete composite.

Scientific studies that proliferate the knowledge base have shown us that for any given program there are responders and nonresponders or, as we see in research papers, error bars around the mean. Thus, the reasons that an individual responds or does not respond to a program are often related to the many context variables that affect a specific target variable. Professionals in each player development team area need to contemplate what might cause a player to deviate from the expected outcome of an intervention (e.g., exercise, nutrition, or skill training). There are many factors, but often it is because the adaptive window is *full*. A great example in nutrition is creatine, which has been shown in many studies to be an effective supplement for performance (Wax et al. 2021). In creatine supplementation, about one in four to five people are nonresponders to the benefits of creatine because they already have genetically high levels of creatine in the skeletal muscle and no room to add more. As we say, the cup is full and giving them creatine does nothing. Still, creatine supplementation is essential to strength and power capabilities, with few, if any, adverse side effects. Additionally, it is not on any banned substance list. What matters, then, is whether the adaptive window is available. As discussed in previous chapters, assessments, monitoring, and managing each variable become the challenge for the player development team members. Individualization is the key to success!

Training Program Variation

A century or more of training theory has taught us that *variation* in the exercise stimuli is vital for the success of a program over time. There are a host of explanations of how variation came about in the different periodization theories. One is that the tracking programs of elite gold medal athletes made by the training theorists in the former Soviet Union used training logs to mimic patterns of changes. Conceptually, this was supported by Dr. Hans Selye's concepts of stress and distress from his research on cells and small animal responses to different stressors from poisons, hormones, and chemicals in the 1940s and 1950s (Selye 1950, 1976). It was also thought to provide a basis for varying training and has since been the underlying concept related to the need for variation. Dr. Hans Selye famously expressed it as the *general adaptation syndrome* (GAS), and it became popular with the lay public in his book *The Stress of Life*.

Today GAS has been analyzed, criticized, evaluated, and modified and still supports the need for variation. The adaptive response to the stimuli is not constant, and unless changed, plateaus will be observed well below the athlete's genetic potential. Even worse declines in performance can continue and lead to what is now called nonfunctional overreaching. One concept that has helped modify the GAS concept term "general" is that stress, while it has general characteristics, is quite specific. This is especially true of exercise workouts. Each workout has a specific fingerprint representing the choices of variables, regardless of the modality. The specific exercise stress will influence the specific adaptations to it (i.e., the SAID principle; see chapter 4).

Understanding the Exercise Stimuli Variables in Workout Design

As noted above, the exercise stimuli in any workout are specific to the choices made to construct the workout itself. In each modality, decisions must be made about the major elements related to the intensity of the exercise, the volume of the training, and the frequency of exercise. Each exercise modality has very specific domains in which choices of exercise stress must be made. The general modalities of aerobic endurance exercise, plyometrics, speed and agility, and resistance exercise have different workout configurations, even within the modality. Acute workouts and chronic sequences of the workouts must be designed in a program.

Programming in Athlete Development

Programming in athletic development is a complex, multivariate challenge encompassing a myriad of factors that inform the crafting of an exercise prescription. This complexity can be seen as a journey with different stages, each requiring unique approaches and insights.

In the early stages of building the foundation for novice athletes, programming is relatively straightforward. The primary training goals are focused on enhancing strength and then power. These adaptations occur swiftly, with beginners often witnessing significant strength improvements within eight weeks. However, while immediate gains in strength are noticeable, other adaptations, such as structural changes like muscle proteins and connective tissue development, require more time (figure 7.1). These changes are more gradual, unfolding over more extended periods, beyond the acute adjustments in the nervous system responsible for rapid strength gains. Implementing programs with basic normative exercises to address joint symmetry and upper and lower-body development is fundamental. Understanding these principles of acute and chronic program variables and principles lays the groundwork for a fundamental programmatic approach.

As we progress to intermediate programming, the situation becomes more nuanced, and this is where the landscape becomes more complex. Structural changes advance to a stage where further alterations demand a deeper understanding of numerous factors. This includes a comprehensive view of all elements of the program, personalized insights into the athlete's specific requirements and potential barriers, and an appreciation of the specific physiological and biomechanical demands of the sport. There's also the need for sophistication in balancing acute- (workout) and long- (periodization) term program variables, as well as recognizing and navigating factors that can interfere with progress. These elements combine to create a landscape where prescribing resistance training workouts and progression requires an advanced set of skills, knowledge, and a more complex and responsive approach to programming.

Programming in athletic development is not a linear task; it is an evolving, dynamic process that requires a keen understanding of the multifaceted interplay between various components. The player development team may have a structured program to follow but must be flexible to accommodate the athlete's current level of fitness, preparation, nutrition, and recovery status. From foundational strength building in novices to the intricate considerations in intermediate programming, it requires both scientific acumen and artistic finesse. The path to peak performance is laden with complexity, but it's this very complexity that makes the journey rewarding and, indeed, essential to the pursuit of athletic excellence. The complexity of intermediate programming, in particular, sets the stage for the next stage of discussion in this journey toward optimal athletic development.

The next steps of intermediate to advanced training program development become a hallmark of elite player development teams. The central goal of any athletic training program is to elevate or evolve an individual's biological capacity to excel in a specific task. Unlike everyday physical development, targeted training propels an athlete beyond what daily life alone can achieve. Sometimes, particular tasks might remain beyond reach due to muscle tissue limitations or physiological hindrances following injuries. Therefore, the careful integration of enhanced physiological understanding with training stimuli becomes a decisive factor in shaping an athlete's career.

Many people overlook the complex systems involved in even basic tasks. Throughout history, our bodies have adapted to our environment. In sports, adaptation—or lack thereof—occurs at an accelerated pace, where resources are constrained.

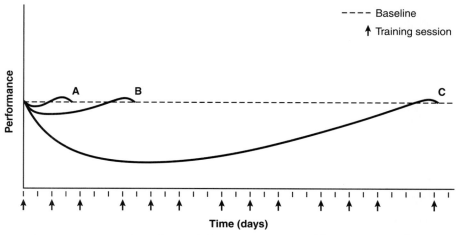

FIGURE 7.1 A longer stress-recovery adaptation cycle is necessary as an athlete progresses from novice to advanced. (A) novice athletes; (B) intermediate athletes; (C) advanced athletes.

Reprinted, by permission, from M. Rippetoe and A. Baker, *Practical Programming for Strength Training*, 3rd ed. (Wichita Falls, TX: The Aasgaard Company, 2017).

The interaction between rapid- and slow-reacting systems not only sustains life but also nourishes an athletic career, setting apart elite athletes from the rest.

In the early stages of athletic development, adaptations occur quickly, from instant changes to those manifesting over 24 hours. These immediate adjustments are predominantly attributed to improved cognitive-motor coordination, optimizing existing resources for efficient task execution. A critical phase emerges when muscle cross-sectional areas and bioenergetic systems, such as the bicarbonate buffering system, reach their upper thresholds. Athletes might then face a plateau, which often becomes the central focus of training. Truly transformative athlete development, however, relies on practitioners proficiently training intermediate athletes—those requiring a week's training and recovery to achieve supercompensation and advancement.

This intermediate stage demands acute awareness of external disruptions. Many athletes exhibit extraordinary progress, advance to an intermediate level, and then encounter injuries due to mishandling in weight training or overambitious sport coaches unfamiliar with their increased abilities. Nearly every head coach can recall a time when an injury in weight training cut short a promising athlete's career. Such incidents often prompt a cautious approach to weight training, focused on injury prevention—a perspective that strength coaches may view with skepticism. However, such caution usually stems from valid concerns created from previous poor program management.

In nearly all of these unfortunate situations, one or more of the following criteria are found:

- an unexpected spike in total tonnage and pounds per rep within a specific movement pattern in a short time frame
- insufficient preparation in the prior 8 weeks of conditioning for the team's intended player load in the practice plan

Most maladaptation results from failing to account for both expected and unexpected stressors. Aspiring practitioners must recognize that even within a structured college training environment of 8 to 10 hours per week, nearly 150 hours remain beyond the staff's oversight. These hours might include unplanned disruptions that should be incorporated into the performance or recovery plan.

In our technologically advancing era, the spotlight will shift toward those capable of unlocking the potential of intermediate athletes. We are now equipped with technology that can revolutionize the training experience, allowing for truly personalized training approaches. The era of outdated, static training methods is drawing to a close, ushering in a new age of sophisticated, individualized, and evidence-based training that can reshape the world of sports.

Understanding the stimuli is vital. Some of the basic constructs for a few of the modalities are covered in this section.

Aerobic Endurance Exercise

Aerobic endurance exercise prescription evolved from the long-distance exercise at lower intensities popularized in other sporting worlds by the term *road work*, which arose from boxing. The concept of a necessary aerobic base for all athletes led to issues identified in the 1980s and 1990s involving incompatibility when simultaneously trying to develop maximal strength and power. Interval training using sprints of various lengths and with exercise-to-rest ratios started to replace the required element of aerobic endurance for athletes who were not in long-duration sports. Even sports like soccer, lacrosse, and basketball were susceptible to too much training with running. Both conditioning and competitions created incompatibility and potential nonfunctional overreaching. Each sport must carefully construct the frequency, duration, and intensity of aerobic endurance training in player development programs.

Plyometrics

The basis of plyometrics is the concept of the *stretch-shortening cycle* of muscular activity, in which an eccentric stretch is followed by concentric shortening (Knuttgen and Kraemer 1987). This takes advantage of the elastic component in the body's connective tissues, from the tendon and ligaments to the muscle itself. When the stretch-shortening cycle is active, it should produce about 15% to 30% more power in a movement, especially in vertical jumping. Its effect can be observed in all exercises, from jumps to the bench press. Basic guidelines have been developed in a position stand by the National Strength and Conditioning Association (NSCA 1993):

1. The stretch-shortening cycle, characterized by rapid deceleration of a mass, followed almost immediately by rapid acceleration of the mass in the opposite direction, is essential to performance in most competitive sports, particularly in those involving running, jumping, and rapid changes in direction.
2. A plyometric exercise program—which trains the muscles, connective tissue, and nervous system to effectively carry out the stretch-shortening cycle—can improve performance in most competitive sports.
3. A plyometric training program for athletes should include sport-specific exercises.
4. Carefully applied plyometric exercise programs are no more harmful than other forms of sports training and competition and may be necessary for safe adaptation to the rigors of "explosive" sports.
5. Only athletes who have already achieved high levels of strength through standard resistance training should engage in high-intensity plyometric drills.
6. Depth jumps should only be used by a small percentage of athletes engaged in plyometric training.
7. Plyometric drills affecting a particular muscle or joint complex should not be performed on consecutive days.
8. Plyometric drills should not be performed when an athlete is fatigued. Time for complete recovery should be allowed between plyometric exercise sets.
9. Footwear and landing surfaces used in plyometric drills must have good shock-absorbing qualities.
10. A thorough set of warm-up exercises should be performed before beginning a plyometric training session. Less demanding drills should be mastered prior to attempting more complex and intense drills.

Yuri Verkhoshansky, the sport theorist from the former Soviet Union, popularized jump training as part of the "shock training method" for improvements in power or so-called speed-strength, coined as plyometrics in Western vernacular. The origins of plyometrics resided in the concept from the 1960s and 1970s of depth or rebound jumps. Classic plyometrics should be based on a solid squat strength for the athlete of 1.25 to 1.5 × body mass capability (for the back squat exercise) before adding higher-intensity plyometric exercises. The variables involved in the configuration of plyometric jump workouts have been detailed in a meta-analysis by de Villarreal and colleagues (de Villarreal et al. 2009). The following choices must be made for the different types of plyometrics:

Major decisions:
- Duration of session
- Frequency of sessions (per week)
- Program duration (in weeks)
- Number of sessions
- Drop height
- Change in jump height
- Number of jumps per session
- Number of exercises per session
- Rest between sets
- Unilateral and bilateral exercises

Combination with other types of exercise or conditions:
- Plyometric exercise + resistance exercise
- Plyometric exercise + electrostimulation
- Plyometric exercise + aerobic exercise
- Plyometric exercise + flexibility exercise
- Plyometric exercises in water

Intensity of the session:
- High
- Moderate
- Low

Type of plyometric exercise:
- Squat jump (SJ)
- Countermovement jump (CMJ)
- Drop jump (DJ)

- SJ + DJ
- CMJ + DJ
- SJ + CMJ + DJ

Many other upper-body exercises are used, including ones involving medicine balls. The medicine ball is especially important for sports or positions with a high rotational component. Earp and Kraemer have overviewed the different exercises and components of medicine ball training (Earp and Kraemer 2010). In brief, the need for rotational power is important for sports, and the medicine ball is a great conditioning tool. The ball exercises should be adapted to the requirements of the athlete's sport, and attention should be paid to the plane of movement and body positioning mechanics of the swinging or throwing movements. The speed of movement and the amount of countermovement are also essential concerns. Progressive resistance with the size of the medicine ball is also necessary to hit each range of the force–velocity curve. Readers are referred to the following resource for further study on the many upper and lower-body plyometric exercises that can be used to augment a training program (Ratamess 2022).

Resistance Exercise

William J. Kraemer, as a doctoral student in the early 1980s, was taking a multivariate statistics class. As a former college athlete and coach, he was still fascinated with the multitude of workouts, which he came across in the popular strength training and muscle magazines, but less so in the literature that was starting to see this line of research become more accepted in the scientific community. Nevertheless, there seemed to be many resistance exercise workouts arising from the other fitness and lifting worlds. When his class started to cover the statistical approach of cluster analyses, he saw the opportunity to bring his passion for resistance exercise front and center. He saw how one might quantify a resistance exercise workout. He decided to quantitate every resistance workout protocol he could from the research literature and popular muscle magazines used by different levels and types of lifters and athletes. From this analysis, five clusters were identified. When he looked at the common features in each cluster, he had to give the cluster a name. What were the main features of the workouts contained in the cluster? As typical of a cluster analysis, one had to name each of the clusters; they only described one given workout, so he called them the "acute program variables." Each cluster was a domain of variables that could describe one specific workout. The acute program variables were named by the choice of exercise, the exercise order, the intensity or resistance used, the number of sets, and the rest periods between sets and exercises, which we discussed over the four editions of his book (Fleck and Kraemer 2014). Any resistance exercise workout could be described by the choices made in the domain of each different acute program variable. As time went on, research would show that each of these variables affected a workout's biomechanical, physiological, and psychological fingerprint.

Choice of Exercise

The choice of exercise is fundamental to the biomechanics of the movements. Its effect on the activation of the neuromuscular system is dramatic in how it activates motor units. Simplistically, one can compartmentalize the choices into free-form exercises, in which multiple degrees of freedom control the movements, and fixed-form exercises, in which the equipment will set up the path of the exercise movements and thereby reduce the number of activations typically needed to stabilize and perform the same movements in free-form exercises (e.g., machine bench press versus free weight bench press). The weight that can be lifted in a fixed-form movement may be greater than in a free-form movement for some individuals (depending on the exercise and familiarity with that exercise). Fixed-form exercises were popularized by the fitness industry in the 1970s to quickly allow athletes to learn exercises and create various circuit training protocols. Also, bodybuilders were interested in isolating exercise movements to better target specific hypertrophy of a given area, and machines were thought to do this effectively. Every machine is biomechanically different. But most importantly, each athlete must be positioned correctly in relation to the machine because only some athletes fit certain machines. An inappropriate fit can result in an inadequate range of motions, unintentional stops with variable resistance machines, and so on.

Order of Exercise

The order of exercise is the sequence of the workout. Classically, large muscle group exercises were put at the beginning of the workout to promote the quality of exercise loading when heavier loads were used. Fatigue continues through the exercise order, so the technique needs to be monitored, especially as the rest periods are shortened in typical circuit workouts or superset protocols. This domain sets up many opportunities for developing protocols and workouts that affect the training of *buffering capacities* in the body, which are crucial for anaerobic glycolytic sports and events (e.g., wrestling and the 800-meter run). However, athletes can benefit from training their buffering capacity to handle extreme exercise demands.

Intensity (Resistance)

The *intensity* (commonly referred to as the *resistance* or *load*) used in an exercise is the most studied domain in resistance training. It also reflects the size principle because resistance dictates the number of motor units recruited to produce force. The motor units that are recruited adapt to the stimuli of the workout. Historically the repetition maximum (RM) was coined in part and made popular by the work of Dr. Thomas Delorme in his early work on the progressive resistance training model with the use of a 10RM and then percentages of the 10RM in rehabilitation programs (Todd, Shurley, and Todd 2012). Thus, resistance has been prescribed in workouts by a *percent of a repetition maximum* (RM) (e.g., 1RM or 10RM) or later by trial and error using an RM zone in which one tries to stay in a three-repetition range without going to failure. The percentages of the 1RM became well known in the worlds of weightlifting and powerlifting. The classic 80% of the 1RM was almost monumentalized as heavy since this loading typically resulted in about 10 repetitions reflecting earlier work (Delorme, Schwab, and Watkins 1948; Delorme and Watkins 1948; Delorme, West, and Shriber 1950). However, studies came along that showed how the percent of the 1RM varies between muscle groups depending on whether a machine or free weights are used. This further supports the use of the RM zone for training many muscle groups where repeated updated testing is inefficient. Finally, *velocity-based training* (VBT) became very popular; it uses velocity cutoffs for repetitions with different loads across the force–velocity curve (Zatsiorsky, Kraemer, and Fry 2020).

Number of Sets

The number of sets determines the volume of work or exercise. The resistance used is a vital part of this equation and must be modulated within the context of the program sequence used and the recovery capabilities of the individual. Volume became a vital parameter in the periodization of workouts. High volume–high intensity to low volume–low intensity is the continuum for this interaction. Care is needed in choosing because of the potential for nonfunctional overreaching when mistakes are made at different training phases.

Rest Between Sets and Exercises

The amount of rest between sets and exercises and the resistance used are what many call "metabolic accelerators," which rely on the body's buffering capacities (e.g., blood bicarbonate system, muscle carnitine, phosphate, and respiratory system buffering) to cope with the acidic effect (Kraemer, Fleck, and Deschenes 2021). As the load gets heavier with multiple sets and the rest periods get shorter (e.g., less than 2 minutes), the lactate production representative of the acid-base system reduces to a greater extent compared to moderate 10RM loads for multiple sets (Kraemer et al. 1990; Kraemer et al. 1993). Thus, higher reps and short rest intervals are conducive to higher blood lactates, although long rest periods are recommended for maximal strength training to reduce lactate response. Short rest periods with moderate loads and higher volume can dramatically elevate blood lactate and cause a dramatic drop in pH and increases in $H+$, creating a very acidic environment that must be buffered. If it is not buffered, symptoms such as unease, dizziness, and vomiting can occur. Such short rest workouts also create more chemical damage from free radicals and the inhibition of the immune system, requiring more time for recovery from the workout during the training week. One must watch for side effects, such as nausea, dizziness, and vomiting, that are representative of an insufficient rest period. If these symptoms occur, workouts should be stopped. The next training session then must extend the rest periods, while assessing for symptoms. Such symptoms indicate that an athlete has not yet adapted to the stress of the workout. It points to an important concept in sports medicine, that an athlete should not take on too much too fast.

Rest and Recovery

In athletics today, one of the more unappreciated prescriptions is rest. This includes total rest on a given day and during longer periods of recovery (e.g., 2 to 4 weeks) and active rest, away from the training modality, but using low-intensity activities to allow for recovery of the different physiological systems, most importantly the neuromuscular system. Other periodization training models have underscored the importance of rest and recovery learned from many decades of theory and practice in strength and conditioning. Rest is an important element of physiological and psychological recovery. What is done during the recovery time frame has also become a topic of intense interest in relation to what interventions may enhance recovery beyond pure rest, from nutritional supplements to various other therapeutics. Recovery technologies are used during training days, as are rest and active recovery days.

Complete Rest

The need for a complete day of rest has been underestimated in its importance. What is an entire day of rest from training? Typically, a full day of rest is where one only does appropriate stretching and uses a recovery intervention but avoids external stressors, from heat to vigorous activities, that limit the repair and recovery processes of cells, tissues, and organs. Over the past ten years, the use of complete rest has been combined with various recovery interventions that can enhance the normal recovery processes. A day of rest is typically placed within a 7-day training and competition cycle.

Even today, one observes athletes who do not know how to take a day off from training. As a friend once said, "we have trained the idea of being a couch potato right out of them." So, in a periodized training program, taking time for a full rest day is essential, especially when dramatic amounts of muscle damage and remodeling are occurring. Rest, nutrition, and sleep are important parts of recovery and the remodeling of the body's structures and physiological functions. I (WJK) used to tell athletes that they are remodeling organisms. This means that what they do after a workout or competition will affect how well their bodies remodel and repair the cells, tissues, and organs that have been stressed.

Additionally, one needs to give the mind time to rest and recover from the stress of training and competition. Psychological recovery is often more critical than physical recovery because the mind drives the passion and effort needed for optimal training and performance. This can be difficult if academic demands, other work demands, or

The Penn State Experiment

We learned about complete rest when Dr. Andrew Fry, then a doctoral fellow, and I (WJK) were studying overtraining, now called *acute overreaching*, of maximal force production at Penn State in the late 1980s and early 1990s. In an overreaching pilot study, we had lifters do the unthinkable: perform ten 1RMs of the squat each day for 7 days, taking Sunday off before starting the next 7-day cycle. We did not think this overreaching stress would affect the downward cycle of their strength, but to our amazement, it did—one day of complete rest. We had to go to 14 straight days of maximal 1RM efforts to create an overreaching effect to study. Still, even then, 27% of the lifters did not drop their 1RM, pointing to the genetic variability in the recovery capabilities of some individuals (Fry et al. 1994). This pointed to the need for individualized training and recovery programs, even for athletes in team sports. However, to do so would require hard work and effective and ongoing testing and monitoring programs to differentiate the needs of each player and to understand the recovery processes and conditions. Nevertheless, individualization is the only answer to this problem (see chapter 5).

further preparations for competition are part of the recovery day.

Scheduling rest days within a microcycle is in part an art and can be difficult since not every athlete on a team needs the same recovery plan (see the sidebar on page 190). This is where hits and misses can occur and a testing program (e.g., psychological perceptions, force plate power assessments, and workout assessments in real-time during the next training session) comes into play. These are of great importance in understanding the acute recovery of the athlete (see chapters 4 and 5).

Active Rest

Active rest takes many different forms and durations to allow the body to gain both physical and psychological recovery. Active rest can be dangerous when the activities or recreational sports have the potential to cause injuries. Wrestlers, for example, who play basketball can sprain an ankle or jam a finger. Thus, the activities used for active recovery need to be carefully considered. Essentially rest should involve low-intensity activities with a minimum of remodeling needs during recovery and exercises that differ from training or competition. Much depends on the timing and role of the rest and recovery period in the training plan. Resting the day after a competition or a significant workout is obvious. Rest and recovery after a specific training cycle, such as the peaking and competition phase, is another question. The length and duration of the active rest phase over the macrocycle involves testing and monitoring each athlete on a day-to-day, week-to-week, and month-to-month basis.

Overemphasis on Recovery without Adequate Testing or No Real Recovery

Although rest and recovery are key elements to the player development program, a significant oversight in mismanagement of recovery days may occur in some sports. For example, in professional baseball an athlete may be scheduled to take a game off with the intention of optimizing rest but may instead spend hours that same day in the batting cage or engaging in intense throwing. One may argue that these players did not adequately rest as they performed similar motions to the sport itself.

Recovery becomes more difficult when players are performing the same motions they are attempting to recover from (even though the intensity may be lower). Far from providing the intended respite, this approach may actually result in a more stressful experience than participating in the game itself depending on the positions played by these players. This practice not only fails to give the athlete the required time off but also violates the principle of active rest, where gentle and restorative activities should replace strenuous sport-specific skills training. Thus, what is done with recovery days becomes a critical consideration. Misuse of these rest periods can be a true disruptor to genuine recovery, hindering the athlete's ability to restore energy, repair tissues, reduce injury risk, and, ultimately, enhance performance. Attention to the true nature and purpose of recovery is essential to prevent this common yet costly mistake, underscoring the necessity for thoughtful, individualized, and evidence-based recovery planning.

- *Lack of individualization:* Without proper assessments, recovery strategies may be generalized and not tailored to individual needs. Athletes may undergo unnecessary treatments or interventions, leading to suboptimal results. Without tailored recovery plans based on proper assessments, athletes may undergo interventions that don't match their unique physiological needs. This lack of personalization can lead to inefficient training and recovery plans, resulting in wasted time and resources. It highlights the importance of employing individualized assessment tools that take into account various factors such as genetics, training history, and specific metabolic responses.

- *Potential for over-recovery:* An excessive focus on recovery might lead to prolonged rest periods, which can reduce training stimulus and potentially hinder performance adaptations. Excessive focus on recovery might decrease the training stimulus required for adaptation, potentially hindering athletic development. Understanding the balance between training and recovery is crucial. Over-recovery might lead to decreased fitness levels and readiness to perform, undermining long-term progression and peak performance.

- *Missed opportunity for optimal interventions:* The lack of proper testing and assessment might overlook specific issues like inflammation or muscle damage, thus missing the chance for targeted interventions. Targeted interventions could be employed to address specific issues. Missing these opportunities might delay recovery or exacerbate underlying issues, impacting both short-term performance and long-term athlete health.

- *Psychological impact:* An overemphasis on recovery without understanding the exact physiological need can lead to anxiety and a lack of confidence in training, which may impair performance. Overemphasis on recovery without clear understanding may lead to uncertainty and anxiety, negatively affecting an athlete's mental state. Addressing the psychological aspects of recovery is vital. Coaches and professionals must foster clear communication and trust, integrating psychological assessments and interventions alongside physical ones to promote optimal mental well-being.

Recovery Overview

The science of athletic recovery has progressed significantly, emphasizing the multifactorial nature of recovery and the importance of personalized strategies tailored to individual needs. This consensus among researchers reinforces the need for a multidisciplinary approach that combines insights from physiology, biochemistry, and neuromuscular science. The legendary stories of athletes in various sports who rarely miss games or plays during games, despite intensive competition schedules, speak to the effectiveness of individualized recovery plans facilitated by modern technology.

A nuanced and comprehensive understanding of recovery requires recognizing that it is not a general concept. Specific assessments must identify what variables in an athlete's composite need recovery from training or competition. The Player Development Team model, as proposed, serves as a beacon for this individualized approach.

Many practitioners are now striking a balance between training and recovery, using advanced tools such as heart rate variability (HRV), force plate assessment, workout log monitoring, and biochemical markers. These assessments guide personalized recovery strategies, allowing for targeted, evidence-based interventions that support both immediate performance goals and long-term athlete development. For example, many athletes have used strength and conditioning programs and recovery strategies to elongate careers and come to play each time.

These examples further illustrate the critical role of individualized recovery strategies in achieving exceptional durability and performance in professional sports. The tailored approaches of these athletes, rooted in scientific understanding and innovative methodologies, reveal a profound awareness of the multifaceted nature of recovery. This awareness, combined with their relentless pursuit of excellence, offers valuable lessons for sports professionals and scientists in constructing personalized recovery plans that facilitate enduring peak performance. Whether it is a lineman in football or iconic figures in baseball, these individual stories illuminate the intricate balance between training, competition, and recovery, affirming the necessity of a nuanced approach guided by evidence-based assessments and interventions.

A tailored approach to recovery, which encompasses various domains like nutrition, physical therapy, sleep management, and conditioning, has enabled these athletes to sustain top performance levels over extended careers. It emphasizes the multifaceted nature of recovery and the importance of personalized, evidence-based strategies.

However, there's a growing awareness of potential discrepancies in applying these strategies. The challenge lies in ensuring that recovery methods are not only understood but effectively implemented by athletes. Even with the best intentions and the most advanced technology, gaps may still exist between what is known by scientists and coaches and what is applied by athletes.

Emphasizing the need for education and collaboration, a translational approach can bridge these gaps, fostering continuous dialogue and collaboration between scientists, coaches, and athletes. This synergy ensures that the broad spectrum of assessments employed leads to the most effective and efficient recovery strategies, enhancing athletic performance.

In conclusion, while recovery is undoubtedly vital, an excessive focus without adequate testing may lead to suboptimal outcomes. Modern approaches increasingly recognize the significance of individualized and evidence-based recovery strategies. The examples of men and women across various sports demonstrate that with the right combination of technology, multidisciplinary collaboration, and education, recovery can be tailored to meet the unique needs of each athlete, leading to remarkable performance and resilience in the most demanding competitive environments.

Sleep

Over the past ten years, sleep has become essential for high performers, from those in the military to front-line professionals and athletes. Specific attention has been given to sleep in sport science (French and Torres Ronda 2022). Additionally, monitoring systems have evolved the ability to assess sleep more effectively to provide insight to athletes regarding their sleep behavior. This is an essential element for the player development team to address for each sport and each athlete.

Sport performance depends on quick reactions and brain function at high speeds of movement. One study tells a cautionary tale about the effect of sleep loss or poor sleep behavior. The effect of sleep loss and the difficulty of making it up in a day or two was reported in a classic study from the division of neuropsychiatry at the Walter Reed Army Institute of Research. Investigators demonstrated that the body could adapt and recover quickly from sleep loss, but brain function is compromised in its rate and ability to respond and takes much longer to recover from accumulated sleep loss (Belenky et al. 2003). It also takes several days to return to normal function, even with 8 to 9 hours a night (figure 7.2). It has also become evident that 7 hours is not enough sleep per night, and athletes are getting far less. Sleep has become the new ergogenic aid of the 21st century.

Effective Interventions for Enhancing Recovery

Various recovery interventions, from nutrition to recovery technologies, have been developed and promoted with exponential advances in engineering and technology (figure 7.3). Elite sport organizations are now creating recovery centers or units, a concept put forth many years ago at the United States Olympic Training Center in the 1990s. The player development team must evaluate each athlete for expense, time demands, acceptability, and scientific evidence for effectiveness in producing enhanced recovery of a particular variable (e.g., soreness, performance, and biological variables). Counterproductive to recovery, especially because

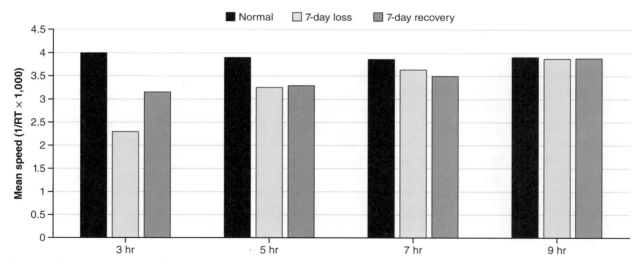

FIGURE 7.2 Mean speed of brain recovery reaction time. Black bars = normal 8 to 9 hours of sleep; light gray = 1 week of sleep loss; dark gray = after 7 days of recovery sleep of 8 to 9 hours. Sleep loss can affect the brain's reaction time. Even 7 days of recovery with a normal 8 to 9 hours of sleep per night may not be adequate to recover the brain function that is so important for performance and cognitive functions. While other performance functions may recover more quickly or be tolerated, sleep loss and brain function do not track on the same recovery timeline.

Adapted from Belenky et al., "Patterns of Performance Degradation and Restoration During Sleep Restriction and Subsequent Recovery: A Sleep Dose-Response Study," *Journal of Sleep Research* 12 (2003): 1-12.

Dry float	Cryotherapy	Thermotherapy	Pneumatic compression
Wet float	Mindfulness	Contrast water therapy	Compression garments
Sleep	Yoga	Therapeutic ultrasound	Massage
Water	Foam rollers	Phonophoresis	Instrumented soft tissue manipulation
Cryocompression	Massage	Bone stimulators	Cupping
Electrical stimulation	Hydro baths	Photobiomodulation	Dry needling
Nutritional supplements	Stretching	Iontophoresis	Hot therapy

FIGURE 7.3 Different recovery technologies enhance the body's abilities to repair and remodel structures and functions.

of high levels of blunt force trauma to the tissues, are alcohol and aspirin, which can delay healing and promote bleeding.

Popular Recovery Technologies

The cost of many new recovery intervention technologies exceeds the budgets of athletes and player development programs. Many coaches look first at less expensive recovery techniques (e.g., stretching or foam rollers) (Pernigoni et al. 2022). Yet the study of recovery and the field itself are quickly moving toward technologically advanced tools, especially at elite levels of competition. Awareness and assessments by the player development team when discussing new innovations are vital. Many of these interventions are still early in their scientific study but still deserve awareness. Each unit in the player development team must know where to find expertise for the many different recovery technologies. This is an overview of the many passive recovery technologies athletes use for recovery (Cullen, Casazza, and Davis 2021). The player development team must make decisions about which innovations to invest in, how the athletes will be educated on their use, and what unit will implement and manage the technology. Again, evidence-based practices will be necessary along with team communication as these technologies are implemented. Many times, different recovery strategies and technologies will be used by each team. Due to the rapid lines of communication among athletes in an organization, each team must know why they are or are not using a particular recovery technology.

As shown in figure 7.3, there are many different technologies and programs to enhance recovery processes in athletes. Knowing about these interventions is vital. Coaches often attempt to "throw everything but the kitchen sink" at the problem or process, hoping to see a positive effect. Trial and error is discussed in this book, but the player development team should use evidence-based practices to determine what technological investments might be appropriate and how and for what they should be used in the recovery or treatment processes.

In another example, an athletic trainer dealing with a large team of athletes after practice gives each athlete coming into the training room a cup of ice and sends them over to a table or corner to rub the ice on their injured limbs as a type of triage until the athletic trainer can take care of each athlete, knowing that the ice will not be very effective, but demand can outweigh the availability of support staff

While beyond the scope of this book, it is vital to be aware of some of the popular recovery technologies increasingly used in player development as important additions to the recovery process. Each targets a different system in the recovery process. The literature base for each is different, and there is a need to evaluate what is being recovered from (e.g., the amount of damage, type of damage, sex, age, and training level) in any evaluation by the player development team.

Stretching

One of the most studied and essential phases of training and recovery is stretching (Ratamess 2022). Stretching focuses on movement ranges of motion and affects muscle and connective tissues (Culav, Clark, and Merrilees 1999). Static, proprioceptive neuromuscular facilitation (PNF), and dynamic stretching are used to improve flexibility and help break up damaged lesions in recovery. Stretching is a hallmark of treatment in physical therapy and athletic training. Various stretching protocols that have been extensively studied can be used and are essential during any recovery phase after workouts and competition. The type of stretching and forms of warm-ups and cooldowns with stretching have been challenged, regarding the importance, use, and context (Afonso, Olivares-Jabalera, and Andrade 2021). While controversial, the use of static stretching as a warm-up prior to power or speed training has usually been discouraged (Nelson et al. 2005; Nelson, Kokkonen, and Arnall 2005; Shrier 2004; Shrier and McHugh 2012). It is generally a prudent approach when the stretch-shortening cycle is highly operational and when the velocity of movement is key because static stretching may well stretch the non-contractile elements (it can take about 10 minutes to reconfigure the different matrices in muscles, tendons, and ligaments) (Torres et al. 2008). Dynamic stretching should be used in warm-ups and static stretch and PNF approaches in cooldowns for recovery.

Massage

In the late 1970s, massage became popular and a demand for licensed massage therapists arose. The demand for a single massage therapist on an American football team became so great that the coach said, "OK, when you are as good as [an All-American and Heisman Trophy candidate], then you can have a massage," showing how the demand for therapeutic intervention can dramatically outweigh the supply for an entire team. There are many types of massage (e.g., Swedish, deep tissue, sport, reflexology, and Shiatsu), many of which have not been scientifically studied in the context of exercise or athletic performance. The player development team must put its findings into context when studying massage and evaluating what type to use. To date, a variety of massage techniques have been used in training rooms because such therapies have been shown to help the athletes feel better after exercise, which, as noted in a review, is one of the evidence-based positive outcomes (Sriwongtong et al. 2020). While they have not been shown to improve performance directly, different massage techniques may help to improve flexibility and delayed onset muscle soreness (Davis, Alabed, and Chico 2020). Any physiological benefits at the neurological, cellular, or tissue levels remain to be demonstrated. Still, the positive psychological benefits of athletes "feeling good" have supported massage as a helpful recovery technique.

Foam Rolling

Often thought of as a type of self-massage, foam rolling has gained popularity over the past twenty years. Foam rolling has been a staple in every conditioning facility and is used before, during, and after exercise. There are many foam rollers of various sizes (e.g., smooth, textured, vibrating, and heated). A review took an in-depth look at foam rolling and its effect on exercise performance and recovery benefits (Wiewelhove et al. 2019). Its use as a recovery tool has been questioned, with research indicating that it may be more of a warm-up tool (Wiewelhove et al. 2019). A further in-depth review of its performance effects shows that it has little effect on performance measures (Konrad, Nakamura, and Behm 2022). Nevertheless, foam rollers as recovery interventions are used in conditioning programs during cooldowns with flexibility training.

Foam rolling is a form of self-massage called a *self-myofascial release* technique (Michalski et al. 2022). Essentially foam rolling is thought to help prevent muscle adhesions, help blood flow, and theoretically reduce inflammation and soreness in muscles and joints. While more research is needed on the mechanisms, it appears to affect the nervous system receptors in the various tissues and helps relaxation for improved movement. It can sometimes be uncomfortable, and thus vibration, heated, and cold foam rollers have been technologically developed as a prophylactic influence when used.

Nutrition

The diet of the athlete is a vital aspect of player development, and the nutritional experts on the player development team must deal with this area that is so important for optimal recovery. The amount of work in sport nutrition is overwhelming: There are over 30,000 citations on this term alone in PUB MED and multitudes of books. For a review of the basics of sport and exercise nutrition, refer to these books (Campbell 2020; Kraemer, Fleck, and Deschenes 2021; Ratamess 2022).

The essential aspects of a nutritional program are related to the number of calories and the quality of the dietary intakes. Diets for weight loss and weight gain also need to be carefully constructed by the sport nutritional dietetic unit. Variations in diet, such as vegetarian, vegan, and keto, also need to be carefully examined for proper implementation and supplement needs. Mistakes can be made in these diets despite their scientific validity. The ketogenic diet is popular, especially for aerobic endurance events and long-distance events, and its applications in other sports is also starting to become apparent insofar as it relates to concussion and cognitive therapies (Volek and Phinney 2012; Volek et al. 2016). Athletes use vegetarian and vegan diets, which have been observed to provide some physiological advantages for aerobic endurance performance but may not be optimal for resistance training for maximal strength and performance (Pohl et al. 2021). Such diets alter molecular signaling via leucine, creatine, DHA, and EPA, directly altering skeletal muscle adaptations (Pohl et al. 2021). The nutritional unit of the player development team must examine the diet pattern of each athlete carefully. Again, individualization is essential.

Hydration

Hydration has been a focus in sports for some time now, combined with concerns about sudden death from heat illness. A review examines in depth the practical strategies for hydration in athletes (Belval et al. 2019). Again, each athlete has a personalized hydration strategy for optimizing performance, training, and safety. The strategy will be specific to the environment, the event or conditioning workout, and what practices need to be employed. The role of hydration, as well as the management of heat toleration and heat illnesses that can lead to injury or sudden death, has been extensively examined by inter-association task forces and requires careful examination by the player development team (Casa et al. 2013; Casa et al. 2012).

Nutritional Supplementation

It is crucial that the player development team carefully vet nutritional supplements for banned substances per the sport organization's governance body (e.g., WADA, USADA, and NCAA). The team must ensure that validated entities have tested commercial products (e.g., Informed Choice for banned substances). Over the past decades, the study of nutritional supplements to assist in recovery from exercise, including resistance exercise and aerobic endurance exercise, has been overwhelming in scientific literature. Supplements have been studied extensively, and the most effective supplements have been protein supplements, creatine, multiple vitamins (especially vitamin D), omega-3, L-carnitine, beta-alanine, and hydration and electrolyte drinks (see the sidebar on page 197). Supplements have timing elements for optimal use. They have been shown to augment recovery after workouts, practice, and competition.

A wide variety of sports medicine interventions can play a role in recovery processes, which can include anything from recovery of soreness and tissue damage from regular training and competition to actual injury that would be taken care of by the sports medicine unit of the player development team. See the list below taken in part from (Statuta and Pugh 2019). Each member of the player development team must be trained and qualified to administer treatments. These interventions are readily available and commonly used, but each intervention or modality still requires informed clinical judgment before application. Interventions include the following:

- *Cryotherapy:* ice bags, cold-water immersion, and cold-water circulating units
- *Thermotherapy:* to increase tissue temperature (e.g., moist heat pack, warm water immersion, and paraffin bath)
- *Contrast water therapy:* alternating extremity or full-body immersion in hot and cold water
- *Therapeutic ultrasound:* acoustic energy, delivered at particularly high frequencies,

> ### Yale Bulldogs Protein Smoothie
>
> During the 2018 American football season, the sport performance staff at Yale University took steps to address the nutritional needs of their athletes by implementing smoothies during the season. With the help of Dr. Cathy Saenz, PhD, RD, from The Ohio State University, a smoothie recipe was developed. Affectionately known by the Yale Bulldogs football team as "Puppy Chow," this involved the production of over 210 16-ounce (473 mL) cups of smoothies each day. The sport performance team would eventually streamline the process so that a trained group of coaches could make 210 smoothies in just 15 minutes. This lightning-fast production was central to integrating the administration of the shakes in the time allotted by the coaching staff. Data from previous seasons had indicated that some athletes were experiencing decreases in body mass, power production, and lean muscle tissue as a result of insufficient caloric intake. The success of this protocol was evident in the improved athletic performance and body composition of the team members. In fact, the smoothie production protocol was so effective that other teams began to implement similar shakes as part of their nutrition plans. Overall, the protocol played a key role in the success of the Yale football team by helping to support the nutritional needs of the athletes and optimize their performance. According to Dr. Saenz, "it is important to start slow [in incorporating the smoothie in a diet] as it is made with fresh or whole ingredients so it may be higher fiber than the athletes are used to. Plus, coconut oil and avocado should be started in lower dosages since they can impact the GI, especially if the athlete isn't used to them. Both reasons are why I recommend they start with small amounts to avoid any potential GI distress in the beginning. They can make up the calories by just breaking them up throughout the day as opposed to all at once." (Cathy Saenz, PhD, RD, CSCS, personal communication).
>
> **Recipe and Nutritional Information**
>
> | Ingredient | Quantity | Calories | Carbs (g) | Fat (g) | Protein (g) |
> |---|---|---|---|---|---|
> | Peanut butter | 2 tablespoons (32 g) | 180 | 8 | 15 | 7 |
> | Banana, medium | 1.5 | 158 | 41 | 1 | 0 |
> | Whole milk (3.25% milk fat) | 1 cup (237 mL) | 146 | 11 | 8 | 8 |
> | Rolled oats | 0.5 cup (40 g) | 150 | 27 | 3 | 5 |
> | Cinnamon | 1 teaspoon (2.5 g) | 6 | 2 | 0 | 0 |
> | Olive oil | 1.5 tablespoons (22 mL) | 180 | 0 | 21 | 0 |
> | Ice | 0.5 cup (118 cc) | 0 | 0 | 0 | 0 |
> | Water | 1 cup (237 mL) | 0 | 0 | 0 | 0 |
> | Totals | | 820 | 89 | 48 | 20 |

to create thermal or nonthermal changes in tissue
- *Phonophoresis:* using sound energy to drive medication—commonly some form of anti-inflammatory medication—through the patient's skin
- *Bone stimulators:* low-intensity pulsed ultrasound stimulators
- *Electrical stimulation:* transcutaneous electrical nerve stimulation [TENS] applies an electrical current to target specific tissues in the body
- *Iontophoresis:* direct electrical current to deliver medication to the target tissue
- *Photobiomodulation:* new technology using red and near-infrared light (non-ultraviolet)

transmitted through the skin to reach intracellular structures, stimulating a chain reaction to accelerate healing by stimulating biological reactions, ranging from metabolic to blood flow and neurogenesis

- *Compression:* application of compression to limit local swelling and edema
- *Pneumatic compression device:* commercial units use compressed air to provide compression through an extremity-specific wrap or sleeve
- *Compression garments:* athletic clothing marketed by companies, often for the lower body
- *Massage:* a variety of manual therapies used to promote soft tissue healing
- *Instrumented soft tissue manipulation:* specially designed instruments to mobilize soft tissue
- *Cupping:* myofascial decompression, commonly known as cupping therapy, applies suction to the skin through the use of a hollow container
- *Dry needling:* insertion of thin monofilament needles, such as those used in acupuncture, in the treatment of myofascial trigger points

Compression Garments

Compression has traditionally been used to treat athletic injuries (e.g., an ankle sprain) or offer support (e.g., hosiery) for aging populations. Some groundbreaking investigations found that compression garments (e.g., shorts) had performance benefits, including improving proprioception and helping in recovery from exercise damage resulting from resistance training workouts (Kraemer et al. 2010; Kraemer et al. 1996). Long-wear compression garments constructed with the optimal Lycra or Spandex content (e.g., 24% to 28%) became more than a fashion statement. The impact on actual performance was less clear for running events (da Silva et al. 2018). Super suits with very high compression worn by powerlifters added significant mechanical support, allowing for higher lift totals (Wilk, Krzysztofk, and Bialas 2020). Using long-wear garments was then found to benefit recovery from long-distance jet travel stress and exercise damage (Kraemer et al. 2016). This may be important since an increasing number of competitions span time zones, and travel stress can last a few days.

Cryocompression

Compression alone can cause pain and discomfort in the early phases of the repair and remodeling process as edema (i.e., water) is pushed back into circulation, protecting the integrity of the muscle cell membranes (Kraemer et al. 2001). Circulating ice water allowed for a prophylactic effect while the compression prevented the structures from swelling. The acute use of 20 minutes of cryocompression using compression apparel with circulating ice water after a workout and again the next day has been effective (DuPont et al. 2017). It has demonstrated reductions in soreness, pain, muscle damage markers, and power performance 24 and 48 hours after a resistance exercise workout (DuPont et al. 2017). However, with the use of pneumatic cryocompression after acute exposure, performance is reduced; thus, the timing of cold exposure is vital in the use of the intervention (Alexander et al. 2022).

Cold-Water Immersion and Light and Heat Therapy

Various cryotherapies have been used, from rapid freezing of the entire body to ice water baths, to theoretically enhance neuromuscular recovery. Research on cold water baths shows it is fantastic for dealing with heat stress or after a hot environmental workout, along with being an obvious treatment for heat illnesses. Our experience with whole-body cold-water immersion, so popular in athlete culture over the past decade, has shown it to be effectual. Still, its use under exercise conditions in which heat is not a factor has been questioned because it causes in men acute reduction in testosterone concentrations, which is important for anabolic signaling after a resistance training workout (Earp et al. 2019).

Furthermore, full-body cryofreezing is still in its early phases of study regarding its possible benefits and how to use it (Cullen, Casazza, and

Davis 2021). Petrofsky and colleagues showed that strength recovery is demonstrated at different time frames with cold and heat therapies, with cold being superior to heat when used immediately after exercise and 24 hours later to reduce pain. Still, both appear to help in reducing muscle damage (Petrofsky et al. 2015).

A review of cryotherapy and the relatively new therapy of photobiomodulation (a form of light therapy that uses light sources, including lasers, LEDs, and broadband light for the relief of pain and muscle recovery) showed no observed differences in oxidative stress and inflammatory levels (Ferlito et al. 2022; Ailioaie and Litscher 2021). However, their findings suggested that the use of photobiomodulation in muscle recovery after high-intensity exercise is beneficial, provides a clinically significant effect, and seems to be a viable option.

Examining heat and cold therapies in another comprehensive review, Wang and colleagues (Wang et al. 2022) concluded that more research is needed due to limitations in the current literature but found that meta-analysis results showed the following:

- Within 24 hours after exercise, the hot pack was the most effective for pain relief, followed by contrast water therapy
- Within 48 hours, the ranking was hot pack, followed by the novel modality of cryotherapy
- Over 48 hours after exercise, the effect of the novel modality of cryotherapy ranked first

In a comprehensive review, Kim and colleagues showed that local heat therapy could accelerate recovery of exercise-induced muscle damage. Local heat therapies include a variety of modalities (e.g., shortwave diathermy, water-circulating garments, heat wraps, and whirlpool therapy) (Kim, Monroe et al. 2020). These methods allow for specific muscle groups or body parts to be heated with minimal or no changes in core temperature. Heat before exercise may protect against muscle damage and enhance tissue remodeling. It has been shown that heat may increase anabolic and cellular signaling (Kim, Reid et al. 2020).

Flotation Therapies

The use of flotation therapies, or flotation-restricted environmental stimulation therapy, has gained popularity in commercial settings to promote relaxation and reduce stress. Anecdotal data found that elite military special operators and elite athletes benefited from the therapy. Therefore, elite athletes and special operators in the military have gravitated to this modality for similar reasons having to do with training and competition stress (Drillera and Argusbc 2016). It has gained acceptance in the medical community and has shown reductions in pain and anxiety and increased relaxation in patients (Loose et al. 2021).

"Wet float" and a new form called "dry float" are based on the concept that one can promote sympathetic and parasympathetic balance and promote deep relaxation and recovery by eliminating all external stimuli. Research on this modality is in the early phases of study, and has yet to answer many questions, including how long to float, what stimuli in the session are allowed, how many sessions are needed, when to float, and differences between float types. The most common float therapy is wet float. Ideally, the wet float is accomplished in a tank made soundproof and dark to remove all stimuli. The tank or room must be big enough for the individual so that one's body parts do not touch the walls of the tank or room while floating. The high saline water content allows one to float with the head above the water line effortlessly. Ideally, the room is dark and the individual floats nude with water equal to the body temperature to remove all mechanical stimuli. This quickly leads to a euphoric state of relaxation. Float times have ranged from 25 to 90 minutes, with 60 minutes being the most common.

Dry float has gained popularity because one only has to lie on a dry membrane filled with warm water that is then lowered into a twin-sized bed. One can wear clothing but should remove all jewelry and objects from pockets. Thus, one floats without getting wet. There is no lid, so one does not feel encapsulated, as in some wet tanks. Again, there is an attempt to simulate the feeling of zero gravity and move one into a state of deep relaxation. At this point, comparisons of float types have been limited, but anecdotal data indicate that they provide similar perceptual experiences for some people. Still, the underlying physiological changes between the two are unclear at best.

Few studies have examined athletes and even fewer have studied performance effects, but its primary benefit is improved recovery of mind and body. A study in our laboratory of highly resistance-trained men showed a reduction in perceptual soreness from training (Caldwell et al. 2022). There was also a reduction in norepinephrine and higher testosterone levels when compared to controls, indicating physiological signaling effects from 60 minutes of wet float. In our continued work, we have found that familiarization is needed to calm any fears. Athletes quickly learn how to float effectively in one session. In one survey, we found that only 4 people out of 2,000 felt worse, most likely due to starting in a balanced state. We have seen a few negative float experiences, such as in subjects who heard their heart rate for the first time or were claustrophobic in the tank or room. We have used 60 minutes of floating in the nude and in the dark to remove all external stimuli. We have also found that floating in the morning before any exercise or practice beneficially reduces cortisol and sympathetic drive. We have also found that if, from other measures, there is no increased sympathetic drive and everything is in balance, the wet float can drive up the sympathetic system. Differences between wet and dry float appear similar but no definitive studies have been done.

Meditation and Mindfulness

Various meditation types (e.g., mindfulness, transcendental, spiritual, mantra) are used to reduce stress and help the athlete's mental recovery. Again, training in each method, including deep relaxation, is necessary to succeed. Sport meditation is gaining increased interest and is evolving for athletes by using theoretical insights into imagery, relaxation, and self-talk. This may help develop a new form of meditation program, apart from conventional meditation approaches (Kim and Kim 2021). Mindfulness (e.g., focused on the moment) is another popular form of meditation used by athletes. It has been shown to be most helpful in recovering from mental fatigue (Cao et al. 2022).

Training Approaches for Different Elements in Player Development

A multi-modality training approach works best for all athletes. Whether the athlete is an aerobic, anaerobic, or hybrid athlete, the proper integration and periodization of multiple training modalities is highly recommended for optimal player development. These modalities include training for maximal strength, power, balance, hypertrophy (when necessary), speed, agility and change-of-direction ability, flexibility and mobility, muscular endurance and buffering capacity, and aerobic endurance ($\dot{V}O_2$max, lactate threshold, and exercise economy).

The basic underlying tenets of designing strength and conditioning programs for progression in any fitness component for any athlete are progressive overload, specificity, and variation. These tenets can be applied to all training programs in numerous ways provided that they form the template of design. In addition, the importance of proper supervision cannot be overemphasized; we have shown that direct supervision of training leads to greater improvements in fitness components (Mazzetti et al. 2000).

Progressive overload refers to the gradual increase in stress placed on the body during training and may be accomplished by the following:

- The loading may be increased.
- Repetitions may be added to current loading.
- Lifting velocity (and the intent to lift fast) may be increased once the technique is mastered. For velocity-based training, one may increase velocity per loading scheme, alter the percentage of velocity loss to terminate a set, or change the load-velocity prescription.
- Rest intervals may be altered depending on the goal (e.g., lengthened to enable greater loading or reduced to decrease recovery and target muscular endurance).
- Training volume may be increased within reasonable limits (2% to 5%) primarily in the progression from novice to intermediate training (advanced to elite training encompasses a range of training volumes that depend on the goals of the phase).

- The source of resistance can be manipulated, or exercise selection can be altered to stress muscles in different ways. For example, one may add bands or chains to barbell exercises, use equipment that provides unstable resistance, such as sandbags or kegs, and cycle different exercises into the program.
- Advanced techniques (described later in this chapter) or methods of supramaximal loading may be used for trained athletes.
- For flexibility training, the intensity (level of discomfort), volume, duration of stretching, and frequency can be increased. One can also use progression—from isolation-type stretches to multiple-joint and total-body stretches and movements—and PNF stretching (see the section on flexibility for a description).
- For foam rolling, one can use denser objects or place more body weight on the roller during each repetition, as well as increase repetitions, duration, and the number of sets.
- For power, speed, and agility training, the intensity, volume (and frequency), and rest intervals can be altered. More complex exercises can be introduced and resistance (e.g., weighted vest, bands, and sleds) may be used. Increased and longer or higher jumps (and boxes) or throws may be used to increase intensity. For plyometrics, transitions from bilateral exercises to unilateral exercises can be used. Rest intervals can be altered to target speed, agility, and power or high-intensity endurance (e.g., repeated sprint ability and power endurance). Heavier balls could be used for throws.
- For aerobic endurance training, one may increase volume, duration, and intensity and decrease rest intervals. For time trials, greater distances can be covered. Higher-intensity intervals are very effective for improving conditioning. Each modality, which can be altered, provides the athlete with a unique conditioning stimulus.

Specificity refers to the fact that each training adaptation is specific to the stimulus applied. Although nonspecific improvements or transferred training effects take place, most improvements will be specific to the stimuli. Training adaptations are specific to the muscle actions involved, velocity of movement and rate of force development (RFD), ROM, muscle groups trained, energy metabolism, movement pattern, and intensity and volume of training.

Variation entails alteration of one or more program variables over time to keep the stimulus optimal. Because the human body adapts rapidly to exercise, variation is critical for long-term improvements. Workouts can be varied in infinite ways and the variation should match the athlete's training phase. The player development team should have a wide array of strategies for progression and individualization for each athlete. Periodized training programs are designed for planning variation in the form of different training phases. The best training programs include multiple forms of progressive overload, specificity, and variation in the program design.

Training for Maximal Strength

Training to maximize muscular strength is best accomplished by an integrated approach that targets multiple levels of force generation. The foundation of strength training is increasing 1RM strength in key structural exercises while gaining as much strength as possible for other assistance exercises. In addition, muscular strength is multidimensional, so coaches and athletes should target specific elements of strength (e.g., speed strength, reactive strength, ECC, and ISOM strength) around 1RM strength. As discussed in chapters 2 and 3, muscle strength, or the highest level of force produced, is specific to the:

- velocity
- muscle action (ECC > ISOM > CON)
- movement or exercise
- type of limb activation (unilateral, bilateral)
- ROM
- transition from ECC to CON action (reactive strength)

Comprehensive resistance training for strength entails targeting all elements of force production in a periodized manner. The ability to generate strength is important for all types of movement. Muscular strength is dependent on the size and arrangement of muscle fibers, the neural drive to muscles (e.g., increased motor unit recruitment based on the size principle and the rate and timing of discharge), musculotendinous stiffness, and possible adaptations to increased metabolites.

Multiple training modalities can increase various strength dynamics. However, resistance training is the best way to maximize strength development because it provides numerous exercises and equipment, is easily quantifiable, and enables many ways to progress. The critical component to optimal resistance training is the design of the program, in addition to the motivation and dedication of the athlete in following the program consistently. As discussed previously, a resistance training program is a composite of the acute program variables that interact with each other to provide a stimulus for adaptation. Because there are infinite ways to vary and design resistance training programs, many programs can be successful if they adhere to the general training guidelines already discussed. In this section we discuss manipulating the program variables to target maximal strength development in accordance with the latest scientific guidelines (American College of Sports 2009; Kraemer and Ratamess 2004). These guidelines and the finer points of program design are discussed in a way that will give the coach and athlete a framework from which to build a template.

The foundation of resistance training for maximal strength is the proper selection of exercises. The exercises play a large role in the transfer of gains in muscular strength to athletic performance. Each exercise variation needs to be treated as a separate exercise because any change will affect muscle activation and leverage, resulting in differences in the amount of weight lifted and number of repetitions performed. Exercise selection is affected by a number of factors, such as the following:

- The targeted muscle actions (CON, ECC, ISOM)
- Size and number of muscle groups targeted
- Goals of each exercise (e.g., maximal strength, functional strength, and imbalance correction)
- Equipment availability, source of loading, and loading vector
- Posture and body position
- Widths and positions of grip and stance
- Unilateral, bilateral, or alternate movements
- Intent to isolate muscle groups or target specific movements with resistance
- Biomechanics, with reference to using progressions for body weight exercises
- Efficacy of the exercise for strengthening muscles based on the needs of the athlete

Dynamic exercises consist of CON and ECC muscle actions with brief ISOM periods in between phases. Ultimately, all loads selected for conventional sets are based mostly on the CON phase of the ECC/CON rep, which is the weakest of the muscle actions and ROM-specific (i.e., affected by a sticking point or point where bar velocity is minimal). Special emphasis must be given to ECC and ISOM actions when needed, and there are a number of ways to do so:

- Slowing the ECC phase prior to performing the CON action
- Using heavier loading on the ECC phase and less loading on the CON phase (with devices such as hooks or special machines)
- Using heavy *negatives* or only performing the ECC phase with heavier loading
- Using forced negatives with partner resistance added to the weight
- For an exercise such as the pull-up or pistol squat (where one repetition is challenging and the athlete is working on building strength to perform multiple repetitions), the athlete may lower their body during the ECC phase and use a machine, partner, or assistance device to be lifted during the CON phase
- Using unilateral negatives (performing the CON phase with two arms or legs but lowering the weight with one arm or leg, usually on a machine or device that allows the loading to remain balanced)
- Use of variable resistance devices such as bands and chains (which also target CON phase as well)

Athletes new to resistance training should focus on the light to moderate loading when learning new exercises so that loading matches the CON strength level. As each exercise is performed with greater loading and the athlete develops higher levels of maximal strength, some sets may emphasize and target the ECC phase. This is particularly helpful for total strength development because greater ECC strength assists in increased musculotendinous stiffness and the mechanical efficiency needed for power development. ECC training is also effective as a treatment for tendinosis and for increasing connective tissue strength.

ISOM muscle actions exist in many forms during resistance training, and ISOM strength is an element needed by many athletes in certain sports. Examples of ISOM actions and the need for high levels of ISOM strength include the following:

- Stabilizer muscles contract ISOM to maintain posture and stability during an exercise.
- ISOM actions occur in between ECC and CON actions for the agonist muscles, and vice versa. For example, the bench press has ISOM actions during the lockout position and when the bar is on the chest. Pausing at the top may assist slightly with intra-set recovery, while pausing at the bottom makes the exercise more difficult by reducing stretch-shortening cycle (SSC) activity (an action trained for by a powerlifter or other athlete targeting ROM-specific ISOM strength).
- Grip training for support, especially during pulling exercises.
- ISOM actions can serve as the primary exercise actions in a specific area of the ROM, such as plank, overhead squat (upper body), mid-thigh pulls, and other anti-gravity or anti-rotation exercises.
- Position-hold ISOM exercises for a number of exercises (loaded or body weight) where a position within the dynamic ROM may be held for several seconds (e.g., ISOM push-up, wall squat, and pull-up).
- Functional ISOM training, such as lifting a barbell (as hard as possible) in a power rack a few inches until it is pressing or pulling up against the rack's pins (set at a desired position) for approximately 2 to 6 seconds.

ISOM training is accomplished by performing pulling exercises or using the aforementioned techniques. Coaches should incorporate ISOM training according to the needs of the athlete. For example, American football players, gymnasts, and athletes in grappling and strength performance sports require high levels of grip strength. Grip training exercises must be included for complete athletic development. Athletes involved in jumping sports (where Olympic lifting variations are used) benefit from the mid-thigh pull, not only as an assessment but as an exercise with the ability to transfer to total-body power. Strengthening the core region for all athletes is paramount in training; thus, including ISOM core stability exercises is necessary because of the relationship between core strength and other performance measures. In some cases, ECC- or ISOM-targeted exercises may be overlooked, but they are important and highly recommended for training progression (American College of Sports 2009).

Historically, traditional resistance exercises were prescribed to target specific muscle groups or regions of the body. In the last several decades, exercise selection has expanded to include loading exercises that mimic sport movements rather than specific muscle groups. These movement-specific, or functional, exercises are intended to have high transfer of training effects to athletic movements. Thus, both types of resistance exercises are recommended for athletes and may be further classified as single- or multiple-joint. *Single-joint exercises* target one joint action or major muscle group, whereas *multiple-joint exercises* target more than one joint action or major muscle group with the potential to stress several major muscle groups. In reality, every exercise stresses many muscle groups, due to the role of stability, even when one muscle group is isolated. However, the classifications are based on the targeted actions. The load distribution on the body is more dispersed when multiple muscle groups are involved. Both single-joint and multiple-joint exercises lead to strength gains, but multiple-joint exercises should form the core of the resistance training program. They are more complex and involve greater technical efficiency, but they also enable the athlete to move greater loading, which is paramount to training for maximal strength. Exercises (and variations of them) such as the squat, bench press, shoulder press, deadlift, power clean, snatch, lunge, and various rowing and pulling movements have formed the basis of successful strength and conditioning programs targeting strength and power athletes. Their benefits extend to aerobic endurance athletes as well. Multiple-joint exercises may be subclassified as basic strength (e.g., squat and bench press), total-body (e.g., Olympic lifts and Turkish get-up), and combination (two or more exercises combined into a sequential movement used to increase muscle mass involvement, energy expenditure, and oxygen consumption) exercises. Total-body exercises are the most complex and take the longest to learn correct technique. In addition, Olympic lifts are highly effective for increasing power because they require rapid force production and fast bodily movements (Comfort et al., 2023). They are best taught in logical progressions rather than all at once (see Comfort et al., 2023 for more detail).

Figure 7.4 depicts a basic progression with associated goals for each exercise variation. It is important to note that other exercise variations can be used to assist in teaching or fixing a technical issue. Coaches should always stress proper technique for all phases of each exercise, especially as weight is added during progression.

Exercise selection is affected by other factors as well. For example, performing exercises unilaterally or bilaterally adds another dimension to resistance training. Skeletal muscle recruitment patterns vary when exercises are performed unilaterally, bilaterally, alternating, and when they involve limb movements that work in opposition or cross the midline of the body. Training unilaterally can increase muscular strength in both trained and opposite limbs, while training bilaterally increases strength on both sides. Unilateral exercises require greater balance and stability and require greater activity from the trunk muscles due to asymmetric loading. Both bilateral and unilateral exercises should be included in the training programs of athletes. Another consideration is the type of training equipment available. Figure 7.5 depicts a strength and conditioning toolbox in which different pieces of equipment are at the disposal of the player development team. All have potential advantages for use in strength and conditioning

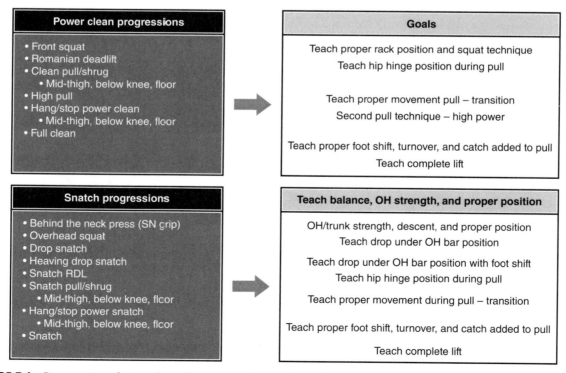

FIGURE 7.4 Progressions for teaching the power clean and snatch exercises.

programs (Ratamess 2022). The coaches may use several of these to provide the athlete with training variation. Collectively, these pieces of equipment provide the athlete with the following:

- Multiple levels and styles of loading
- Unbalanced resistance and shifting resistance (fluid and sand)
- An unstable surface to perform exercises on
- Controlled ROM and movement trajectory
- Variable resistance
- Sport-specific loading
- Oscillations and vibration
- Multiple or varied loading vectors
- Multi-planar movement capacity
- Altered leverage, diameter, and gripping to enhance grip strength or alter exercise dynamics

A comprehensive resistance training program for athletes will be focused on structural free weight multiple-joint exercises. Assistance and sport-specific exercises (single- and multiple-joint) can be performed with free weights, body weight, or any of the pieces of equipment mentioned previously, in an auxiliary manner. The key for the player development team is the selection and subsequent periodization of exercises for the training program. Although some key structural exercises may remain throughout the macrocycle, athletes benefit from exposure to multiple stimuli. Exercises may be varied within a periodized cycle plan to avoid plateaus and target movements and muscle groups in different ways to match training goals and sport demands. Coaches may identify key structural exercises (e.g., squat, bench press, and Olympic lift variations) and focus the program on them as key strength builders. These same exercises are often selected for strength testing. It is not advisable to remove these exercises for extended periods of time, given their importance in development. For example, some coaches form off-season training around the back squat but then remove it during in-season training. There may be a detraining effect from removing such exercises

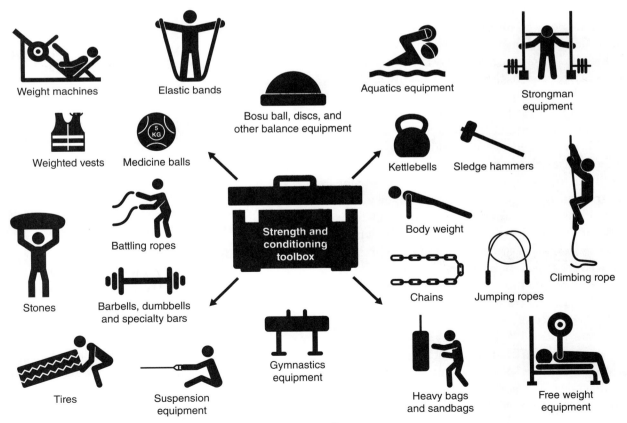

FIGURE 7.5 The strength and conditioning equipment toolbox.

(if there is not an adequate replacement, similar in technique and loading parameters) that could transfer to sport performance. Detraining effects from multijoint exercise removal could carry over to other resistance exercises as well. Thus, key multijoint exercises form the base of the program and exercise periodization may prosper in the orbit of exercises selected for assistance. Including an assistance exercise in a period of 4 to 6 weeks or more allows for progression and may be sufficient for adaptation. Some exercises are more easily maintained or resistant to detraining than others if the intensity of training is moderately high to high. These exercises can be cycled without fear of performance reduction so long as structural exercises are emphasized. Thus, the player development team has numerous effective exercises to choose from to complement structural multijoint resistance exercises.

Exercise selection is a critical component of resistance training, but the exercises need to be structured in a logistic manner to develop a workout and program. Many athletes incorporate exercises that target all major muscle groups. These workouts are referred to as *total-body workouts* (where single- and multijoint exercises target the entire body in sequence or total-body exercises are included). Some athletes may divide workouts into separate sessions that predominately consist of upper or lower-body exercises using a *split routine*. Total-body workouts are advantageous because they stress large muscle mass, allow greater load distribution, and enable the performance of complex exercises that stress many muscle groups. Within a total-body workout, segments can be designated that target a specific region or movement of the body. Variation may also occur from workout to workout in a microcycle in which structural exercises are emphasized early and are followed by assistance exercises. Various workout structures can be used effectively if the variables are systematically prescribed over time.

The sequence of exercises within a workout is important because it determines which exercises are performed in a fresh state and which are performed with some level of fatigue. Exercises performed early in the workout generate higher repetition number, power output, and load lifted because there is less fatigue. Thus, structural exercises are given priority. When exercises that stress similar muscle groups are performed in sequence, a decline in performance may be expected, which requires the coach to select loading accordingly (Ratamess et al. 2012a). This is particularly true when sets are terminated at failure or near failure. In some cases, exercise performance may be augmented if the opposing muscles are targeted in a preceding set (Baker and Newton 2005). Maximal strength is best trained in a nonfatigued state, which makes the sequencing of exercises critically important, especially for highly trained athletes. Although some exceptions can be justified, basic resistance training recommendations include the following:

- Large muscle exercises should be performed before smaller muscle exercises.
- Multiple-joint exercises should be performed before single-joint exercises.
- The Olympic lifts and total-body exercises should be performed from most to least complex (e.g., the most complex is the snatch, since the bar must be moved the greatest distance, followed by cleans and presses) and before basic resistance training exercises.
- Upper and lower-body exercises or opposing exercises (i.e., agonists and their antagonists) can be alternated when applicable.
- Some exercises targeting different muscle groups can be staggered in between sets of other exercises to increase workout efficiency.
- When applicable, higher-intensity exercises should be performed before lower-intensity exercises. The sequence can proceed from heaviest to lightest exercises.

Intensity describes the amount of weight lifted during resistance training. Light to moderate loads (50% to 60% of the 1RM) can increase strength in novice athletes and may be useful when learning techniques for new exercises. Moderate loading can increase strength in athletes, especially if the exercises are performed at a high velocity (Jones et al., 2001). However, high (moderate to very heavy) intensities (more than or equal to 80% to 85% of the 1RM) are needed to increase maximal strength as one progresses to advanced training. Strength increases will be greater with fewer repetitions of heavy weights (1 to 6 repetitions) than with moderate loading and repetitions (8 to 12 repetitions). Heavy lifting produces a neural pattern that is distinct in light to moderate loading. Training the nervous system is important to resistance training for maximal strength. Maximizing strength can only occur when the maximal numbers of motor units are recruited. Heavy loading is necessary at times, but the periodization of intensity is what is most critical to resistance training. Every exercise in a program will have distinct goals. For exercises designated as structural, athletes who are sufficiently trained to tolerate it can benefit from handling heavy to very heavy loading periodically throughout their training macrocycle. In elite Olympic weightlifters, approximately 8% of training encompassed loads of 60% or less of their competition best, 24% was dedicated to 60% to 70%, 35% was dedicated to 70% to 80%, 26% was dedicated to 80% to 90%, and only 7% was dedicated to lifting maximal loads for their competition exercises (Zatsiorsky, Kraemer, and Fry 2020). Another study in powerlifters showed the most commonly used intensity range was 71% to 80% of the 1RM, followed by 81% to 90% of the 1RM for the bench press, squat, and deadlift (Shaw et al. 2022). Interestingly, only about 20% of the powerlifters surveyed reported using supramaximal loads in training (Shaw et al. 2022). Elite lifters frequently lift heavy to very heavy loads in training but only during specific cycles and for a fraction of total training time. Often, loading begins at a moderate to heavy relative intensity and progresses over time until peak strength is attained.

As discussed previously, not every exercise in a program may be designated to maximize strength; some are meant to increase strength to sufficient levels. For example, low to moderate intensities for corrective exercises, or body weight exercises, may be preferred, especially when training scapular, rotator cuff, spinal, and some core muscles. Other assistance exercises may be loaded in a range from moderate to heavy depending on the goals. Some exercises may be included to fix mechanical issues seen during multiple-joint exercise performance. These can enhance technique but also specific strength in a way that may transfer to a larger strength exercise. Long-term heavy loading with the same exercises may lead to plateaus over time, but periodization of loading and of exercises can prevent plateaus and potential overreaching or overtraining. Most elite strength athletes have a base target for maximal strength. The subsequent peaking strength cycle that occurs over months yields maximal strength gains that may be only maintained for a short period of time. A strength phase may begin with loads that are closer to the athlete's base but then progress to maximal strength or competition-best loads by the end of the cycle. The duration of peaking depends on the number of competitions and the sport. For example, a team-sport athlete may reach peak strength preseason but then shift to maintenance training, which may be >90% to 95% of that load. A strength athlete who peaks for a competition may unload for a few weeks afterward and then switch to a more hypertrophy-based phase to begin preparing for the next training cycle for another competition. Novice to intermediate trained athletes are less susceptible to declines; they are quite capable of maintaining maximal strength because they are at a lower segment on the theoretical maximal strength curve. In figure 7.6, athletes with strength levels corresponding to the steep incline from novice to intermediate can more easily maintain their maximal strength (regardless of training phase) because they still have not approached their upper limits of genetic potential. Advanced to elite strength athletes have to train to target peak strength but may only maintain for a period of time. Thus, heavy loading is a must for resistance training for maximal strength, but it must be done systematically so that the athlete peaks at the right time.

With heavier weights come fewer repetitions and vice versa. The number of repetitions performed relative to the 1RM varies depending on the exercise and the level of muscle mass involvement (Shimano et al. 2006). In addition, the velocity of lifting affects repetition numbers. Figure 7.7*a* depicts the relationship between repetitions performed and lifting velocity. Loading and repetition zones are shown with corresponding training goals. For each level of loading, faster repetitions yield greater repetition numbers, whereas intentionally slow velocities yield fewer repetitions. Figure 7.7*b* depicts the continuum where high

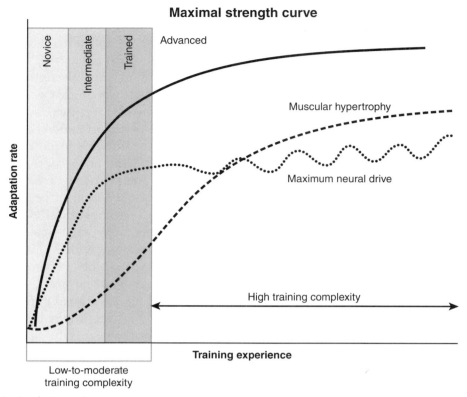

FIGURE 7.6 Maximal strength curve.
Adapted from M. Rippetoe and A. Baker, *Practical Programming for Strength Training*, 3rd ed. (Wichita Falls, TX: The Aasgaard Company, 2017).

intensity and low repetitions are most conducive to maximal strength development. Strength becomes less targeted and muscular endurance becomes the predominant goal as load decreases and repetitions increase. Although maximal strength can increase with moderate to moderately heavy loading, the rate of maximal strength increase is highest with heavy weights and low repetitions. Hypertrophy is targeted in all three zones. Although each training zone on this continuum has its advantages, an athlete should not devote 100% of training time to one general zone but rather use the continuum in accordance with the goals of the training cycle. Many types of resistance training programs and techniques have been successful over the years. The sidebar on page 210 depicts some common systems and techniques used by strength athletes.

The progression of loading or determining the starting load for an exercise may be accomplished in a variety of ways. Determining starting loads can be done based on a percent of maximal strength (if the 1RM or multiple RM values are known for key exercises) or through a trial-and-error approach. If the current loading for a training phase requires 75% intensity, then the coach may multiply the 1RM value by 0.75 and round up or down to the nearest 5-pound value (if using weights in pounds). In some cases, starting loads may be determined by using percentages for a similar exercise. For example, loading for a ballistic exercise like the jump squat could be determined based on the 1RM for squat performance (e.g., 30% of the 1RM squat). For several exercises, the trial-and-error approach may be used. The athlete performs a designated number of repetitions with good technique. If the weight is lifted easily, more weight can be added, and vice versa, until an acceptable starting load is determined. The weight determined serves as the weight coaches can use to progress from as training ensues. This is an effective way of determining starting weights for new assistance exercises. For *velocity-based training*, a load-velocity profile can be determined for an exercise. Using technology such as a linear position transducer, mean and peak CON velocities are measured for at least five to six intensities (e.g., 45%, 55%, 65%, 75%,

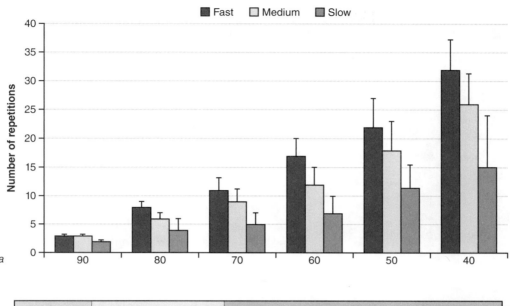

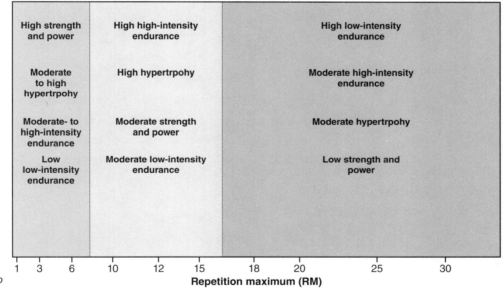

FIGURE 7.7 *(a)* Relationship between percent of the 1RM and repetitions performed at various lifting velocities; *(b)* RM continuum.

Figure 7.7a Adapted from Sakamoto and Sinclair (2006).

Figure 7.7b Adapted by permission from S.J. Fleck and W.J. Kraemer, *Designing Resistance Training Programs* 2nd ed. (Champaign, IL: Human Kinetics, 1997).

85%, and 95% of the 1RM or predicted 1RM) for three repetitions per set. The velocity of the fastest repetition per set per intensity is plotted against the corresponding relative load (as a percent of the 1RM), and the data form the basis for training progression. The athlete selects the load at the specified intensity and attempts over time to increase the velocity at which the load is lifted.

The most common methods to increase loading during resistance training are to (a) increase relative percentages, (b) increase weight within an RM zone, (c) increase absolute amounts of weight for an exercise, and (d) use velocity-based training as a guide to selecting loads. Increasing relative percentages is common in periodized programs, especially for structural exercises such

Heavy Loading Systems and Examples

Constant-Load-Rep Schemes
- 5 × 5 reps
- 5 × 3 reps
- Texas method: 5 × 5 reps; 2 to 3 × 5 reps (light); 5RM day
- 5 × 1 to 3 reps
- 5 × 4 to 6 reps
- 3 × 5 reps
- 8 × 3 reps
- Dynamic method: 10 × 2 to 3 reps (explosive reps with moderate loads)
- Maximal effort: work up to 1RM
- 6 × 4 reps

Ascending Pyramids (heavy to very heavy)
- 3 × 6, 4, 2 reps
- 5 × 5, 4, 3, 2, 1 reps
- 3 × 3, 2, 1 reps
- 4 × 6, 5, 4, 3 reps

Step Sets
- 5 × 3 reps with progressively heavier weight each set

Descending Pyramids (Very Heavy to Heavy)
- 3 × 2, 4, 6 reps
- 5 × 1, 2, 3, 4, 5 reps
- 3 × 1, 2, 3 reps
- 4 × 3, 4, 5, 6 reps

Undulating Pyramids (Combinations)
- 6 × 5, 5, 3, 3, 2, 2 reps
- 4 × 5, 3, 2 reps
- 5 × 5, 5, 3, 3, 1 reps
- 4 × 2, 2, 4, 4 reps
- 5 × 1, 3, 3, 5, 5 reps

Heavy Breakdowns (Drop Sets)
- 2 to 3 × 3 to 5 reps + 1 to 2 drop sets with load reduction

Rest-Pause Training
- Cluster sets
  - 3 to 5 × 1 to 3 reps with an intra-set rest interval length of 10 to 30 seconds
- Wave loading
- Maximal functional isometrics
- Multijoint isokinetics

Supramaximal Techniques and Examples
- Heavy negatives
- ECC load release
- ISOM-dynamic release
- Forced negatives
- Forced reps
- Partial reps
- Overloads and walkouts
- Specialized gear
  - Squat suits
  - Bench press shirts
  - Slingshot®
  - Briefs

as the Olympic lift (and its variations), squat, and bench press. Percentages can be used to vary intensity from set to set or to quantify a training cycle. Training within an RM zone requires an increase in repetitions of a load until a target number is reached. In a 6RM to 8RM zone the athlete selects a 6RM load and performs six repetitions. Within a few workouts, the athlete increases repetitions with that load until eight repetitions are performed on consecutive workouts. Loading is increased by 2% to 10% (with a lower percent for small mass exercises and a higher percent for large mass exercises), and the athlete returns to performing six repetitions (American College of Sports 2009). A practical way to increase loading is by increasing the weight in absolute amounts. For example, an athlete may perform four sets of six repetitions with 200 pounds (91 kg). Over the next two to four workouts five to ten pounds are added and the athlete performs four sets of five or six repetitions with 210 pounds (95 kg) (the target is six repetitions, but five repetitions may be performed initially). When the athlete is stronger, an absolute amount of weight is added. The absolute increase depends on the exercise: A large muscle mass exercise can tolerate a greater increase than a small mass exercise. For velocity-based training, loading can increase at a specific percentage as velocity increases. Coaches can alter the targeted training percent at various phases, from workout to workout, or from set to set, but velocity improvement is the predicate that determines whether to change or increase loading. All of these methods are effective, and it is the preference of the player development team that decides which one or combination to use. It is important to note that loading increases can be made for non–free weight or machine modalities (e.g., increasing intensity with elastic bands can be accomplished by stretching them further or using thicker, stronger bands).

Training volume is a summation of the number of sets and repetitions performed during a workout. A better term to use is *volume load*, which is calculated by multiplying the load lifted by the number of sets and repetitions, because it takes into account the amount of weight lifted. Volume load is an effective means of quantifying total loading in the weight room and is commonly used to quantify training cycles. Previously, we discussed *tonnage* as it relates to pounds per repetition because it provides insight into hypertrophy and muscular endurance and is another useful monitoring tool. Manipulating the volume load can be accomplished by changing the number of exercises performed per session, the number of reps performed per set, the number of sets per exercise, and the loading. There is an inverse relationship between volume and intensity such that volume should be reduced if major increases in intensity are prescribed. Resistance training for maximal strength is synonymous with low to moderate training volume because a low to moderate number of repetitions are performed per set for structural exercises. The set number may be moderate to high if fewer repetitions are performed per set. Training volumes of athletes vary considerably and depend on factors besides intensity, such as training status, number of muscle groups trained per workout, nutrition practices, practice and competition schedule, and goals. Current recommendations for athletes include multiple sets per exercise with systematic variation of volume and intensity (based on training phase) for progression into intermediate and advanced training (American College of Sports 2009). Not all exercises need to be performed with the same number of sets; whether a higher or lower volume is emphasized depends on the program objectives. There are no specific recommendations for the total number of sets performed per workout; these values vary greatly and depend on numerous factors. For example, many total-body workouts have been used successfully with 10 to 40 sets per workout or more (Ratamess 2022). Clearly, athletes benefit the most from multiple-set training. Across multiple sets, the loading and volume patterns can be varied to stimulate maximal strength increases.

Critical to resistance training for maximal strength are the rest intervals between sets, exercises, and potentially repetitions. Strength performance is limited when short rest intervals are used because recovery will be more diminished than if the rest intervals were longer. We have shown the magnitude of performance reduction (repetitions and load) in several studies (Kraemer 1997; Ratamess et al. 2007; Ratamess et al. 2012a, 2012b). These studies show better lifting performance with long (3 to 5 minutes) versus short (less than

2 minutes) rest intervals. Long rest intervals help maintain volume load, while larger reductions in performance with short rest intervals may be seen in stronger athletes (Ratamess et al. 2012a, 2012b). We also found less performance drop-off with short rest intervals in women. It appears that the physiological and biomechanical factors that enable an athlete to lift a heavier load may not translate into muscular endurance or recovery ability in between sets. In addition, training studies have shown greater strength increases (2% to 8%) with long (2 to 5 minutes) versus short (30 to 60 seconds) rest intervals between sets (Ratamess 2022). Thus, long rest intervals in between sets of structural exercises are recommended for resistance training for maximal strength in athletes (American College of Sports 2009). The goal of each exercise may determine rest interval length; for example, some assistance exercises do not require as much rest in between sets. Coaches should select rest intervals that are long enough to enhance recovery in between sets so that athletes can train effectively with heavy weights. Other nonstructural exercises can be performed effectively with short or moderate rest in between sets. Intra-set rest (in the form of cluster sets; see the sidebar on page 210) can increase force and velocity during each repetition since partial recovery is gained. This gives the coach an additional option in designing set structures. Overall, each set of each exercise may have its own specific rest interval to target the goals of the training phase.

Lifting velocity is another variable affecting strength outcomes. The key to resistance training is to attempt to maximize the velocity of each repetition, regardless of the load. With heavy loading, net velocity will be unintentionally slow (based on the force–velocity relationship). For submaximal loads, the athlete has greater control over the velocity of the weight. Since force = mass × acceleration, force and acceleration increase proportionally when mass is constant. For CON phase, lifting velocities of up to 1 to 2 seconds has been recommended for resistance training for maximal strength (American College of Sports 2009). The ECC phase can be 1 to 2 seconds, or slightly longer, to accentuate the negative. The relationship between force and acceleration is the underlying rationale for velocity-based training where bar velocity is measured and maximized with each repetition across a loading spectrum.

Figure 7.8 depicts some linear velocities attained at different intensities of multijoint exercises. The athlete attempts to increase velocity as strength improves. Subsequently, load modifications can

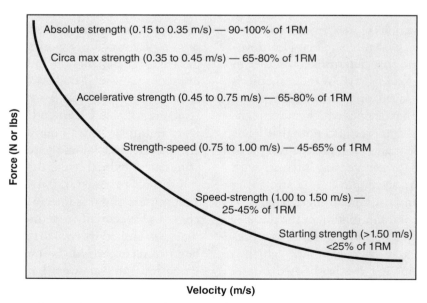

FIGURE 7.8 Concentric force velocity curve and associated exercise prescription loads.
Adapted by permission from D.N. French, "Advanced Power Techniques," in *Developing Power*, edited for the National Strength and Conditioning Assocation by M. McGuigan (Champaign, IL: Human Kinetics, 2017), 101.

be made. In velocity-based training, the repetition scheme can be determined by the percentage of velocity loss. Often, sets may be terminated with a threshold velocity loss of 20% for resistance training for maximal strength, 10% for power training, and 30% for hypertrophy training (Weakley et al. 2021). Both velocity-based and traditional resistance training programming can increase maximal strength in athletes.

Another consideration for the player development team is to determine when to conclude a set of a resistance exercise. Should the set be performed until failure or concluded prior to failure with a specific number of repetitions in reserve? The rationale for concluding sets at failure is to attempt to maximize motor unit activity and muscular adaptations but sets performed to failure cause a higher level of fatigue and can reduce set performance thereafter. A meta-analysis concluded that resistance training not performed to failure increased muscular strength by 23% to 24% while resistance training to failure increased strength by approximately 23% (Davies et al. 2016b, 2016a). Both approaches, then, work when used correctly. Complex exercises that require high force and velocity production and proper technique, such as the Olympic lifts and their variations and ballistic exercises, are best performed with minimal fatigue, so training to failure may be counterproductive. Muscular failure should be distinguished from a missed Olympic lift, which is usually due to a technical breakdown, but resistance training with multiple-joint, basic strength exercises to failure, at least part of the time, may be beneficial. Not every set is performed to failure, but it does appear that at least a few sets can be performed to failure to maximally increase muscular strength at various points in training. The challenge for the coach is to designate the proper number of failure sets while still minimizing overuse. Figure 7.9 depicts the use of RPE in estimating *repetitions in reserve* (RIR) during resistance training. A higher RIR means the athlete is further away from failure when concluding a set. This method has increased in popularity as *auto-regulation* (i.e., an approach to adjust training based on daily performance fluctuations) in resistance training has increased in popularity.

Rating of Perceived Exertion (RPE)	Repetitions in Reserve (RIR)
10	0
9.5	0
9	1
8.5	1 or 2
8	2
7.5	2 or 3
7	3
5 to 6	4 to 6

FIGURE 7.9 Repetitions in reserve perceptual scaling.
Adapted by permission from B.J. Schoenfeld and R.L. Snarr, "Resistance Training Program Design," in *NSCA's Essentials of Personal Training*, 3rd ed., edited for the National Strength and Conditioning Association by B.J. Schoenfeld and R.L. Snarr (Champaign, IL: Human Kinetics, 2022), 408.

Frequency includes the number of workouts per week, or the number of times certain exercises or muscle groups are trained per week. It is dependent on several factors, such as volume and intensity, exercise selection, level of conditioning and training status, recovery ability, nutritional intake, and training goals. Training frequency for resistance training may vary considerably. Many athletes resistance train 3 to 5 days per week. Advanced athletes, such as weightlifters, bodybuilders, and powerlifters, use high-frequency training (e.g., 4 to 6 sessions per week or more if multiple workouts are performed per day). High-frequency training may use either a variation of a split routine or low-volume total-body workouts (e.g., Olympic lifting). Heavy training increases the recovery time needed prior to subsequent training sessions involving similar muscle groups.

Training for Maximal Power

Maximal power production is produced when a greater amount of work is performed in a shorter period of time. It is the product of force and movement velocity. Maximal power contributors include maximal rate of force development, strength at slow, moderate, and fast contraction velocities, and SSC performance, all of which are cohesively tied to skill and technique (American College of Sports 2009). Because power is the product of force and velocity (or force $\times$ displacement/time), both components need to be emphasized in a comprehensive power development training program. Training for maximal power involves multiple modalities, including resistance, plyometric, speed, and agility training. Heavy resistance training (i.e., training for strength) improves maximal strength, while power training (using light to moderate loads at high velocities) increases force output at higher velocities and RFD.

As discussed in the previous section of this chapter, maximal strength is a critical component of power development. Heavy resistance training is needed for the athlete to maximize gains in power. However, traditional resistance exercises (including exercises performed at high velocity) are limited by the deceleration phase common to an exercise in which a reversal of action is needed before reversing motion for the next phase or terminating. For example, during the squat the athlete ascends from the bottom position with high intended velocity but then decelerates near the end for approximately 25% to 50% of the phase (depending on load since deceleration phases are longer with lower intensity and vice versa). The presence of the deceleration phase limits complete power development throughout the ROM. The solution is to maximize acceleration and limit or eliminate deceleration through *ballistic resistance exercise* that enables the athlete to safely release the weight (e.g., a bench press throw) or leave the ground (e.g., a jump squat) to maximize acceleration. For example, a loaded jump squat is one of the most effective exercises for increasing vertical jump performance. A key measure to prescribing ballistic resistance exercise is loading; it should encompass a spectrum from low to moderately high depending on the athlete's need. For example, high jumpers may benefit from light loads since they compete against the force of gravity of their body weight. However, since a lineman in American football must develop power in combative moves against large opponents, moderate to moderately heavy loading may benefit this type of athlete. Central to load assignment is knowledge of where peak power is produced. For example, some studies have shown the following peak power ranges (Ratamess 2022):

- 0% to 60% of the 1RM squat for the jump squat (note: 0% equates to body weight without external loading)
- 30% to 60% of the 1RM bench press for the bench press throw
- 40% to 70% of the 1RM for the bench press and squat
- 70% to 80% of the 1RM for selected Olympic lifts

Specialized equipment may help with ballistics, but exercises may also be performed with basic resistance training equipment. For example, the bench press throw is safe when performed on a Smith machine–type device with a hydraulic braking system to control bar descent. A similar device can be used for the jump squat, although this can also be performed with dumbbells, bands, kettle bells, weighted vest, hex bar, and other free weight equipment. The use of suspension or pendulum straps attached to a power rack also enables performance of ballistic bench press unilaterally or bilaterally. All repetitions are performed at maximal velocity per given load. Augmented ECC loading is present as well. For example, the athlete will land with greater force during the jump squat due to external loading (compared to no loading), thereby targeting increased ECC strength as well as SSC efficiency when the athlete lands, yields, or brakes, and then reverses action to an explosive CON phase. The same concept applies to the bench press throw. Thus, the augmented ECC phase provides a shock-like stimulus that maximizes SSC activity and subsequent power development.

Power training via resistance training entails a two-concept approach to program design. Basic resistance training recommendations apply (e.g., multiple-joint basic strength and Olympic variation exercises, multiple sets of 1 to 6 repetitions with sufficient 3-to-5-minute rest intervals or more in between sets). The intent to lift the weights as fast as possible is recommended. For ballistic resistance training added to a resistance training program, light to moderate loading (30% to 60% of the 1RM for upper-body exercises, 0% to 60% of the 1RM for lower-body exercises), performed at an explosive velocity for three to six sets for one to six repetitions in a periodized manner, is recommended (American College of Sports 2009). Loading for Olympic lifts and derivatives varies from light loads of 30% to 60% of 1RM when targeting speed-strength and heavier loads of 70% to 90% of 1RM for strength-speed (Comfort et al., 2023).

A critical component of power development is plyometric training. Plyometric exercises target plyometric actions (emphasizing the SSC) and embody a range of exercises from low (e.g., double leg hops) to very high (e.g., depth jumps and single-leg hops or jumps) in intensity. Some plyometric drills may be considered low or moderate intensity. They are still performed explosively but with less ECC loading than in more intense exercises. The quality of each repetition is what is most critical. That is, it should be performed with a minimal *amortization phase* (i.e., the time between beginning of ECC to beginning of CON phases) and *coupling* (length of the ISOM phase between end of ECC to beginning of CON phases, preferably less than 0.15 seconds) times. The CON phase is augmented by neuromuscular mechanisms analogous to the stretch and release of a rubber band. Collectively, plyometric training consists of jumps, hops, skips, bounding, and upper-body throws, tosses, and passes, in addition to power-specific exercises from specific sports (e.g., throws and swings in baseball and kicks, blocks, and strikes in martial arts). In addition, plyometrics include yielding exercises that involve high-level ECC muscle actions. Plyometric training increases power, jumping ability, strength, speed, agility, and numerous elements of sport performance.

Plyometric training program design is multifactorial and should include planned progressive overload, specificity, and variation. The proper integration of plyometrics with other training modalities is another key design mechanism. Exercise selection should be as specific to the demands of the sport as possible and consist of bilateral and unilateral exercises. Proper technique should always be emphasized, especially when fatigue manifests. Sufficient rest interval lengths should be used to minimize fatigue when peak power is the goal. Gradual progression should be used and should be based on the training level of the athletes. Progression entails increasing intensity through the addition of more complex exercises and external loading. Volume can be increased within reasonable limits. Low- and moderate-intensity drills should be mastered before progressing to high-intensity drills. High-intensity workouts require greater recovery time in between workouts, so frequency must account for this.

The intensity of plyometrics is defined by the magnitude of stress placed on skeletal muscles, joints, and connective tissues. It depends on the exercise complexity, loading, body weight and muscle mass involved, speed, and the size and length of boxes or barriers used. Complexity relates to the type of drill used and the technical involvement. On the intensity continuum, double-leg jumps-in-place are low to moderate in intensity, followed by standing jumps, multiple hops and jumps, bounding, box drills, and single-leg exercises (Chu 1998). The height attained during a standing jump is critical. Landing forces can exceed that of a depth jump for athletes with high jump capacity so some exercise intensities are performance-based (Ebben 2006). Depth jumps are very intense, especially when large boxes are used. Drop heights of 20 to 110 centimeters (8 to 43 inches) are common, but conservative heights of 20 to 40 centimeters (8 to 16 inches) are a good starting point when an athlete is first introduced to depth jumps. Loading increases when the mass of the athlete increases (from external loading with weighted vests or weights) and when the velocity of impact increases (from higher jump heights). Single-leg jumps are more intense than comparable double-leg jumps. Single-leg plyometric training may provide more comprehensive increases in jump performance, as well as development in the rate of force, compared to bilateral-only training (Bogdanis et al. 2019). Plyometric training programs begin with low- and moderate-intensity exercises and progress to higher-intensity exercises over time. This progressive shift often entails a larger proportion of unilateral drills toward the end of the training cycle than the proportion of mostly bilateral drills early in the cycle. Intensity is increased by using larger barriers or boxes or by setting cones or barriers farther apart. This requires the athlete to jump higher or farther for each repetition.

Plyometric exercises can be sequenced in many ways within a workout. Most sequencing patterns are beneficial when adequate recovery is allowed between sets and exercises. Low-intensity drills can be included anywhere in the sequence, but usually preference is given early on to moderate- and high-intensity drills for which fatigue is minimal. If upper and lower-body plyometric exercises are performed within the workout, the coach may choose to alternate between lower- and upper-body drills to facilitate recovery. Another option is to incorporate plyometric exercises into a comprehensive strength and power workout consisting of resistance exercises. All of these sequencing and structural strategies are effective for increasing power in the athlete; which approach or combination is used depends on the preference of the coach. Adequate rest intervals are needed when maximizing power is the goal. Intra-set rest intervals (e.g., 5 to 15 seconds) are useful for noncontinuous jumps and some variations of throws. For very high and intense depth jumps, intra-set rest intervals of 2 to 3 minutes may be needed. Rest intervals between sets should allow maximal recovery when maximal power is the goal. Rest intervals of at least 2 to 3 minutes may be needed for intense sets, while less rest may suffice for low- or moderate-intensity exercises. Work-to-rest ratios of 1:5 to 1:10 are recommended (Ratamess 2022).

The volume of plyometric workouts may vary considerably depending on the cycle goals and training status of the athlete. For lower-body plyometrics, the number of foot contacts or distance covered denotes training volume. For upper-body or core plyometrics, the number of repetitions (e.g., throws, passes, or tosses) represents training volume. Few guidelines regarding plyometric training volume are available. Analysis of the literature has shown a positive relationship between the number of jumps per session (when more than 50) and performance enhancement (de Villarreal et al. 2009). For advanced athletes, 120-to-200-foot contacts have been recommended for off-season training and 150-to-450-foot contacts for in-season training (Chu 1998). Plyometric training typically takes place 1 to 4 days per week, with 2 to 3 days being the most common. In-season training necessitates a low training frequency since sport practices and competitions are plyometric in nature. Because of the intense nature of plyometric training, approximately 48 to 72 hours of recovery in between training sessions is recommended.

Training for Hypertrophy

Training to maximize hypertrophy involves an integrated approach. Hypertrophy is consequent to both mechanical and metabolic stress and hypoxic (i.e., reduced oxygen availability) stimuli. Mechanical factors are related to force production.

Thus, resistance training is a potent stimulus for hypertrophy. Metabolic stress and hypoxic stimuli result from a variety of loading and repetition schemes that are primarily performed with short rest intervals. Training for muscular endurance helps maximize the metabolic stress and hypoxic-induced anabolic pathways augmenting muscle growth. Maximal hypertrophy training may be viewed as a combination of strength and muscular endurance training performed using many exercises, stressing muscles at different angles, and using a continuum or large range of loading and repetition schemes, rest interval lengths and velocities, and advanced strategies to optimize muscle growth.

Maximal hypertrophy training entails the use of heavy loads in combination with moderate and light loads and a wide range of repetitions. Multiple- and single-joint exercises should emphasize multiple-joint exercises for the resistance training element. Hypertrophy training must be viewed in the context of the effects of the interaction between intensity, volume, rest interval length, and velocity and duration. A common load assignment for hypertrophy training is the 6RM to 12RM zone (65% to 85% of the 1RM) because this loading range combines mechanical and metabolic stress for growth-inducing responses. Heavy weights used for strength are a good mechanical stress for muscle growth, while moderate or light loads performed for 20 to 30 repetitions or more maximize the metabolic stress component (and endurance) but limit the level of motor unit recruitment seen during heavy lifting. A range of loading and repetition parameters (a multidimensional, periodized approach) is recommended for hypertrophy training, as is an emphasis on strength, given the importance of muscular strength in athletes.

The interaction of intensity and volume must also be viewed within the context of the interaction with rest interval (RI) length. A range of RIs is recommended to accommodate the goals of each set. For example, long RIs of 2 to 3 minutes or more are needed for heavy strength sets, while shorter rest intervals contribute to greater metabolic stress and may suffice during sets specifically targeting endurance or hypertrophy. It has been recommended that a loading range of 70% to 100% of the 1RM be used for 1 to 12 repetitions per set in a periodized manner. Thus, the majority of training should be devoted to 6RM to 12RM and less to 1RM to 6RM loading (American College of Sports 2009) in order to target the mechanical and metabolic stress factors directly and maximize hypertrophy for advanced hypertrophy training. Higher repetitions than noted with light to moderate loading may also be used in conjunction with moderate to heavy loading. The variation of loading, as well as the interaction of loading with other acute program variables, is critical to maximizing hypertrophy. In addition to advanced resistance training techniques, other advanced hypertrophy techniques may be used in cycles to promote long-term growth (see the following sidebar). These techniques, in addition to traditional training approaches, are designed to alter the stimuli to skeletal muscles to induce growth. Although a few studies have addressed some of these techniques, protocols often differ as to how they should be used by athletes. The compounding approach is recommended where these techniques are used to add a new dimension to the previous training phase. Periodization of intensity, volume, rest intervals, exercise selection, and use of techniques is critical to maximal hypertrophy training.

Part of hypertrophy training is muscular endurance training. Basic strategies of endurance training for traditional resistance training involve performing sets to and beyond exhaustion, progressively increasing repetition number with a given load, using high repetition sets, and reducing rest intervals in between sets. For advanced muscular endurance training, it is recommended that various loading strategies be used (10 to 25 repetitions or more) in a periodized manner (American College of Sports 2009). Set duration may be prescribed for some exercises, in which case the total set duration can be increased, or intensity can be increased, while a constant set duration is used for muscular endurance training. Modern muscular endurance conditioning programs have used various

Hypertrophy Training Techniques

- ECC training (e.g., heavy negatives, forced negatives, and accentuated negatives)
- Isokinetics
- Split routine workouts
- Supramaximal loading
- Metabolic (glycolytic) training (high lactate, acidosis workouts)
- Training to failure and beyond
- Increased time under tension (e.g., continuous tension) sets
- High-volume workouts (e.g., German volume training)
- Rest-pause training
- Supersets, trisets, and beyond
- Compound exercises (sets)
- Staggered sets
- Quality training approach (e.g., reduced RI while maintaining loading and reps)
- Descending (breakdown) sets
- Partial reps and stage (segmental) sets
- Pre-exhaustion techniques
- Pause reps
- Cumulative reps
- Isolated "blitz" methods that target an area with high volume
- Blood flow restriction training

"metabolic training" strategies in which multiple modalities are integrated within each workout, intensity and volume are moderate to high, rest intervals are short (in a circuit training manner), and each circuit may progressively decrease in time to completion.

Training for Speed and Acceleration

Speed is the change in distance over time, and maximal speed is a critical component of sport performance. Linear sprinting consists of phases of acceleration (from a static or dynamic position influenced by reaction time), maximal speed, and deceleration (if distance is long enough). *Acceleration* is the rate of change of velocity over time, which involves the athlete's ability to reach high velocities in the shortest period of time after a change of direction, after deceleration, or from a static position. Athletes with an ability for explosive acceleration have a major advantage in sports such as American football, basketball, and baseball. The highest rates of acceleration are seen within the first 8 to 10 strides or 10 yards (or meters). The athlete is capable of maintaining maximal speed for only a short period of time before *deceleration* (reduced velocity) occurs due to fatigue. Sprint speed is the product of stride length and frequency (rate). Stride length is increased by improving the athlete's ability to apply explosive forces to the ground. Plyometric and resistance training are critical for improving acceleration, as are speed-specific and acceleration training. Sprint, agility, plyometric, and ballistic training are the most effective ways to increase stride rate. Training programs designed to increase speed and acceleration are multifactorial, consisting of resistance training, plyometric, flexibility, resisted, overspeed, and nonresisted sprint training.

Speed training consists of form drills at the beginning of a workout, following a general warm-up, and dynamic ROM exercises to help prepare the body for more intense sprints or plyometric exercises performed later in the workout. Form drills also teach proper sprinting technique, a crucial element of speed training. Technique should be the focus of training for youth athletes and should continue to be taught in adulthood while strength and power components are simultaneously trained for. A typical speed training workout should begin with a general warm-up and a specific warm-up that consists of dynamic flexibility exercises and form drills. The main segment of the speed workout should consist of drills for linear sprints (various lengths), overspeed, and resisted sprint. Short linear sprints of 5 to 20 yards (4.6 to 18 m) target acceleration ability, 40 to 60 yards (37 to 55 m) target acceleration ability and maximal speed, and more than 60 yards (55 m) targets all phases of sprinting.

Overspeed training allows the athlete to attain supramaximal speed (up to 10% higher than maximal speed) or an assisted speed that is greater than the athlete's maximal effort without altering sprinting mechanics. Overspeed training increases stride length and rate via downhill running (approximately 1° to 7°), high-speed towing, or high-speed treadmill running. The intensity is high and can result in greater muscle soreness, so adequate recovery in between workouts is essential. For downhill sprinting, the athlete should have access to a training area with a downward slope of at least 50 meters (55 yards). For towing, the athlete is towed or assisted in attaining a supramaximal sprint speed with a harness and elastic cords, although there are several ways of applying towing to a sprint. The towed athlete is catapulted forward while the partner begins the drill in motion. This catapult action creates overspeed. Towing can acutely produce a higher stride length and rate and decreased foot contact times, producing a potent stimulus for speed development. The towing force should be less than 4% of the athlete's body weight to maintain proper sprint mechanics.

Resisted speed training requires the athlete to sprint maximally against a resistance. Resistance may come in the form of sleds, chutes, weighted vests, sand, partner resistance, harnesses, an uphill slope, and wearable resistance. Sleds are dragged posteriorly while the athlete sprints. The amount of weight on the sled expresses the vertical weight; however, the horizontal frictional force needs to be overcome to provide resistance to the athlete. Loading is prescribed based on a percent of body mass or based on the magnitude of velocity loss during a sprint, usually up to approximately 80% of body mass with 10% to 50% being common. For speed training, less than 10% velocity loss is considered light loading, 10% to 20% is moderate,

20% to 30% is heavy, and more than 30% is very heavy. Moderate loads (20% to 45% of body mass) target acceleration, while lighter loads (up to 10% of body mass) target the maximal velocity phase of sprinting. Chutes open as the athlete accelerates and increase resistance, while weighted vests provide loading on the athlete's trunk. Often, up to 40% of body mass may be used. Lighter loads can increase sprint speed during chronic training with weighted vests. Wearable resistance involves applying an external load to specific segments of the body during sprinting (e.g., trunk, forearms, upper arms, lateral or medial thighs, medial or distal thighs, and calves). The position of the external loading is important since applying the same resistance more distally to the thigh (compared to the medial thigh) increases difficulty to a greater extent.

Often, speed and agility (discussed in the next section) may be trained together, and with the inclusion of plyometric exercises as well. When training only speed, novice programs should focus on proper technique using basic drills. Quality is more important than quantity. Linear sprints of varying length, using form drills during warm-ups, are a good place to start. Overspeed and resisted sprint drills are more intense and may be introduced once basic sprint technique is mastered and the athlete has improved sprinting ability (i.e., developed a base). These drills are typically performed earlier in the workout, when energy is high and fatigue is minimal, to facilitate skill acquisition. Many types of speed training programs may be used effectively, but very few comparative studies have been conducted. A typical speed workout sequence (when speed training is isolated from other modalities) is as follows:

general warm-up → dynamic ROM exercises → form drills → resisted and overspeed drills → basic speed (linear) sprints → cooldown

Within each workout, specific speed elements can be targeted in blocks. For example, after warm-ups the segments targeting acceleration and maximal velocity can be grouped. Overspeed and resisted sprint are the most intense drills (more than basic speed drills) and are typically performed soon after warm-ups. Speed is high for each drill, so the quality of effort for each set and repetition is critical. Volume is quite variable and depends on several factors, including intensity, frequency, diet, recovery, and training status. Advanced athletes can tolerate higher training volumes, but caution must still be used. Performing one to three sets for form drills and dynamic exercises is common, while three to five sets is common for workload sets. Data from elite sprinters and coaches have shown that acceleration drills are typically 10 to 50 meters (11 to 55 yards) each, for a total of 100 to 300 meters (109 to 328 yards) per workout, maximal velocity drills are typically 10 to 30 meters (11 to 33 yards) each, for a total of 50 to 150 meters (55 to 164 yards) per workout, overspeed drills are 10 to 30 meters (11 to 33 yards) each, for a total of less than 100 meters (109 yards) per workout, and resisted sprints are 10 to 30 meters (11 to 33 yards) each, for a total of 50 to 200 meters (55 to 218 yards) per workout (Haugen et al. 2019). Rest intervals of 1 to 3 minutes between sets are common but depend on the intensity and duration of the drill. Work-relief ratios of 1:10 to 1:20 may be used. Elite sprinters may use rest intervals of 3 to 5 minutes or longer (Haugen et al. 2019). Training frequencies of 1 to 3 days per week are typically recommended for intense speed training. Higher frequencies can be used with caution in advanced athletes who would typically cycle high speed (more than 95% intensity) and tempo (less than 70% intensity) workouts and integrate other modalities such as resistance training, plyometrics, and agility training.

Training for Deceleration

Deceleration is needed to slow down or stop prior to reaccelerating. Deceleration involves large ECC braking forces applied in short periods of time. Emphasis on deceleration ability is critical to agility and change-of-direction training and injury prevention. It should be a focus early in training and emphasized throughout. Deceleration training involves a multi-modal approach that requires balance, mobility, power, and strength, especially ECC strength to control the athlete's COG. Resistance training can improve deceleration ability by focusing on the ECC component of the repetition. Exercises such as the barbell squat, front squat, split squat, step-up, lunge, and deadlift with an augmented ECC component can enhance strength needed for deceleration. Plyometrics (e.g., squat jump, forward and lateral broad jump, single-leg hop, and jump with various foot landing positions) that emphasize proper soft-landing technique can augment ECC strength and deceleration ability. Holding the landing position is an effective way to increase the strength and balance needed for deceleration. Body weight exercises such as the lunge, lateral lunge, wall slide, and step-up can be effectively used for deceleration training. Deceleration should be emphasized in targeted drills involving forward, backward, or side-to-side movements that use two-foot, one-foot, or lateral braking techniques. Coaches may reinforce deceleration with each drill rather than allowing athletes to slow down at their own pace. Below are a few examples of deceleration drills:

- run 5 to 10 yards (or meters) to a line → lower COG → decelerate to a complete stop
- run 5 yards (or meters) to a cone → decelerate and stop → reaccelerate to the next cone → stop and reaccelerate → repeat to the 3rd cone
- run forward 5 yards (or meters) to a line → decelerate and touch the line → backpedal to the starting line → decelerate and touch the line → repeat

Training for Agility and Change of Direction

Agility is the ability to move rapidly while changing direction in response to a stimulus. It is complex and involves the interaction of several physiological systems, fitness components, anthropometrics, and perceptual-cognitive ability. Agility requires the athlete to coordinate several activities, including the ability to react and start quickly, accelerate, decelerate, move in the proper direction, and maintain the ability to change direction as rapidly as possible while maintaining balance and postural control. The athlete may have a small window within which to accelerate or decelerate before changing direction, and the rapid direction change may take place from a variety of stable or unstable bodily positions, such as standing (unilateral or bilateral), lying (prone or supine), seated on the ground, and kneeling positions, forcing the athlete to react to a number of situations. Agility is a complex fitness component that requires a multimodal training approach (figure 7.10).

Agility requires mobility, coordination, balance, power, optimal SSC efficiency, stabilization, proper technique, bilateral and unilateral strength (in the development of forces applied to the ground for impact and propulsion), flexibility, body control, footwork, metabolic conditioning (to reduce fatigue), and a rapid ability to accelerate, decelerate, and change direction. There are perceptual and cognitive components to agility, such as visual scanning, scanning speed, and anticipation. Agility performance may improve by up to approximately 15% following plyometric training (with a mean increase of 5.3%), up to 12.7% following resistance training (with a mean increase of 3.3%), up to 6.8% following specific COD training (with a mean increase of 2.4%), and up to 8.2% following combined training methods (e.g., resistance training, plyometrics, and COD) (with a mean of 3.2%) (Nygaard et al. 2019). Plyometric training (consisting of bilateral and unilateral jump variations and depth jumps), resistance training (consisting of the squat, Olympic lifts and their variations, and other lower-body exercises), flexibility, and speed training, in addition to specific COD, deceleration, and agility training, are all needed to maximize agility performance in athletes.

The ability to change direction is a critical component of agility performance. Each COD requires a braking force for deceleration, followed by a subsequent propulsive force for acceleration (and reorientation of the body) in a different direction. Smooth and rapid CODs are crucial to maximizing athletic performance. COD ability should be emphasized in youth athletes and further augmented into adulthood. COD ability forms the basis for more complex agility maneuvers. Specific COD training should serve as a basis for agility training. Below are a few examples of COD training drills in which only one COD is emphasized:

- athlete sprints 10 yards (or meters) → performs a 45° V cut for 5 yards (or meters)
- athlete runs 10 yards (or meters) → performs a lateral (90°) L-cut for 5 yards (or meters)

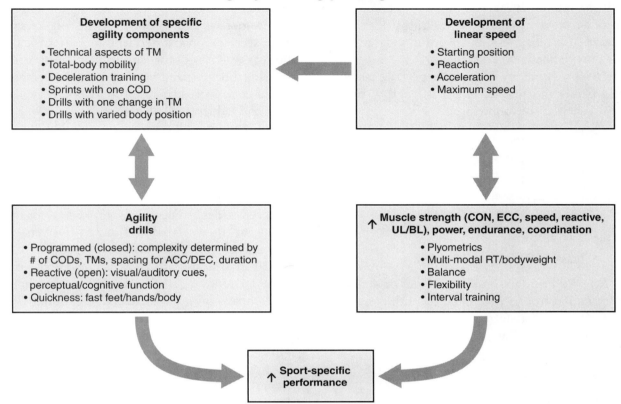

FIGURE 7.10 Agility training paradigm.

- athlete sprints 10 yards (or meters) → decelerates and turns (180°) off of the L or R leg → sprints 10 yards (or meters)

Agility involves a multitude of targeted movements. In addition to linear sprints and COD drills, agility drills involve jumps, backpedaling, side shuffling, side running, cariocas, drop stepping, cross-over stepping, pivoting, and cutting. Cutting is a directional change in as little as a few degrees to 90°. Cutting involves side stepping, cross-over steps, and split steps, each of which involves an initial acceleration, deceleration, COD (with weight acceptance and propulsion in the direction of movement), and final reacceleration. Performing one basic move and adding one COD or targeted movement to stress proper control, technique, and positioning of the COG is a good training strategy prior to adding more complex drills later in training. The following are a few examples of drills involving one COD or one change from basic movement to a different targeted movement:

- athlete sprints 10 yards (or meters) → decelerates and stops → backpedals for 5 yards (or meters)
- athlete sprints 5 yards (or meters) → transitions to backpedaling for 5 yards (or meters)
- athlete side shuffles 5 yards (or meters) → sprints the final 5 yards (or meters)

Agility training begins with the teaching and proper execution of technique during targeted movement patterns, acceleration, deceleration, and COD. Athletes should be able to demonstrate fundamental technique while performing basic targeted agility movements and be able to properly accelerate, decelerate, and change direction when directed to do so. This is why it is so important for coaches to stress proper technique in youth athletes. Agility training may progress from simple to more complex movements (including footwork drills) and from linear sprinting ability to multidirectional movements. Agility training drills can be classified as quickness, reactive, and programmed (i.e., preplanned, closed skills).

Quickness drills are designed to produce fast feet and hands and may include basic agility ladder drills, such as the following:

- Ladder runs (one and two feet in box)
- Double-leg bunny hops
- Lateral ins and outs
- Left-to-right (and reversed) shuffles (side steps)
- Two feet forward
- Icky shuffle

Reactive drills are based on visual or auditory information from a coach, another athlete, or an object such as a ball (e.g., *open skills*). Example drills include the following:

- Partner mirror drills
- Reaction ball drills
- Tag drills
- Reactive sprint drills

Programmed drills are preplanned (*closed skills*) drills in which the athlete is aware of the movements prior to initiating the drill. Examples include the following:

- Proagility (20-yard shuttle)
- T-drill
- Square drill
- 40-yard (37-m) and 60-yard (55-m) shuttles
- Three-cone drill
- X-drill

Many drills will use at least one COD, and some consist of more than 10 CODs. Complex agility drills with several CODs and targeted movements increase the duration of the exercise and are useful as forms of metabolic conditioning. Similar to other training modalities, agility training may be performed on a continuum from simple (i.e., emphasizing the basics) to more complex training, depending on the training status of the athlete.

Drills can be made more complex by adding other targeted movements, CODs, changing the lengths and positions of cones or other agility markers (to affect acceleration and deceleration patterns), and adding a reactive or sport-specific skill. Basic drills stressing linear speed and targeted movements should be mastered first. For footwork, basic line drills and ladder drills that consist of only one or two major footwork components should be mastered before progressing to more complex drills with more foot contacts and motions. Agility training is performed 1 to 3 days per week, but a higher frequency may be used with caution in advanced athletes. Form drills may be performed for one to three sets while three to five sets are common for workloads. Work-relief ratios of 1:10 to 1:20 may be used to allow adequate recovery. A shorter ratio (e.g., 1:5) may be used for short-duration sets or when anaerobic conditioning is a goal. Less rest is needed between sets of form drills. Below is a sample program structure for an agility-only workout:

general warm-up → dynamic ROM exercises → agility form drills → basic COD, deceleration, or transition drills → quickness drills → agility drills: open, closed (most complex to least complex) → cooldown

Training for Flexibility

Flexibility is a measure of joint ROM. *Static flexibility* describes ROM about a joint during movement (where the final position is held), whereas *dynamic flexibility* describes ROM during movement. Training for flexibility involves an integrated approach of myofascial release, static stretching, dynamic ROM movements, and partner-assisted or PNF stretching. Static stretching involves holding a position statically with some level of discomfort for at least 15 to 20 seconds. Static stretches may isolate a muscle group; the advantage is that the stretch in isolation can thoroughly stretch the muscle group. Other stretches target several muscle groups (e.g., several yoga stretches and poses). The advantage is that the complex of muscles and tendons is stretched but so are the myofascial slings that connect muscles to other muscles. This may add an additional mobility component. Dynamic flexibility exercises (e.g., arm circles and trunk circles) involve actively moving a joint through its full ROM without any relaxation or holding joint positions and offer an advantage to static stretching when included as part of a warm-up. These exercises are performed as repetitions in place or in series and cover a specific distance. *Proprioceptive neuromuscular facilitation* (PNF) stretching incorporates passive stretching and combinations of CON, ECC, and ISOM muscle actions. The rationale is to cause relaxation via muscle inhibition of the targeted muscle group to facilitate greater ROM. Several variations of PNF stretching may be performed, such as hold-relax, contract-relax, hold-relax with agonist contraction, and contract-relax with agonist contraction. The term "hold" refers to an ISOM action and "contract" refers to CON contraction of the agonist or antagonist muscle group. "Relax" refers to passive static stretching. Minimum recommendations for PNF stretching include athletes holding a light-moderate contraction for 3 to 6 seconds (at 20% to 75% of maximum voluntary contraction), followed by a 10- to 30-second assisted stretch (American College of Sports 2011).

Myofascial release is a technique used to reduce fascial adhesions, lengthen fascia, alter fluid content, reduce scar tissue and trigger points, restore extensibility to the myofascial unit, increase muscle blood flow and reduce arterial stiffness, augment mechanoreceptor-induced relaxation, and increase pain tolerance. Techniques include massage therapy and self-myofascial release (with foam rollers of various sizes, shapes, and densities, baseballs or softballs, tennis balls, massage sticks, PVC pipes, medicine balls, or devices such as the Peanut). The athlete rolls over the desired area, finding the trigger point, and continues to roll for a number of repetitions or durations to relieve the area. Pressure is controlled by altering body position or controlling the percentage of body weight compressed during loading. One strategy used in myofascial release is to start with a pliable foam roller while the athlete becomes accustomed to the pressure, and then progress to a denser device as tolerance improves. Foam rolling is performed as a warm-up or prior to flexibility exercises to facilitate ROM enhancement and enable the athlete to augment flexibility training.

Stretching to improve flexibility should follow a workout (e.g., resistance training, aerobic endurance, plyometric, or speed and agility) or follow a general warm-up (where flexibility or corrective exercises are the sole modality for that training workout). Unlike other training modalities, flexibility training can be performed with high to very high frequency. Basic flexibility training guidelines include the following:

- Selection of stretches that work each major muscle group. Isolation, multiple-joint, and total-body stretches are recommended.
- The program should last at least 10 minutes and include at least 2 to 4 repetitions per muscle group for at least 2 to 3 days per week. Greater gains in flexibility may be achieved with higher frequency.
- Dynamic, static, and PNF stretches may be selected. Dynamic exercises and myofascial release serve as good, specific warm-up exercises prior to static and PNF stretching.
- Static stretches should be taken to the point of mild to moderate discomfort and held for at least 10 to 30 seconds, although 30 to 60 seconds is better for athletes.
- Progression for flexibility training involves gradually increasing stretch ROM, duration, and repetition number and possibly progressing to more complex stretches or PNF stretches.

Anaerobic Buffering Capacities

One of the more important aspects of sport performance is the status of the athlete's buffering capacity. This becomes paramount in sports or events that challenge the body's acid-base balance and results, if not addressed, in fatigue in many of the body's functions, from physical power output to brain function. This has been discussed extensively in exercise physiology; for further details see (Kraemer, Fleck, and Deschenes 2021). In brief, sports or events that depend on glycolysis produce high hydrogen ion (H+) and lactic acid concentrations.

Lactate is not involved in the change in pH, but it does act as a significant correlate to acid-base status (Roberks, Ghiasvand, and Parker 2004). Although we have known this for twenty years, we still hear people erroneously blaming lactic acid or lactate for fatigue and soreness. In fact, lactate contributes to the energy needed for the body in the Cori cycle and has many other positive influences. This has been related by George Brooks and his lifetime of work on the lactate shuttle and anaerobic threshold concepts (Brooks 2020; Poole et al. 2021).

It is the drop in pH and the increases in H+ ions that contribute to the fatiguing process and a decrease in pH in tissues in the body (e.g., blood and muscle). The H+ ions in part interfere with the contractile muscle process and reduce strength and power production of the neuromuscular system, in addition to signaling fatigue to the brain and affecting decision-making and cognitive functions. Three buffering systems can address these changes to modify the severity of the changes in the body's pH: the proteins that bind hydrogen and hydroxyl ions and thus function as buffers, the bicarbonate buffering system observed primarily in the blood, and the phosphate buffering system in the cells such as those of skeletal muscle. These systems are trainable (with RT, HIIT, speed, agility, plyo training, etc.) and can be improved to minimize the changes in the body's acid-base status and keep the H+ ions from interfering with physical performance.

Methods of Program Variation

Strength and conditioning professionals must be intimately knowledgeable about the different types of variation methods. There are many approaches, and we want to present our approach in this jungle of methodologies. As discussed in chapter 4, it is important to underscore that one of the general findings of sport training theory over the past hundred years has been that variation is an important element in any training progression. In today's training programs, the time used for workouts is directed at the mutable aspects of the player's development. Thus, the effectiveness of the strength and conditioning program is affected by the number of days that can be used over the different cycles of the macrocycle. The concept of "quality over quantity" is more critical than ever here. Individualizing strength and conditioning programs is more critical than ever. Mountains of books, magazine articles, scientific studies, reviews, and blogs have been written on training periodization. However, as Dr. Greg Haff, former president of the National Strength and Conditioning Association (NSCA), once stated in a presentation, "periodization is a tool." He also noted that one needs a plan to implement variation in a program. We agree that variation with no fundamental basis in theory or testing of its sequencing makes no sense. While beyond the scope of this book on player development, all members of the player development team must be aware of the basic concepts concerning vital periodization in player development programs. Aligning with fundamental principles is crucial for the athlete's success and the clarity of the messaging to members of each team.

Classical Linear Periodization

As noted in chapter 4, the two classifications of periodization models that schedule the volume and intensity of resistance exercise workouts have been called *classical linear* and *undulating* but are now called *nonlinear*. The opposite of the classical model, termed *reverse periodization*, has been used for aerobic endurance athletes and athletes such as bodybuilders. In this model, high-intensity, low-volume training takes place early in the cycle, while intensity tends to decrease as volume increases over the training progression.

Classic Linear Periodization

For years, professor and biomechanist Michael Yessis of California State University, Fullerton published the *Yessis Review*, which translated many research and training theories from the former Soviet Union, including periodization. He was renowned for translating, adapting, and implementing sport training methodology from the former Soviet Union, including work by famous sport training theorists Yuri Verkhoshansky, Anatoliy Bondarchuk, and Vladimir Issurin. After the book by Russian physiologist and sport theorist Leo Matveyev was translated and published in 1981, more American strength and conditioning professionals became interested in the topic. A host of different sport training theorists, including Romanian-born and national sport team member Tudor Bompa, now a professor emeritus at York University in Toronto, were all involved with developing and promoting various periodization models arising from the more classical linear model. Eventually, sport-specific models were developed using the basic principles of periodized training from the macrocycle, mesocycle, and microcycle contents (Plisk and Stone 2003).

The typical progression of classical, or linear, periodization models is a decrease in the volume of work as the intensity increases to peak and competitive cycles. The famous Matveyev progression of cycles became synonymous with linear periodization progression (Matveyev, 1965). As time went on, with the continued development of periodization models, the starting intensities became higher and microcycles decreased from about 4 weeks to 2 weeks to gain more variation in the exercise stimuli. Interestingly, while we call it linear periodization (although it is not linear in structure), variation exists from workout to workout. The addition of a hypertrophy high repetition day can also be used in the cycles.

Drs. Stone, O'Bryant, and Garhammer popularized what was coined as the "American style" of periodization with recognizable names for the different cycles in periodization theory (Stone, O'Bryant, and Garhammer 1981). They also added a first transition between the preparatory and competitive cycles in their theoretical development of Matveyev's model. Their theory of periodization was further discussed, as were results from studies showing the advantages of periodized training, as members of the NSCA gained interest in the topic (Stone et al. 1982). In 2003, a variety of periodization strategies were overviewed, with these basic concepts in mind, for different sports and training outcomes (e.g., team sports, strength, speed, power, and agility) (Plisk and Stone 2003).

The proliferation of books and periodization articles has grown over the past twenty years. The explanations and use of approaches to sport training from former Soviet and Eastern Bloc countries have fueled the development of many periodization models or derivatives from the original forms. Bompa and Haff have detailed the multiple methods using various block periodization models, which have become very effective and popular (Bompa and Haff 2009). Vladimir Issurin has also published books on its application, especially to different sports (Issurin 2008).

Conjugate Periodization

Conjugate periodization models involve training different elements of neurophysiological function and evolved most notably from the core concepts of Medvedyev and Verkhoshansky (Medvedyev 1986; Verkhoshansky 1977). They range from models for youth readiness training to mature adult models, ultimately training high-force development and power velocity optimization as separate entities (Verkhoshansky and Siff 2009; Plisk and Stone 2003). Concurrent training of different features of the neuromuscular system was used to optimize the physiological potential of athletic movements. Popularized in the United States by Louie Simmons and Westside Barbell in Columbus, Ohio, for powerlifting, the program devotes two training sessions per week to focus on maximal effort training, one on the squat and deadlift and one on the bench press (Simmons 2007). This was influenced by Dr. Vladimir M. Zatsiorsky, who wrote that "lifting a maximal load against maximal resistance ... should be used to bring forth the greatest strength increments" (Zatsiorsky, Kraemer, and Fry 2020). This is combined with days of maximal velocity effort training in each exercise as well as additional exercises to gain other angular musculature development (e.g., back reverse hyperextension and triceps pushdown).

Block Periodization

A great deal of information has emerged on block periodization from the work of Tudor Bompa and Greg Haff over the years (Bompa and Haff 2009). The term was coined in the 1980s and was based on Verkhoshansky's conjugative successive system (Issurin 2008; Verkhoshansky and Siff 2009). The blocks include an *accumulation block* or concentrated loading that focuses on one of the elements of physical fitness, such as power, muscular endurance, and strength, for anywhere from 2 to 6 weeks. The length depends on the targeted goal and the level of fitness progression over the cycle. This block is fundamental and is typically of a higher volume in order to develop base characteristics of the targeted goal. The next block is the *transmutation block*, where the volume is reduced. It can be from 2 to 4 weeks, has very specific goals, and uses a higher intensity with a reduced total training load. The *realization block* is next, tapering the total training load even further while maintaining the frequency as one leads up to a peaking or event point in time. This phase is typically not much longer than two weeks. The accumulation block focuses on hypertrophy, transmutation develops strength, and realization targets power. This is then organized over the macrocycle for the preseason competitive season, and off-season when training starts again.

Nonlinear Periodization

One of the reasons for nonlinear periodization is that the body can become stale and not adapt, whether due to the stimulus not being practical or from nonfunctional overreaching. Variation allows the stimuli to change and more effectively stimulate other systems each time. The basic construct for nonlinear periodization arose from several sources and used varying intensities and volumes over time with short training periods. Yuri Verkhoshansky (1928 to 2010), Charles Poliquin (1961 to 2018), and Dr. Matthew Rhea have all used variation, although their intensity loading was not as dramatic as Kraemer's group proposed it should be in the early 2000s (Poliquin 1988; Kraemer and Fleck 2007; Kraemer et al. 2003; Kraemer et al. 2000; Rhea et al. 2002).

Early on in different linear periodization models, it was found that by shortening the microcycles from 4 weeks to 2 weeks, greater variation could be achieved, with exposure to repetitive stimuli while allowing for recovery. Variation of the stimuli thereby again became more evident to practitioners.

Flexible Nonlinear Periodization

Sport performance, sport science, and strength and conditioning professionals must match a type of periodization model to each athlete and sport. At the University of Connecticut in the early 2000s with Coach Jerry Martin and Coach Andrea Hudy, we used the flexible nonlinear approach to periodization, which allowed us to use any of the different models for different periods of time over the macrocycle to meet various opportunities for training or to deal with disruptors to the strength and conditioning programs.

The keys to flexible nonlinear periodization are in assessing the athlete's quality of training each day. Quality is more than just going through the motions for a workout, which will not effectively stimulate a change in a targeted variable like strength, local muscular endurance, or power. This is vital because there are a limited number of training sessions for an athlete over a macrocycle. The macrocycle is developed over the entire year, depending on the sport. Different durations of mesocycles are then placed within the macrocycle with specific targeted goals (Kraemer and Fleck 2007). Typically, there is a targeted goal for a particular mesocycle. The mesocycle has specific microcycle days that are also targeted for specific workouts that stimulate different physiological components. The difference from a typical nonlinear program is that rather than just continuing with the next type of workout in line, the flexible nonlinear program changes up the sequence of the mesocycle or changes the workout based on how the athlete is performing on a given day. There is a continual potential for rearranging the mesocycle. If too many defaults occur, that mesocycle's targeted goal is quickly reevaluated for a given athlete. Another key component is that all of the programs should be individualized for each athlete in their progression and targeted goals over particular phases of the training program.

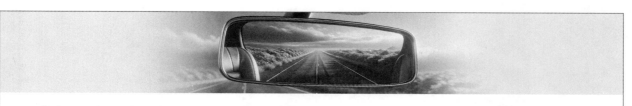

LOOKING IN THE REARVIEW MIRROR
- The most successful strength and conditioning programs use planned variation (periodization), progressive overload, and specificity, and are best when individualized to the needs of the athletes.
- We have established specific guidelines for maximal strength, power, hypertrophy, muscular endurance, plyometrics, speed and acceleration, deceleration, change-of-direction ability, agility and mobility, flexibility, and anaerobic capacities. The player development team should carefully integrate proven training methods to maximize athletic development.
- Several models of training periodization exist. The player development team should select the most appropriate models for their athletes in order to maximize performance and have them peak at the right times.

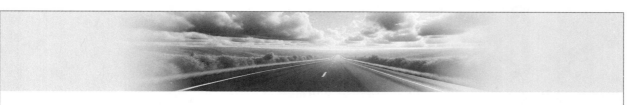

LOOKING AT THE ROAD AHEAD
The road ahead comes with many decisions and efforts of the player development team to work with athletes of all ages. Training should be monitored and adjusted based on what has worked or has not worked across time. The pillars of a program will be determined by the ability to surround athletes with professionals who can evaluate and respond to the fast-paced rhythm of their athletes' development and performance.

8

Looking Back and Ahead at the Road for Player Development

The road ahead for a player development program's success in delivering accurate information to the individual athlete is daunting without a paradigm or model to work from. In chapter 1, we provided a multi-unit model that can be used as a programmatic process. In this final chapter, we look at the road behind us and discuss some historical models that act as object lessons and that have evolved to help athletes reach their potential. We propose that the optimal model is one in which each of the different unit areas of expertise works together to deliver the most effective scientific and evidence-based approaches to each athlete in a given sport. Our proposed model has yet to be fully achieved in practice, usually due to alignment problems with sport coaches, but some organizations have come close. Even in those cases, however, historical memory and structures can be lost with coaching and athletic administration changes. Thus, challenges exist at each level (i.e., from youth to professional) in optimizing player development. In this process, as noted during an NSCA conference keynote presentation by Meg Stone, director of the Center of Excellence for Sport Science and Coach Education at East Tennessee State University, the work starts with educating sport coaches about the importance of the multiple dimensions of sport science and where the content expertise resides. This is necessary for the various interventions from the player development team, as well as the evidence-based approaches for the care and development of athletes, to be valued.

The challenges for player development reside in the need for alignment between the different units that contribute to improving the athlete's composite. Further challenges are funding, the need for professionals, and maintaining the three Cs in each unit. The stability of a program and its need for historical institutional memory are also important. Proper evaluation of each unit must be ingrained into the organizational fabric to ensure cutting-edge competence. Timely delivery of factual information to the athlete from each player development unit requires innovation to make it work. Developing a player development team model that reflects the needs outlined in this book is necessary to prevent injury and enhance each athlete's inherent potential as well as the athlete composite brought to each competition. Finally, funding to support the model designed by an organization is also paramount to success.

The Conceptual Model of Player Development

The player development concept has existed since humans created games and sports. With the driving motivation being to win the game, the development of skills and strategies evolved in each sport and became the responsibility of the sports coach. While its evolution has been slower, attention has also been given to developing the athlete's physical and psychological elements to enhance performance. Equipment and technologies also evolved to improve the sport, as did other factors related to enhancing performance. Various individuals with different skill sets now influence each sport. Today's elite level has a gargantuan platform related to player development and sport business.

As noted in chapter 1, sport participation in youth can have positive benefits on player development. At every level and age, the athlete is exposed to a staggering amount of information. Thus, mechanisms for evaluating information (i.e., evidence-based practices) must be in place as part of the player development team's mission. Volunteer coaches who have no background in the areas affecting player development are a threat to healthy and safe participation in a sport. The lack of input from a player development team of professionals also causes many issues that challenge the safety and efficacy of sport participation. Some of these issues include but are not limited to the following:

- Young athlete's body not strong enough to play the sport
- No age-appropriate strength and conditioning programs
- Too many competitions on a given day for adequate recovery
- Poor nutrition to support the sport participation
- Inadequate hydration for practices and competitions
- Not enough sleep or recovery time
- Injuries not managed properly
- Inadequate teaching progressions for sport skills
- Inadequate psychological management of athletes
- No understanding of practices and games stresses
- Misinformation on training, nutrition, etc., allowed to spread
- Inadequate equipment for safe practices and competition
- Inadequate practice venues and space

Often, the elaborate environment and money involved with success at the elite level of a sport misrepresent the reality of an individual journey for a young athlete. Optimal player development seeks to help athletes realize their potential for success at the competitive level. Because health is not equal to sport participation, everything must be done to diminish the physical and mental costs of participation in a sport, especially later in life after a competitive career. Optimal coaching and player development can teach athletes important life lessons without hijacking the entire landscape for social, psychological, and physical growth.

Historical Models Can Provide Object Lessons for Implementation

In the modern era, with the development of Olympic training centers in the United States and worldwide, almost every country with a significant emphasis on Olympic sports has provided a basis for player development models. The global development of training centers proliferated in the 1970s and was motivated by the pursuit of gold medals. The origin of this drive can be traced back even earlier to the cold war of the 1950s, a geopolitical struggle between the United States and the Soviet Union that in sports used medal counts rather than bullets to show which form of government was superior (Guttmann 1988). Technology was on the rise with the concomitant "space race" between the two nations, and the use of science and technology to advance athletic performance was accelerated during this time. Even today, exercise technologies have been influenced by the space race to Mars and beyond (English et al. 2019; English et al. 2020). While the historical development is beyond this book's scope, it set the basis for the various fields of physical education, which morphed into sport science over time.

The pioneering work of various laboratories, institutes of physical cultures, and centers accelerated interest in the scientific basis of exercise worldwide in the 20th century (Massengale and Swanson 1996; Tipton 2014). Sport science has evolved over the past century to where it is now part of the sport coaching vernacular. The training centers and institutes developed around the world grew out of the field of physical culture and physical education. In the 1970s, the fields of exercise sciences were starting to break into the different specialty areas in the physical education of exercise physiology, biomechanics, motor learning, and sport psychology. Eventually, these areas developed multiple subdisciplines because of the many technological advances in biology, medicine, and engineering, to mention a few.

Training centers with facilities, coaches, and other exercise and sports medicine professionals were needed to meet the demand of developing and training large numbers of athletes of all ages in each sport. By the 1960s, countries worldwide were competing to build multimillion-dollar Olympic centers. For the massive funding needed for such centers and their facilities, as well as to find sport scientists who would work effectively in them, each country drew upon its culture of physical education. Essentially, each Olympic training center or institute was developed to have core facilities for the specific training of each sport, food and nutrition services for resident athletes, conference and educational facilities, specific strength and conditioning facilities, sports medicine facilities for the care of athletes and management of injuries, specific testing facilities for athlete testing and management, and multiple professionals in every area supported by the center. Essentially, this was the extraordinary dream everyone working in sports in the 1970s was jealous of and wanted to bring to a local level. With progress in education and the large number of professionals in sport sciences, it is now possible to deliver a player development team in a virtual or real format that reflects the model used in this book.

The key to all these centers and institutes revolves around science and the team approach to training an athlete for competition. This has been the approach used by many organizations in their attempts to optimize the athlete composite, but it has often failed due to some of the issues we have addressed in this book, including a lack of alignment, not using evidence-based practices, a lack of sport coach education, and a lack of funding for developing a structure to enhance player development.

Academic and Research Influences

Academic research and teaching in universities and institutes around the world influenced the development of athletes over the years. As the 20th century progressed, many former athletes continued to become scientists to help other athletes in their sports. In many countries, especially in Eastern Europe, sport training theorists provided paradigms for player development. With the creation of the American Association for the Advancement of Physical Education in 1885 (later called the American Alliance of Health, Physical Education, Recreation, and Dance, and then later called SHAPE America), the development of different aspects of education and research in physical education began in the United States (Means and Nolte 1987) (https://en.wikipedia.org/wiki/SHAPE_America [2022]). Stemming from Scandinavian and German laboratories in the 19th and 20th centuries, along with the Harvard Fatigue Laboratory (1927 to 1947) in the United States, the specialized development of the fields of exercise physiology and biomechanics in physical education departments in the 1950s and 1960s became the epicenter for the embryonic field of sport science (Tipton 2014). Historically, funding for sport research was limited at best. Most college and university laboratories interested in such research depended on the medical field to support its efficacy or to translate it to health issues for the lay public. With the founding of the American College of Sports Medicine in 1954, a group of physicians and physical educators took up the mission to study the medical and exercise aspects of sports, with exercise being a greater focus of the organization (Berryman 1995; Tipton 2014).

At the first meeting in 1978 of the National Strength Coaches Association (later, in 1983, renamed the National Strength and Conditioning Association), many of the speakers were top exercise physiologists, but their topics and message did not hit home for attendees who were hungry for more information on resistance training and workouts relative to strength and power development for sports (McQuilkin and Smith 2005; Shurley, Todd, and Todd 2019). While documented elsewhere, this led the organization to evolve to provide more information for individuals interested in strength and conditioning with journals and research related to the field. The *NSCA Journal* (now the *Strength and Conditioning Journal*) and later, in 1987, the *Journal of Applied Sports Science Research* (later, in 1991, renamed the *Journal of Strength and Conditioning Research*) were two pillars that supported this need, leading to the further development of the sport science professional (Shurley, Todd, and Todd 2019).

With many former athletes leading the charge in such fields, more young scientists were trained to keep the momentum going. Interestingly, the sports examined were typically those that the individual scientists had experienced in their youth. Olympic sports were common, but track-and-field, aerobic endurance sports, and swimming moved forward the most quickly, with studies examining their different dimensions of training and performance. Sports medicine played a significant role in the field, and sport science and exercise often joined forces to give efficacy to its research.

Influence of the Strength and Conditioning Coach

The origins of sports science, at least in the United States, were probably stimulated by strength and conditioning coaches (now typically called strength and conditioning professionals) who worked with athletes daily and tried to improve their physical capabilities. At the same time, sport nutrition emerged as a significant area that supported the growth and development of muscular fitness. In the late 1970s, Dr. Bob Ward, who worked with the Dallas Cowboys, tried to bring more science into the field, having been influenced by the Cowboys' prevalent use of computers and technology to test and draft players (Ward and Engel 2015). After earning his doctoral degree at Indiana University, he was exposed to the work of James Edward "Doc" Counsilman, of swimming and coaching fame, which influenced his career in the field and his ideas about how sport science could enhance the performance of athletes. The founding of the NSCA in 1978 also started a process in which education and the need for science became part of the fabric of strength and conditioning. The emphasis of the early NSCA on equipment to help strength and conditioning professionals was a natural fit, and, by the late 1990s, computer-mediated assessment technologies and record-keeping software were being developed for use in collegiate strength and conditioning and personal training venues. To date, there is a need to integrate such technology into programs more quickly. This is a significant concern for optimal player development apart from highly funded organizations. Collaboration with local universities and other facilities that can provide help and assistance is needed and poses a significant challenge in today's field of sport science and player development programs.

Player Development Models in the United States

There is often an incorrect perception about how available and knowledgeable strength and conditioning professionals are to athletes trying to improve their potential to prevent injury and improve performance. The strength and conditioning profession has made tremendous progress since the 1970s, but it still has a long way to go to become a pervasive and positive experience for many athletes. The availability of sport science and player development programs is even more uncertain.

The Classic Model

As strength and conditioning evolved, the typical player development model came to include a head strength and conditioning professional and assistants who were responsible for different teams. Historically, the head strength and conditioning professional in the United States was responsible for American football and maybe basketball, which are highly funded sports at all levels. There has long been a concern that women's teams at the collegiate level do not get the same attention as men's sports. This inequality was brought to national attention in 2021 at the NCAA National Basketball Championships, when the women's teams were presented with weight room facilities inferior to those given to the men's teams. Anecdotal data indicate that the gender gap in many institutions is far from being closed. Many times, the role of a strength and conditioning professional is taken on by one of the assistant coaches who has experience from college or was a recreational or amateur lifter in different strength sports. The three Cs are compromised by this kind of insufficient support. This approach resembles the state of things in the 1970s, despite the NCAA now requiring professionals to be certified to work with athletes. Even today, in many smaller colleges, a certified strength and conditioning professional may not even exist, or there is only one professional responsible for training all the athletes at the school. Often in these situations, the training of athletes spills over to recreational fitness facilities for the general population, where professionals working with the entire student population substitute for strength and conditioning programs for athletes on various teams. This is almost unbelievable for today's world of collegiate sports, but it occurs even in programs at the level of smaller colleges that have won national championships.

It became evident at many of the larger universities that the strength and conditioning professional working with athletes needed more help in player development. Most of these professionals depended on sports medicine and team physicians to gain peripheral information for the care of the athletes who were trying to develop their inherent potential. The fundamental model used in player development is shown in figure 8.1, and it still predominates in collegiate programs today, where models exist at all. Any ancillary support for such elements as sport nutrition or testing arises from the academic unit at the institution. With the rise in certification programs in sport science, one may see dual roles played by one or more strength and conditioning professionals. For all those involved with athletes, to adhere to the three Cs is vital for the optimal success of a program.

Advanced Models

As time passed, more advanced models for player development were developed due to the continued demands of the modern athlete for performance enhancement and for the readiness of the composite at the time of competition. Numerous models are available for player development, and I (WJK) have firsthand experience with these. I have utilized these models as experimental frameworks in the early stages of creating player development programs. By treating them as experiments, I was able to analyze their effectiveness and application, providing valuable insights into the embryonic development of player development initiatives.

Historically, a novel and daring approach to player development at the Pennsylvania State University in 1989 led to the creation of its Center for Sports Medicine. It was created to comprehensively address the care and development of the university and club athletes in different sports. The idea came from legendary exercise physiologist Dr. Howard Knuttgen from Boston University as well as the president of Penn State, Dr. Henry Bryce Jordan; his administration; the college deans; and the athletic director. It was the first time a player development team was conceived from the top down, rather than originating from within an athletic department. As shown in figure 8.2, this center still represents a viable paradigm for a player

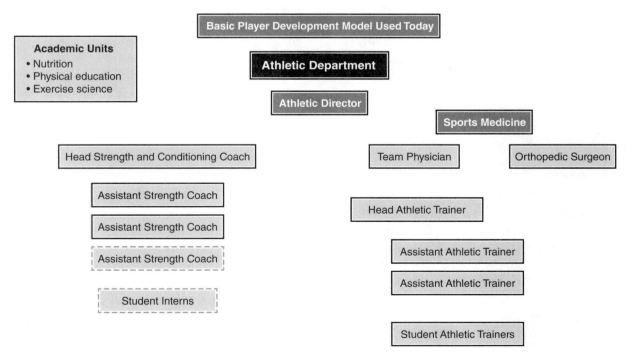

FIGURE 8.1 A basic model for player development used in the United States.

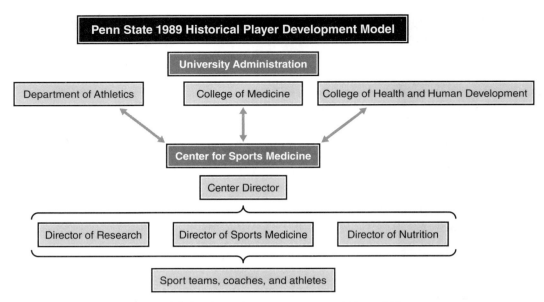

FIGURE 8.2 Player development model developed at Penn State in 1989 to 1998.

development team. The challenge at the time was one of program alignment among the different units and sport coaches, a subject outlined in this book.

In this model, the director of the center supervised a number of units, including the director of sports medicine, an orthopedic surgeon, who oversaw all of the team physicians and athletic trainers for the different athletic teams; the director of sport nutrition, who addressed the nutritional needs of the athletes, oversaw research and engaged in day-to-day interactions with athletes and coaches, and collaborated with dietetics; and the director of research (WJK), who was the first sport scientist hired at the university level to oversee the applied sport science research programs and to coordinate research with the college of medicine and the college of health and human development for collaborative research projects and grants. This model depended on alignment among coaches from different sports, which was a major issue at the beginning of this player development model. The Penn State model often served more as a theoretical resource than an effective tool for implementing and optimizing player development. This limitation stemmed from a lack of alignment between the various sport coaches and the strength and conditioning coaches. Lacking the three Cs, optimal training programs for various sports were only implemented in research programs or when training with the Director of Research (WJK). Unfortunately, during the years of the Penn State model, many athletes remained mired in antiquated machine circuit strength training paradigms of the 1970s that had been discredited in contemporary research literature of the time. A transformative overhaul occurred around 2014, involving sweeping changes in academic and athletic administrations, coaching staffs, and sport conditioning units. This shift allowed for a transition to a more modern, evidence-based approach to athlete development. The experience with the Penn State model underlines the crucial role of departmental alignment and competent personnel in achieving an optimal athlete development team and model.

Another advanced model developed was the bottom-up model that existed for about 13 years at the University of Connecticut (figure 8.3). This program was the brainchild of a collaboration in 2001 between Mr. Jerry Martin, the head strength and conditioning coordinator in athletics, and Dr. William Kraemer, who was a kinesiology professor at that time. Different from the prior model, this particular model was developed by the academic unit, the department of kinesiology, in collaboration with the strength and conditioning and sports medicine units in athletics. This collaboration started with grassroots professional and personal linkages within the departments as well as inter-

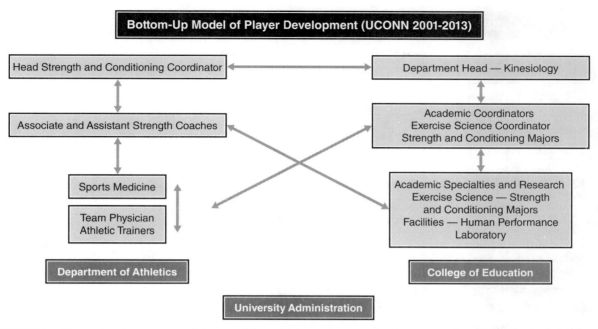

FIGURE 8.3 Player development model started from the bottom up at the University of Connecticut and developed between 2001 and 2013.

facing with the sport coaches and teams. At the start, the higher-level administrators in academics and athletics did not interfere with the relationships or the development. Academic programs and curricula were initiated and developed in exercise science, where undergraduate and master's students were trained in strength and conditioning with a specific academic curriculum. Integrated internships and research were promoted that focused on sport performance and related issues, including sport nutrition, tracking of sport team biomarkers, athletic injuries, and strength and conditioning research, making it the most productive sport science program created to date. It was the first integrated player development athletic–academic model to graduate applied sport performance and strength and conditioning professionals at the undergraduate and master's levels. However, the lesson learned from this bottom-up model in player development was that when upper-level administrations and American football coaches are changed, alignment is disrupted with the personnel changes. With no respect for the three Cs or historical memory, the approach failed, and the program collapsed.

Another interactive collaborative model, developed at The Ohio State University and probably the most innovative model to date, is shown in figure 8.4. Taking advantage of much evidence-based programs, the model creates a collaboration of university athletics and academics. This human performance collaborative model was headed up by the efforts of Dr. Josh Hagen in the department of integrated systems engineering and central administration, along with Mr. Mickey Marotti, the assistant athletic director and head of sport performance in the department of athletics at The Ohio State University. The goal was to build a leading, multidisciplinary team of researchers, sport scientists, data scientists, and practitioners with the unified goal of optimizing human performance. This collaborative model involved the applied science units in athletics, including sport performance, strength and conditioning, sport nutrition, sport psychology and sociology, and athletic training professionals, working with each team. The other side of the model involved a human performance collaboration between scientists from engineering, exercise science, psychology, nutrition, genetics and biology, and rehabilitation sciences. The interface between the two entities is the performance innovation team (WJK), which allows for global interactions between two major elements of the model for planning, education, testing, database

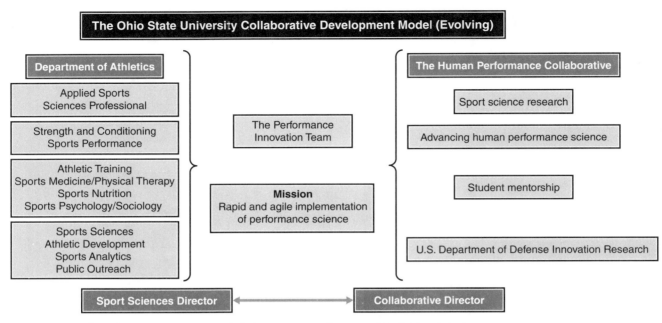

FIGURE 8.4 The Ohio State University Collaborative Development Model (evolving).

management, technological interventions, rapid response to applied questions, and integration of the latest science and technology interventions. This model is stable enough for the dynamic changes in personnel that come with program dynamics and collaborative approaches. It may be the model of the future and, at present, the closest model to what is needed in sport science and player development.

High School Model

A high school model for player development has been developed and may predict a new way of defining physical education and strength and conditioning. This model typically consists of a strength and conditioning professional or a sport coach, making it a challenging and long developmental process for a school system. Virtual linkages to experts and involvement with national organizations such as the NSCA are vital to this process. In a high school physical education program, Coach Mike Nitka (figure 8.5a) of Muskego High School in Wisconsin developed what he called the Human Performance Center (figure 8.5b) for many years (Kraemer and Nitka 2022).

Classes, in what was conventional physical education, now revolve around concepts and principles related to strength and conditioning and, ultimately, human performance. With 50-minute classes, organization, movement efficiency, and effective teaching and messaging are vital to success. Following a semester-long syllabus, the course and the development of the students go beyond activity to teach knowledge about human performance and skill sets in strength and conditioning for both students and student-athletes alike. The class in the physical education program was the beginning; these efforts then resulted in two after-school weight club classes where more advanced programs in strength and conditioning were offered, teaching proper techniques to student-athletes participating in sports. Ultimately, with administrative support, the Muskego strength and conditioning program flourished with the acceptance of students and sport coaches. In the classes, students track their own workout progress. Coach Nitka supports, guides, and supervises each student as they implement a training program. He and his staff give corrective directions to those using improper techniques or inappropriate workout designs. "I sincerely want them to succeed in here so they can succeed in their respective sports," Nitka says. The 12-week session is broken into four-week tiers and the students' progress in training over that period of time. The following quote from Nitka appeared in a newspaper article: "It happened because a lot of people around the country were sharing their ideas on what would

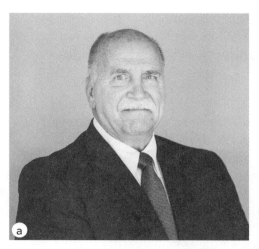
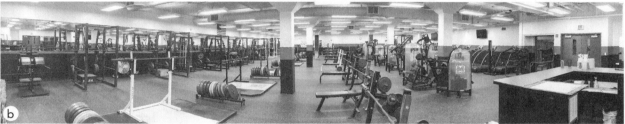

FIGURE 8.5 *(a)* Coach Mike Nitka, *(b)* the human performance model at Muskego High School, Muskego, WI.
Photos courtesy of Coach Mike Nitka.

happen if we could set up the perfect high school physical education class, and we're getting pretty darn close to it." The use of a class that instructs students and student-athletes in proper techniques, workout programs, and testing metrics is the key to this approach in strength and conditioning because it brings the science of player development to the high school athlete. With the help of collaborative fundraising and PEP grant funding, the necessary training facilities were developed over the years, allowing the athletes to have one of the best high school strength and conditioning experiences in the United States and resulting in multiple conferences and state-wide championships in men's and women's high school sports.

Virtual Models and Their Communication Linkages

With the pandemic and our experiences using virtual environments to communicate, a virtual model for player development may now be a pivoting point in athletics, from youth to the collegiate level. The issue, however, with communication over the Internet is the need for evaluating the information presented for its evidence-based veracity. One also has to examine the information's context to see whether it translates to the field the individual is working in. Here again, evidence-based practices and collaborations with research-based scientists are vital, but challenges still exist in this wild west of information flow coming from a host of pseudo-experts on the Internet. There are many nonprofit membership organizations that are based on educational and research aspects of the player development field (e.g., NSCA and the American College of Sports Medicine), which link to important knowledge bases for each of the different units. This is useful if one is starting out as a strength and conditioning professional, athletic trainer, or both, looking to put a player development team together in virtual form.

Another issue, often not given enough thought, is athletes' safety. The University of Connecticut's Korey Stringer Institute provides free (or cost-effective) and accurate information, resources, and professional interactions that are invaluable for learning more about various sports medicine topics such as the prevention of injuries and sudden death in sports. There is a need for science and evidence-based practices in each of the player development areas. Even when school resources are minimal, it is important to meet the needs of the athletes for the sake of both the professional and moral obligations of their management.

Other Models

For the many different professional sports teams, such as the National Football League, National Basketball League, Major League Soccer, and Major League Baseball, sport-specific models typically include strength and conditioning, sport rehabilitation, sport performance research, draft analytics, and sport data analytics (Coleman 2012; Weldon, Duncan, Turner, LaPlaca et al. 2022; Weldon, Duncan, Turner, Lockie et al. 2022). The testing and conditioning phases of the different athletes is often set by player union rules and contracts.

Sport Analytics and Technology: The Good, the Bad, and the Ugly

Any player development model should incorporate both the expertise of the player development team and improvements in technology. Every element of athlete development should be assessed, monitored, and modified based on data acquired from various technologies. In previous chapters, we discussed the roles of technology in the coaching and strength and conditioning professions. In coaching, the rise of sport analytics has led to a decision-making process based more on computers than pure intellect. The sport analytics team compiles vital statistics on player and team performance with the hope that detailed data will give the team or player a competitive advantage. Most professional teams employ an analytics team to provide the coaching staff with the most relevant data available. Several teams have large databases of statistics used for coaching and making organizational decisions, but they are also now likely to use *machine learning* (e.g., artificial intelligence that targets data and algorithms to make decisions) to guide some coaching decisions. Advanced data can positively influence coaching ability and player performance, but it can also enhance player development and help recruit the type of player that best fits the team's system. However, coaches still need to know which statistics are most valuable to team success and understand that analytics cannot be viewed in a vacuum but must be seen in the context of game strategy. The human element cannot be replaced when the actual game is played on the field. Coaches must use data wisely and ultimately make the tough decisions needed for team success. They should apply advanced data to the on-the-field environment during gameplay to make the best possible team decisions. Games will be won or lost based on player performance, but coaches must put players in the best possible positions, and that takes a combination of intuition, expertise, planning, strategy, and feedback combined with data analytics to maximize player performance.

Technology has also become important to strength and conditioning as an increasing number of organizations have invested in technological advancements and allocated a larger segment of the budget to research and development. The sport science of monitoring athlete training has greatly expanded over the past twenty years. As discussed in previous chapters, technology (e.g., wearables, watches, force plates, and apps) used to test and monitor training load, KPIs, and talent identification is commonly employed by player development teams. Technology helps the player development team improve athletic health and performance, and it becomes easier to implement as innovations allow devices to become smaller, faster, less expensive, and capable of advanced analyses. Similar to sport analytics, the player development team must understand how to wisely select and use technology for athlete monitoring. The most critical variables of the program can be measured and used in decisions related to training. Given the abundance of data collected, the player development team must accurately assess the data and make informed decisions while taking context into account. Likewise, data collected should be complementary to the objectives of the training program and help steer modification, when necessary, in a manner beneficial to the athlete. Clearly, technological advancements have the ability to streamline the decision-making process; however, members of the player development team should use the data wisely, ultimately making the key decisions in program design themselves.

Historically Proven Programs to Fit Any Paradigm

Regardless of the paradigm an individual operates in, it is essential to have a set of programs to set the foundation for the future. Over the last 50 years, athlete development has undergone an incredible evolution, but great care must be taken to honor the past and build upon the lessons learned through trial and error in the research labs. Reinventing the wheel is not evolution but ignorance, and ignorance creates vulnerability. Knowing what we know about the science of training, how can we use it to our advantage? Contextual limitations aside, there are, in fact, several programs that have demonstrated reliable and repeatable results relating to the mutable traits of athletes across all domains. If the guidelines and principles outlined in this book are followed, these programs are likely to continue to grow, and practical application will become more refined.

At the time of writing this book, we are just beginning to discover the adaptations that can be elicited from formal resistance training interventions. Significant progress is being made in the research and understanding of the human brain and its interaction at both the gross motor and epigenetic levels of interconnectivity. Practitioners now have access to state-of-the-art sensors to measure even the most minute changes in the biological status of an athlete. However, as the speed of disseminating information increases, so does the risk of misinformation and the threat of corporate exploitation to efficacy and accuracy. We would like to provide several approaches to this problem that have proven to be highly effective. While rooted in scientific research, these approaches have been repeatedly implemented to win countless championships and an untold amount of national individual awards. Many of these programs serve as a starting point on a program's roadmap for development. Please build upon these foundational training programs by using the skills and approaches outlined in this book to push the industry to even greater heights.

The Metabolic Circuit

Boyd Epley, previously the director of strength and conditioning for the University of Nebraska's American football program, initially developed the survivor circuit, which was meant to motivate players to survive the workout and simulate a football game, especially the fourth quarter. It was developed as a complementary workout to heavy resistance yet used higher intensities (approximately 80% of the 1RM) than typical circuit weight training protocols at the time, which used around 40% of the 1RM. The workout progressed from a 3-exercise circuit to a 10-exercise circuit using short rest periods and targeting high-intensity muscular strength, power, and endurance. It was also intended to help athletes cope with the higher physiological and psychological stress (i.e., fight-or-flight stress) of competition.

Eventually the optimal program became 9 stations of 3 sets of 10 at approximately 75% to 80% of the 1RM, done twice a week, with slow progression in reducing the rest periods. Early on, we learned that great care was needed with very short rest period lengths, even in trained athletes, because adverse symptoms (e.g., nausea, vomiting, and dizziness) were occurring that were counterproductive to proper training and risked development of rhabdomyolysis (Kraemer et al. 1987). Such symptoms led us to shut the workout down and increase rest. It was also shown that the relative resistance used under shorter rest conditions was dramatically lower than under long rest conditions in both men and women (Kraemer et al. 1993; Kraemer et al. 1990). The 10-exercise metabolic circuit produced a continuing elevation of perceptual demands over the workout in both circuit-trained and strength-trained athletes. However, it was observed that stronger athletes who did not have this type of prior metabolic circuit training could not attain as high of a percent of the 1RM. A major reason to use the metabolic circuit was to train the body's buffering capacities to offset fatigue related to the drop in pH and increases in H+ ion concentrations that interfere with muscular contractions. In addition, allowing the body to better tolerate increases in adrenaline (i.e., epinephrine), so typical of intense arousal and competition, was important for training adaptations in the proper progression of the metabolic circuit.

These and other studies showed that metabolic circuits increased endocrine signaling, which helps to develop underlying mechanisms for muscle hypertrophy (Kraemer et al. 2020). Here again, the bottom-up model promoted interactions on programming, promoted the use of metabolic circuits both in the military and in the work with Coach Jerry Martin at the University of Connecticut, and contributed to improved player development in the area of improving muscularity.

Modifications to the circuit were made in 2016 at Yale by Tom Newman, where the sport performance staff used various technologies and data analytics to engineer the first successful defeat of the Harvard Crimson football team in 10 years. The circuit was also used with the men's lacrosse program, resulting in the first ever national championship against the Duke Blue Devils in 2018. At this time, the strength and conditioning staff at Yale could quantify exercise and movement pattern-specific loads and intensities for every player, exercise, and repetition. This allowed them to optimize the circuit for each athlete and achieve unprecedented results.

Affectionately called the "nuclear bomb" at Yale University in the weight room, this workout requires great care in its practical application. Below are the operational considerations that should be applied when administering it:

- *Prerequisites:* Athletes should be able to demonstrate exercise technique competency in the 80% to 90% 1RM strength band. Within their training program, athletes are required to gradually reduce rest periods from an initial 2 to 3 minutes to a more challenging 1-minute rest interval. It's essential to recognize that not all athletes are prepared to immediately undertake this 1-minute challenge, especially with high-intensity loading. A thoughtful training progression, typically spread over about sixteen workouts, is needed to slowly decrease the rest periods without symptoms. This progression must occur without any signs of illness or maladaptive responses. Consequently, the implementation of short rest programs must be approached with caution throughout the training period. Proper progression is essential, allowing these programs to be used effectively as a training modality for enhancing the body's ability to buffer stress and perform under conditions of extreme fatigue. They must also be able to sufficiently articulate RPEs during exercises that match the program's desired load and intensity. Additionally, athletes must demonstrate a commitment to proper nutrition and recovery from training, which will be paramount in the recovery process.

- *Rest periods:* Once able to tolerate the 1-minute rest period, the athlete should stick to a strict 1-minute rest period to maximize the endocrine response for this workout routine. However, rest periods should be long enough to allow for the proper execution of each exercise and as noted previously when using this workout model.

- *Loads:* Loads should be carefully monitored and progressed as needed. Loads should not be so heavy that they compromise proper technique, but they should also not be too light to elicit a training response.

- *Progression:* As in any program, progression is critical. The metabolic circuit should be progressed as needed to challenge the athlete and elicit adaptation.

- *Variety:* Variety is essential to avoid boredom and continue challenging the athlete. The metabolic circuit can be modified by changing the exercises, their order, the number of sets and repetitions, and the rest periods.

- *Monitoring:* Careful monitoring of the athlete's progress and recovery is essential for ensuring that the program is effective and for making any necessary adjustments. This can be done through various methods, including subjective self-reports, objective performance measures, and physiological markers.

- *Safety:* Just as with the metabolic circuit, the foremost concern is safety, and measures must be taken to prevent any adverse symptoms, including the potentially severe outcome of rhabdomyolysis if not managed correctly. If, on any given day, an athlete experiences symptoms such as nausea, dizziness, or feelings of faintness, an immediate and dramatic reduction in exercise technique is required, and the set must be halted at once. If rapid acute recovery does not occur, the workout should be stopped and athletic training personnel consulted. The athlete's program is then adjusted, reverting to longer rest periods within their progression toward the 1-minute challenge. This ensures that their advancement toward shorter rest intervals is conducted with the utmost caution, prioritizing health and well-being.

Kraemer's Early Strength Training Progressions

Muscle is the sole mediator of human locomotion and serves as a critical factor for numerous conditioning and metabolic adaptations. Although individuals possess a unique blend of fast and slow muscle fibers, many have yet to fully tap into their muscular potential. Force production is a highly trainable attribute, acting as a catalyst for various physiological changes, including neural adaptations, tendon strengthening, and bone remodeling. The body's physiological subsystems often rely on the force requirements of daily activities and training to either reinforce tissues and pathways or initiate deconditioning. Regulatory mechanisms of downregulation and upregulation play pivotal roles in optimizing athletic performance. Many sport-specific abilities are directly linked to maximal strength: for instance, power is derived from approximately 60% of maximal strength, while speed accounts for 10% to 20%. Strength is fundamental not only for effective tissue recruitment but also for activating hormonal receptors and various signaling pathways.

If strength is so important, then why are people chronically weak? The answer is that developing strength takes consistent commitment and training on the athlete's part and the expertise in administering the workout on the coach's part. Medical considerations aside, the most significant reason for failing to reach maximal strength potential is that programs overtrain people after the initial 6 to 8 weeks of daily training adaptation. Especially when administering plans to intermediate (weekly adaptations) or advanced (multi-week or monthly adaptations) athletes, training without proper program auditing is risky. Sport coaches often lament that an athlete who got better suddenly got stiff and hurt in the weight room. This is not the fault of the program but the practitioner who has created a maladaptation in the athlete composite. This has usually been associated with poor recordkeeping or none at all, a lack of documentation of prior workouts, and the coaches administering a one-size-fits-all program for a team over a set period of usually 3 to 4 weeks. At the intermediate level, great care must be taken with not only the previous exercise results but also the daily readiness on the part of the athlete. A recipe for disaster is a strength and conditioning professional who does not have comprehensive training logs working with athletes who have had great success and do not want to disappoint their coach. The athlete overreaches and is injured due to maladaptation.

Assuming that the procedures in this book are followed, coaches should be able to develop strength safely over the course of an athlete's career. However, during the initial training phase, programs to improve strength can range from effective but years in the making to extreme and short-lived. The following program outlined below is one of the most effective intermediate resistance training programs for developing strength that can be used to train individuals to squat 2 × body mass (men) and 1.75 × body mass (women).

In 1977, while coaching at Carroll College, then Coach Kraemer began to develop various plans for the American football team, attempting to maximize the strength of the players in the off-season. At the same time, he tried various repetition schemes with the players (Kraemer 1997). One specific training pattern would become increasingly more effective at eliciting strength in a shorter period. After painstakingly reviewing the data from the paper training logs, the results became increasingly more consistent. The percentages for the athletes became tighter and tighter with each training cycle. The repetition scheme and accompanying intensities, volumes, and tonnages became reliable.

Over the years, *Coach* Kraemer transformed into *Dr.* Kraemer, and while he was in graduate school, the U.S. Army, and academia, he continued to chase the concept. The mission was simple: develop a resistance training program that increases back squat strength as quickly as possible. Such a program was found for tasks such as ruck marches, load carriage, and virtually every lower-body activity that required total-body strength. Individuals who were stronger stayed healthier and became more effective (Kraemer et al. 1995; Kraemer et al. 2001). Countless strategies were analyzed for optimal training frequencies and a wide range of training implements. Once again, the fabled Carroll College training plan would emerge as one of the top-performing protocols tested. The most significant difference now was that there was a major advancement in understanding just how much the role of strength affected the body and the coordinated neurological symphony that had to occur across the 244 muscles that must contract in harmony for each repetition in the squat. The program hit the targets over the years when properly progressed in each individual, and this was also observed at Yale University.

In the summer of 2019, the third iteration of the Carroll plan emerged during a visit to New Haven. Unlike every other college athletic league, the Ivy sports league does not provide a developmental redshirt freshman year to develop their athletes physically. Athletes are afforded different opportunities than their out-of-league opponents in physically preparing for college athletics. At best, some individuals could arrive in the summer, about 4 to 6 weeks before their first year. However, they could play immediately during the first week of the competition. As expected, many individuals needed help managing both the impacts of practice and competition and the demands that far exceeded high school or club competitions. Again, the mission was to identify the program that produced the greatest increase in strength in the shortest period. At this point, power output assessments and digital training logs were available to fine-tune the programs to a near-mythical level. The typical increase in 1RM squat strength was 80 to 120 pounds (36 to 54 kg) in 4 weeks, thereby effectively elevating the 1RM squat to be between one and two times an athlete's body mass, a sweet spot of athletic development.

Some of the features of the program resided in the periodized sequences of various heavy loadings in different exercises. A study by Hoffman and colleagues showed this to be effective for NCAA Division III American football players (Hoffman et al. 2009). The key to the program is heavy loadings with the triangle programs from yesteryear that stimulate high threshold motor units, necessary for boosting maximal strength and power in whole-body exercises, in a training cycle for intermediately trained athletes.

The following were general features of the 8-week mesocycle program:

- Focus on major muscle group exercises over the 8-week program: for primary exercises, squat, power clean, Romanian deadlift, bench press, push press, seated row, and military (shoulder) press; for ancillary exercises, biceps curl, abdominal exercises, and other dumbbell exercises
- Training 4 days a week—Monday, Tuesday, Thursday, and Friday—with a full rest on Wednesday
- Only three large muscle group exercises per workout with heavy loading
- Loading in power exercises using three sets, varying between at 60% and 80% of the 1RM
- Loading strength at 80% of the 1RM
- Half-triangle workout (5-5-3-3 RMs) and full-triangle workout (6-4-2-4-6 RMs), with a focus on the squat, deadlift, and bench press exercises
- Long rest of 3 minutes or longer for heavy sets greater than 80% of the 1RM, especially for power exercises
- Train symmetrically front and back of body and joints with seated rows and hamstring exercises, using primary and secondary exercise choices over the week

See an excerpt example of such a program in figure 8.6.

Future Challenges for Strength and Conditioning and Sport Performance Professionals

Several components make up any industry. Every industry experiences growth spurts, regressions, and refinement. A customer is looking for a solution to a problem. In its infancy, modern resistance training and rehabilitation was primarily focused on reconditioning the body after operations or injuries sustained during World War II. There is a product, a tangible item, or a service that customers will pay for with the expectation of resolving or improving the current problem. How much they pay, whom they pay, and how often they pay are questions for economics. As every industry grows

MONDAY

Exercise	Workload	1	2	3	4	5	6
Power Clean	3 × 3 @ 80% 1RM						
Push Press	3 × 5 @ 70% 1RM						
Romanian Deadlift	3 × 3 @ 80% 1RM						
Bench Press (6-4-2-4-6)	Rep Max						

TUESDAY

Exercise	Workload	1	2	3	4	5	6
Squat (6-4-2-2-4-6)	Rep Max						
DB Bench Press	3 × 10-12						
Standing Shoulder Press	3 × 8-10						

THURSDAY

Exercise	Workload	1	2	3	4	5	6
Squat (5-5-3-3)	Rep Max						
Bench Press (5-5-3-3)	Rep Max						
Seated Row	3 × 8-10						

FRIDAY

Exercise	Workload	1	2	3	4	5	6
Hang Clean	3 × 3 @ 60% 1RM						
Stiff-Leg Deadlift	4 × 10 @ 80% 1RM						
Side Squat	4 × 8-12						

FIGURE 8.6 An example of the basic exercise plan for major muscle group primary exercises in the 8-week mesocycle for improving strength and power capabilities.

and more capital is applied, expectations increase, competition is formed, and supply and demand take their course as with any other commodity.

What makes any form of training challenging to value, specifically in the team scenario, is that sometimes there needs to be a clear way of attributing value to athlete development, as opposed to effective recruiting or sport skill instruction. Practitioners often need proper recognition to feel more valued and less overworked. While sport coaches can point to win-loss records for validation and ultimately higher-paying contracts, the support staff in performance cannot. This is why, historically, many of the highest-paid coaches directly attribute their relationship with the head sport coach as the driving factor in their professional career track. This is particularly troublesome because the position of performance coach or rehab specialist requires a wide range of experiential knowledge and formal study in the life sciences, advanced exercise sciences, and statistics. Especially as they relate to athlete development, these professions require individuals with a rare combination of high analytical intelligence and extremely high levels of emotional intelligence.

Frustrations typically manifest as each generation of coaches follows the path of education, internship, assistant coach, and then burnout as they exit the industry in their early thirties. Especially with today's financial incentives in the private sector, some of the most talented young professionals are leaving. This brain drain on the industry will likely take several decades to actualize fully and will result in a new structure for the industry. As outlined in this book, there has been tremendous change shifting toward more specialized domain experts as shareholders, whereas even 20 years ago, a single coach general practitioner was expected to oversee all domains.

Flexible Nonlinear Programming—Another Historical Look

Regardless of the future's organizational structure, it is certain that greater emphasis will be placed on producing measurable results that equate to better on-field outcomes. More than ever, the ability to explain the current athlete composite concisely and forecast development potential with accurate timelines will increase in value. Throughout the centuries, there have been numerous programming styles and methodological advancements. Many of these approaches have stood the test of time because of a proven track record of results in specific populations. Any methodology must be passed down by senior coaches via apprenticeships. In theory, the more exposure young coaches have with different methods, the greater will be their range of utility on the market, which makes them easier to place in more sports. Whether linear programming, undulating, tiered, or proprietary, each method functions similarly. Someone is dropped into the program, and the program works its magic. Regardless of the individual, every program has a set of parameters that affects the body's stress responses with varying degrees of effectiveness. Great effort has been placed in researching and developing the best way to train, and in some cases the faith of the devotees to a particular method is almost religious.

Dr. Thomas Delorme was a pioneer of promoting resistance training in the field of medical science and for the lay public (Todd, Shurley, and Todd 2012). In 1951, he published his seminal text *Progressive Resistance Exercise* (Delorme and Watkins 1951). In it, he wrote, "Exercise is a battery of remedial agents. Just as an internist delimits his prescription for 'medicine' to a particular drug or combination of drugs and regulates their dosage in accord with their pharmacological effects, so also must the physiatrist give specificity to his prescription for exercise. It can attain its objectives only when administered with full appreciation of the wide range of effects it can produce and full technical knowledge of how these may be elicited." Fast-forward over seventy years later and the technological equipment and resources are readily available to make this statement a reality.

The concept of individual, unique training programs of nonlinear resistance training for women's tennis and a few other sports began to evolve at Penn State in the 1990s to overcome many disruptors (Kraemer et al. 2003; Kraemer et al. 2000). It continued its evolution during the early 2000s at UConn. This style or language of programming evolved into what is now called *flexible nonlinear programming* (Kraemer and Fleck 2007). It was novel in that instead of placing an individual in a set block programming scheme for 3 to 4 weeks, it was a hyper-focused effort to select a daily dosage of training that would most affect the athlete composite. The idea of emphasizing quality, rather than just going through the motions, became an important aspect due to the limited number of workouts what were available over the macrocycle. Athletes would enter the 12-week training program not with fixed exercises but with a roadmap of directed focus. Coach Jerry Martin, Coach Andrea Hudy, and the other staff worked closely with Dr. Kraemer, his many undergraduate and graduate assistants in strength and conditioning, and the Human Performance Laboratory to objectively monitor the physiological and psychological state of an athlete on an exact day and time, reach into the medicine cabinet of training options, and administer accordingly. Just like a physician, the staff would analyze the intended training load versus the actual load, audit the training effect daily and weekly, and attempt at the end of the 12-week cycle to elevate weakness, slowness, or any other deficient parameter. The on-field results spoke for themselves, with UConn achieving arguably one of the greatest runs of athletic dominance in basketball and leading an American football division from FCS to FBS.

While this programming language showed dramatically better results than traditional programming, it required much more effort to optimally implement. Later memorialized in other work by Coach Hudy at the University of Kansas, back at UConn the program style was there to stay (Hudy 2014). What was formally a once-every-four-weeks roundtable discussion on the upcoming training block turned into a fast-paced game of trying to optimize daily programs.

In 2017, this concept was brought to Yale with much more technological support. The strength and conditioning staff built on the past program results and digitized them for future use. This digitization in the TeamBuildr software platform resulted in a unique training experience that was ahead of its time. An athlete would approach the lifting platform, perform an athlete survey and vertical jump assessment, and be administered one of 26 available programs based on algorithmic logic built for that athlete's specific training goals. The only way to describe the experience was that it was like a packed emergency room managed by an elite NASCAR pit crew. Equipment was swapped out, broken down, and set up for each exercise, ensuring that each individual received the best customized plan at that exact moment. All of this was done within 8 minutes of starting the exercise for up to 45 athletes. History would repeat itself as it had up the road at UConn as Yale's athletic program achieved many first-ever and first-in-a-long-time successes. In football, a 10-year drought against archrival Harvard came to an end, and the men's lacrosse program accomplished what was once considered the impossible goal of winning a national championship. These are just a few of the countless successes across both men's and women's programs, happening almost simultaneously. Flexible nonlinear programming is the most effective known training protocol available to the practitioner. What separates this style from all others is that it has no constraints, as traditional methods do, and it is primed to leverage the power of machine learning and artificial intelligence. As Dr. Thomas Delorme idealistically described the future of modern resistance medicine, we must, as an industry, realize that the time is finally here to make this theoretical concept into an industry standard.

In the face of the multifaceted demands on modern athletes, individualized training within the team context remains a critical and complex challenge, extending even to youth training programs. Without addressing this need, the field risks stagnation, reflecting methods from the 1960s and 1970s when athletes were handed standardized programs on sheets of paper.

The work required to properly implement truly individualized programs transcends mere effort; it necessitates the integration of modern technology. Without embracing technological advancements, professionals in player development may find themselves trapped in outdated practices, and results become inconsistent—a hit-or-miss proposition with a complacent acceptance of "good enough."

Reflecting on the famous words of the late legendary American football coach Vince Lombardi, one might ponder whether "good enough" truly meets the standards we must set for athletes of all ages. Lombardi said, "We will pursue perfection but while we know that is not possible, in the process we will catch excellence." To fulfill this aspiration, every level of the organization must be aligned, from top to bottom, in utilizing the tools that optimize athlete development.

Failing to do so may signify a failure in our responsibility to those who place their trust and well-being in our hands as they participate in sports. The promotion of individualized training programs is not merely a professional challenge; it is a commitment to excellence and a duty to the athletes we serve. Think about it.

The Post-Competitive Career

As we have noted multiple times, health is not equal to participation in sports, especially as the competitive level increases and even more so without a player development team. One of the frequent failures for many sporting organizations is the lack of transition following the athletic career of an athlete. Often, an athlete cannot even get back into the locker room or training facilities. The player development team must prepare athletes for this phase of their careers. Much has recently been written on this topic in white papers (e.g., https://olympics.com/athlete365/whitepaper/life-after-sport-why-athletes-need-to-prepare/). In 1983,

Kraemer identified this as a potential problem for many athletes in sports requiring bulk due to athletes needing to be detrained to more active levels of body mass, which is not an easy change (Kraemer 1983). In some sports, training and conditioning take athletes to levels of physicality that are not healthy, and issues such as obesity, high blood pressure, arthritis, cardiovascular disease, and other maladies may chase these individuals over a lifetime. It has been noted that, after a sports career, a loss of identity, a loss of team, and a lack of purpose can each contribute to psychological stress (Wylleman, Alfermann, and Lavallee 2004). Beyond these physical challenges, the effects of psychological stressors, including the well-established depression syndromes, are cause for each player development program to have a transition team with follow-up procedures in place for each athlete to prepare them for life after a competitive career, no matter the level (McKight et al. 2009; Henriksen et al. 2020). Thus, a transition unit collaborative between psychology, nutrition, and exercise health needs to be in place to address the post-competitive athlete composite.

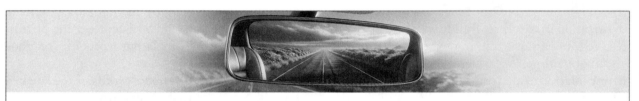

LOOKING IN THE FINAL REARVIEW MIRROR

In summary, player development is a multimodal team approach that should begin when the athlete is young. The following is a list of summary points covered in each chapter to be used as a guide or roadmap for player development:

- Youth should be exposed to multiple sports (*sport sampling*); the conditioning and motor learning gained from participating in different sports contributes to their overall athleticism and assists in the development of their main sport in the future.
- Sport specialization should only occur for those sports that require peak performances at early ages. Caution should be used to prevent athlete burnout.
- Understanding the mutable and largely nonmutable characteristics is very important for placing youth in the most appropriate sports and the right positions within each sport.
- Youth should be exposed to quality physical education programs, coaching, and potentially strength and conditioning facilities that feature youth training and adhere to the long-term athletic development (typically abbreviated to *LTAD*) model.
- Understanding the athlete composite and matching the athlete with the sport is critical. The importance of talent identification, anthropometrics, and their relationships to sport performance is important for sport selection.
- Building the player development team. Coaching staff, athletic trainers, physical therapists, physicians, strength and conditioning staff, sport science and analytics, sport nutrition, sport psychology and sociology, and academic advisers play large roles in the development of the athlete.
- Conducting the needs analysis. Breaking down the kinesiological, metabolic, physiological, and biomechanical elements of the sport and relating them to practice, the strength and conditioning program, and profiling

and benchmarking of the athlete is essential to understanding the sport demands and conditioning needs.
- Developing a testing battery and preparing the staff for appropriate testing procedures. The staff must adopt scientific and standardized procedures to collect the most accurate data during testing. Testing must be valid and reliable.
- Preparing the athlete for testing is paramount (e.g., medical clearance, familiarization, nutrition and hydration, and procedural practices).
- Testing the health-related fitness components, including body composition and anthropometry, muscular strength, muscular endurance, aerobic endurance, and flexibility and posture. The player development team may pick one to three tests per component, depending on the athlete, and implement them with high levels of standardization.
- Testing the skill-related fitness components, including power, anaerobic capacity, speed and acceleration, agility, change of direction, and mobility, balance, and reaction time. The player development team may pick one to three tests per component, depending on the athlete, and implement them with high levels of standardization.
- Developing sport-specific tests for the athletes. This helps the player development team transfer performance from the strength and conditioning program to a specific sport.
- The big three for optimal training adaptation are the training program, nutrition and hydration, and sleep and recovery. They are equally important for maximizing athletic performance.
- The training program mediates the response-adaptation cycle. Proper manipulation of the acute program variables is the key to long-term progression for any fitness component.
- Recovery is a critical component of athletic development. The player development team needs to invest in optimal recovery strategies and technologies to maximize athletic performance, deal with disruptors, and reduce the risk of overtraining and injury.
- Training workouts elicit acute physiological responses that can lead to chronic adaptations over time. The player development team must understand the underlying physiological mechanisms that contribute to long-term player development.
- The player development team must not only test and collect data on athletes; they must also be able to understand the results and apply them in a meaningful way for comparison or intraplayer analysis. This involves comparing data to established norms and previous player data.
- The player development team must have the three Cs of successful player development: appropriate credentials, competence, and commitment to optimize the athlete composite.
- The player development team must select appropriate sources of knowledge and use the scientific method to properly disseminate data and form conclusions.

- Periodic testing of selected health- and skill-related fitness components, as well as sport-specific performance, must occur on a regular basis in order to monitor performance and evaluate the efficacy of the training program. This includes subjective measures for monitoring training load and possibly the measurement of biomarkers.
- The most successful strength and conditioning programs use planned variation (periodization), progressive overload, and specificity, and are best when individualized to the needs of the athletes.
- Specific guidelines for maximal strength, power, hypertrophy, muscular endurance, plyometric, speed and acceleration, deceleration, change-of-direction ability, agility and mobility, flexibility, and anaerobic and aerobic capacities have been established and presented throughout this book. The player development team should carefully integrate proven training methods to maximize athletic development.
- Several models of training periodization exist. The player development team should select the most appropriate models for their athletes to maximize performance and have them peak at the right times.

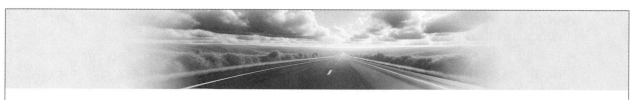

LOOKING AT THE ROAD AHEAD: THE ELEVEN PILLARS OF A PLAYER DEVELOPMENT TEAM

The road ahead in the development of an optimal player development team is left up to the creativity and innovation of each organization to put the necessary units together. There are a number of crucial factors related to the development and transition of the athlete composite over time. The player development team must have the following pillars for the program:

1. A model for implementing programs and constantly challenging their efficacy
2. Alignment with all units and shareholders in the processes of developing athletes
3. Evidence-based practices in decision-making
4. Mechanisms for repaying changes and responding to athlete needs
5. Individualization for optimal results
6. Critical monitoring and accounting procedures in place
7. Valid and reliable testing protocols
8. Using analytics properly with context and human insights guarding for errors in interpretation
9. The three Cs and annual reevaluation for every team member
10. Understanding of the programs and interventions used
11. Transition unit and model for athletes' post-career

References and Suggested Readings

Chapter 1

Amonette, W.E., K.L. English, and W.J. Kraemer. 2016. *Evidence-Based Practice in Exercise Science: The Six-Step Approach*. Champaign, IL: Human Kinetics

Balyi, I., and A. Hamilton. 2004. "Long-Term Athlete Development: Trainability in Childhood and Adolescence." Windows of Opportunity—Optimal Trainability, Victoria, British Columbia, Canada.

Bawa, P.N., K.E. Jones, and R.B. Stein. 2014. "Assessment of Size Ordered Recruitment." *Front Hum Neurosci* 8: 532. https://doi.org/10.3389/fnhum.2014.00532.

Behringer, M., A. Vom Heede, M. Matthews, and J. Mester. 2011. "Effects of Strength Training on Motor Performance Skills in Children and Adolescents: A Meta-Analysis." *Pediatr Exerc Sci* 23 (2): 186-206. https://doi.org/10.1123/pes.23.2.186.

Bell, D.R., E.G. Post, S.M. Trigsted, S. Hetzel, T.A. McGuine, and M.A. Brooks. 2016. "Prevalence of Sport Specialization in High School Athletics: A 1-Year Observational Study." *Am J Sports Med* 44 (6): 1469-74. https://doi.org/10.1177/0363546516629943.

Blimkie, C.J.R. 1989. "Age- and Sex-Associated Variation in Strength During Childhood: An Anthropometric, Morphologic, Neurologic, Biomechanical, Endocrinologic, Genetic and Physical Activity Correlations." In *Perspectives in Exercise Science and Sports Medicine*, edited by C. Gisolofi and D. Lamb, 99-163. Indianapolis, IN: Benchmark Press.

Carder, S.L., N.E. Giusti, L.M. Vopat, A. Tarakemeh, J. Baker, B.G. Vopat, and M.K. Mulcahey. 2020. "The Concept of Sport Sampling Versus Sport Specialization: Preventing Youth Athlete Injury: A Systematic Review and Meta-Analysis." *Am J Sports Med* 48 (11): 2850-2857. https://doi.org/10.1177/0363546519899380.

Duchateau, J., and R.M. Enoka. 2011. "Human Motor Unit Recordings: Origins and Insight Into the Integrated Motor System." *Brain Res* 1409: 42-61. https://doi.org/10.1016/j.brainres.2011.06.011.

Epstein, D. 2014. *The Sports Gene: Inside the Science of Extraordinary Athletic Performance*. London, UK: Penguin Publishing Group

Faigenbaum, A.D., W.J. Kraemer, C.J. Blimkie, I. Jeffreys, L.J. Micheli, M. Nitka, and T.W. Rowland. 2009. "Youth Resistance Training: Updated Position Statement Paper from the National Strength and Conditioning Association." *J Strength Cond Res* 23 (5 Suppl): S60-79. https://doi.org/10.1519/JSC.0b013e31819df407.

Faigenbaum, A.D., R.S. Lloyd, and J.L. Oliver. 2020. *ACSM Essentials of Youth Fitness*. Champaign, IL: Human Kinetics.

Faigenbaum, A.D., J.P. MacDonald, A. Stracciolini, and T.R. Rebullido. 2020. "Making a Strong Case for Prioritizing Muscular Fitness in Youth Physical Activity Guidelines." *Curr Sports Med Rep* 19 (12): 530-536. https://doi.org/10.1249/JSR.0000000000000784.

Issurin, V.B. 2017. "Evidence-Based Prerequisites and Precursors of Athletic Talent: A Review." *Sports Med* 47 (10): 1993-2010. https://doi.org/10.1007/s40279-017-0740-0.

Jayanthi, N.A., C.R. LaBella, D. Fischer, J. Pasulka, and L.R. Dugas. 2015. "Sports-Specialized Intensive Training and the Risk of Injury in Young Athletes: A Clinical Case-Control Study." *Am J Sports Med* 43 (4): 794-801. https://doi.org/10.1177/0363546514567298.

Jayanthi, N.A., E.G. Post, T.C. Laury, and P.D. Fabricant. 2019. "Health Consequences of Youth Sport Specialization." *J Athl Train* 54 (10): 1040-1049. https://doi.org/10.4085/1062-6050-380-18.

Kraemer, W.J., and S. Fleck. 2004. *Strength Training for Young Athletes*. 2nd ed. Champaign, IL: Human Kinetics

Kraemer, W.J., S.J. Fleck, and M.R. Deschenes. 2021. *Exercise Physiology: Integrating Theory and Application*. 3rd ed. Philadelphia, PA: Wolters Kluwer.

Liddell, E.G.T., and C.S. Sherrington. 1925. "Recruitment and Some Other Factors of Reflex Inhibition." *Proc Royal Society of London—Series B* 97: 488-518.

Lloyd, R.S., J.B. Cronin, A.D. Faigenbaum, G.G. Haff, R. Howard, W.J. Kraemer, L.J. Micheli, G.D. Myer, and J.L. Oliver. 2016. "National Strength and Conditioning Association Position Statement on Long-Term Athletic Development." *J Strength Cond Res* 30 (6): 1491-509. https://doi.org/10.1519/JSC.0000000000001387.

Lloyd, R.S., and J.L. Oliver. 2012. "The Youth Physical Development Model: A New Approach to Long-Term Athletic Development." *Strength and Conditioning Journal* 34 (3): 61-72.

McHenry, P., and M.J. Nitka, eds. 2022. *NSCA's Guide to High School Strength and Conditioning* Champaign, IL Human Kinetics.

Myer, G.D., N. Jayanthi, J.P. Difiori, A.D. Faigenbaum, A.W. Kiefer, D. Logerstedt, and L.J. Micheli. 2015. "Sport Specialization, Part I: Does Early Sports Specialization Increase Negative Outcomes and Reduce the Opportunity for Success in Young Athletes?" *Sports Health* 7 (5): 437-42. https://doi.org/10.1177/1941738115598747.

NSCA. 2017. "NSCA Strength and Conditioning Professional Standards and Guidelines." *Strength and Conditioning Journal* 39 (6): 1-24.

Post, E.G., S.M. Trigsted, J.W. Riekena, S. Hetzel, T.A. McGuine, M.A. Brooks, and D.R. Bell. 2017. "The Association of Sport Specialization and Training Volume With Injury History in Youth Athletes." *Am J Sports Med* 45 (6): 1405-1412. https://doi.org/10.1177/0363546517690848.

Post, E.G., S.M. Trigsted, D.A. Schaefer, L.A. Cadmus-Bertram, A.M. Watson, T.A. McGuine, M.A. Brooks, and D.R. Bell. 2020. "Knowledge, Attitudes, and Beliefs of Youth Sports Coaches Regarding Sport Volume Recommendations and Sport Specialization." *J Strength Cond Res* 34 (10): 2911-2919. https://doi.org/10.1519/JSC.0000000000002529.

Raikova, R., V. Krasteva, P. Krutki, H. Drzymala-Celichowska, K. Krysciak, and J. Celichowski. 2021. "Effect of Synchronization of Firings of Different Motor Unit Types on the Force Variability in a Model of the Rat Medial Gastrocnemius Muscle." *PLoS Comput Biol* 17 (4): e1008282. https://doi.org/10.1371/journal.pcbi.1008282.

Ratamess, N.A. 2022. *ACSM's Foundations of Strength Training and Conditioning*. Philadelphia, PA: Wolters Kluwer.

Stricker, P.R., A.D. Faigenbaum, T.M. McCambridge, and Council on Sports Medicine and Fitness. 2020. "Resistance Training for Children and Adolescents." *Pediatrics* 145 (6). https://doi.org/10.1542/peds.2020-1011.

Tucker, R., and M. Collins. 2012. "What Makes Champions? A Review of the Relative Contribution of Genes and Training to Sporting Success." *Br J Sports Med* 46 (8): 555-61. https://doi.org/10.1136/bjsports-2011-090548.

Wade, S.M., Z.C. Pope, and S.R. Simonson. 2014. "How Prepared Are College Freshmen Athletes for the Rigors of College Strength and Conditioning? A Survey of College Strength and Conditioning Coaches." *J Strength Cond Res* 28 (10): 2746-53. https://doi.org/10.1519/JSC.0000000000000473.

Chapter 2

Amonette, W.E., K.L. English, and W.J. Kraemer. 2016. *Evidence-Based Practice in Exercise Science: The Six-Step Approach*. Champaign, IL: Human Kinetics.

Appelbaum, L.G., J.E. Schroeder, M.S. Cain, and S.R. Mitroff. 2011. "Improved Visual Cognition Through Stroboscopic Training." *Front Psychol* 2: 276. https://doi.org/10.3389/fpsyg.2011.00276.

Baker, C. 2020. "Warrior Genes." *Mod Fiction Stud* 66 (4): 775-779. https://doi.org/10.1353/mfs.2020.0050.

Campa, F., T. Bongiovanni, C.N. Matias, F. Genovesi, A. Trecroci, A. Rossi, F.M. Iaia, G. Alberti, G. Pasta, and S. Toselli. 2020. "A New Strategy to Integrate Heath-Carter Somatotype Assessment With Bioelectrical Impedance Analysis in Elite Soccer Player." *Sports (Basel)* 8 (11). https://doi.org/10.3390/sports8110142.

Carter, J.E.L., and B.H. Heath. 1990. *Somatotyping: Development and Applications*. Cambridge, UK: Cambridge University Press.

Davis, D.S., E.E. Bosley, L.C. Gronell, S.A. Keeney, A.M. Rossetti, C.A. Mancinelli, and J.J. Petronis. 2006. "The Relationship of Body Segment Length and Vertical Jump Displacement in Recreational Athletes." *J Strength Cond Res* 20 (1): 136-40. https://doi.org/10.1519/R-16354.1.

Fry, A.C., and W.J. Kraemer. 1991. "Physical Performance Characteristics of American Collegiate Football Players." *Journal of Applied Sports Science Research* 5 (3): 126-138.

Garstecki, M.A., R.W. Latin, and M.M. Cuppett. 2004. "Comparison of Selected Physical Fitness and Performance Variables Between Ncaa Division I and II Football Players." *J Strength Cond Res* 18 (2): 292-7. https://doi.org/10.1519/R-13104.1.

Giannopoulos, N., G. Vagenas, K. Noutsos, K. Barzouka, and N. Bergeles. 2017. "Somatotype, Level of Competition, and Performance in Attack in Elite Male Volleyball." *J Hum Kinet* 58: 131-140. https://doi.org/10.1515/hukin-2017-0082.

Guth, L.M., and S.M. Roth. 2013. "Genetic Influence on Athletic Performance." *Curr Opin Pediatr* 25 (6): 653-8. https://doi.org/10.1097/MOP.0b013e3283659087.

Hoffman, J.R. 2008. "The Applied Physiology of American Football." *Int J Sports Physiol Perform* 3 (3): 387-92. https://doi.org/10.1123/ijspp.3.3.387.

Hoffman, J.R., J. Kang, N.A. Ratamess, M.W. Hoffman, C.P. Tranchina, and A.D. Faigenbaum. 2009. "Examination of a Pre-Exercise, High Energy Supplement on Exercise Performance." *J Int Soc Sports Nutr* 6: 2. https://doi.org/10.1186/1550-2783-6-2.

Hoffman, J.R., N.A. Ratamess, A. Gonzalez, N.A. Beller, M.W. Hoffman, M. Olson, M. Purpura, and R. Jager. 2010. "The Effects of Acute and Prolonged Cram Supplementation on Reaction Time and Subjective Measures of Focus and Alertness in Healthy College Students." *J Int Soc Sports Nutr* 7: 39. https://doi.org/10.1186/1550-2783-7-39.

Kim, T.B., and K.H. Kim. 2016. "Why Is Digit Ratio Correlated to Sports Performance?" *J Exerc Rehabil* 12 (6): 515-519. https://doi.org/10.12965/jer.1632862.431.

Knuttgen, H.G., E.R. Nadel, K.B. Pandolf, and J.F. Patton. 1982. "Effects of Training With Eccentric Muscle Contractions on Exercise Performance, Energy Expenditure, and Body Temperature." *Int J Sports Med* 3 (1): 13-7. https://doi.org/10.1055/s-2008-1026054.

Knuttgen, H.G., J.F. Patton, and J.A. Vogel. 1982. "An Ergometer for Concentric and Eccentric Muscular Exercise." *J Appl Physiol Respir Environ Exerc Physiol* 53 (3): 784-8. https://doi.org/10.1152/jappl.1982.53.3.784.

Kraemer, W.J., L.K. Caldwell, E.M. Post, W.H. DuPont, E.R. Martini, N.A. Ratamess, T.K. Szivak, J.P. Shurley, M.K. Beeler, J.S. Volek, C.M. Maresh, J.S. Todd, B.J. Walrod, P.N. Hyde, C. Fairman, and T.M. Best. 2020. "Body Composition in Elite Strongman Competitors." *J Strength Cond Res* 34 (12): 3326-3330. https://doi.org/10.1519/JSC.0000000000003763.

Kraemer, W.J., B.A. Comstock, J.E. Clark, and C. Dunn-Lewis. 2012. "Athlete Needs Analysis." In *NSCA's Guide to Program Design*, edited by J.R. Hoffman, 1-21. Champaign, IL: Human Kinetics.

Kraemer, W.J., and L.A. Gotshalk. 2000. "Physiology of American Football" In *Exercise and Sport Science*, edited by W.E. Garrett and D.T. Kirkendall, 795-813. Philadelphia, PA Lippincott, Williams & Wilkins.

Kraemer, W.J., J.C. Torine, R. Silvestre, D.N. French, N.A. Ratamess, B.A. Spiering, D.L. Hatfield, J.L. Vingren, and J.S. Volek. 2005. "Body Size and Composition of National Football League Players." *J Strength Cond Res* 19 (3): 485-9. https://doi.org/10.1519/18175.1.

Lijewski, M., A. Burdukiewicz, A. Stachon, and J. Pietraszewska. 2021. "Differences in Anthropometric Variables and Muscle Strength in Relation to Competitive Level in Male Handball Players." *PLoS One* 16 (12): e0261141. https://doi.org/10.1371/journal.pone.0261141.

Monson, T.A. 2018. "Allometric Variation in Modern Humans and the Relationship Between Body Proportions and Elite Athletic Success" *Journal of Antropology and Sport and Physcial Eduction* 2 (3): 3-8.

Moore, C.A., and A.C. Fry. 2007. "Nonfunctional Overreaching During Off-Season Training for Skill Position Players in Collegiate American Football." *J Strength Cond Res* 21 (3): 793-800. https://doi.org/10.1519/R-20906.1.

Moura, T., M. Costa, S. Oliveira, M.B. Junior, R. Ritti-Dias, and M. Santos. 2014. "Height and Body Composition Determine Arm Propulsive Force in Youth Swimmers Independent of a Maturation Stage." *J Hum Kinet* 42: 277-84. https://doi.org/10.2478/hukin-2014-0081.

Orvanova, E. 1990. "Somatotypes of Weight Lifters." *J Sports Sci* 8 (2): 119-37. https://doi.org/10.1080/02640419008732139.

Ratamess, N.A. 2022. *ACSM's Foundations of Strength Training and Conditioning*. Philadelphia, PA: Wolters Kluwer.

Ryan-Stewart, H., J. Faulkner, and S. Jobson. 2018. "The Influence of Somatotype on Anaerobic Performance." *PLoS One* 13 (5): e0197761. https://doi.org/10.1371/journal.pone.0197761.

Scroggs, K., and S.R. Simonson. 2021. "Writing a Needs Analysis: Exploring the Details." *Strength and Conditioning Journal* 43 (5): 87-95.

Shurley, J.P., J. Todd, and T. Todd. 2019. *Strength Coaching in America: A History of the Innovation That Transformed Sports*. Austin, TX: University of Texas Press.

Smith, J., and P. Smolianov. 2016. "The High Performance Management Model: From Olympic and Professional to University Sport in the United States." *The Sport Journal* (February 4).

Sterkowicz-Przybycien, K.L., S. Sterkowicz, and R.T. Zarow. 2011. "Somatotype, Body Composition and Proportionality in Polish Top Greco-Roman Wrestlers." *J Hum Kinet* 28: 141-54. https://doi.org/10.2478/v10078-011-0031-z.

Stewart, A.D. 2011. "Self Selection of Athletes Into Sports Via Skeletal Ratios." *Journal of Contemporary Athletics* 5 (2): 153-167.

Vaeyens, R., M. Lenoir, A.M. Williams, and R.M. Philippaerts. 2008. "Talent Identification and Development Programmes in Sport: Current Models and Future Directions." *Sports Med* 38 (9): 703-14. https://doi.org/10.2165/00007256-200838090-00001.

Chapter 3

Abadie, B.R., G.L. Altorfer, and P.B. Schuler. 1999. "Does a Regression Equation to Predict Maximal Strength in Untrained Lifters Remain Valid When the Subjects Are Technique Trained?" *Journal of Strength & Conditioning Research* 13 (3): 259-263.

American College of Sports, M., L.E. Armstrong, D.J. Casa, M. Millard-Stafford, D.S. Moran, S.W. Pyne, and W.O. Roberts. 2007. "American College of Sports Medicine Position Stand: Exertional Heat Illness During Training and Competition." *Med Sci Sports Exerc* 39 (3): 556-72. https://doi.org/10.1249/MSS.0b013e31802fa199.

Amonette, W.E., L.E. Brown, J.K. De Witt, T.L. Dupler, T.T. Tran, J.J. Tufano, and B.A. Spiering. 2012. "Vertical Jump Power Estimations in Youths and Young Adults." *J Strength Cond Res* 26 (7): 1749-1755. https://doi.org/10.1519/JSC.0b013e3182576f1e.

Amonette, W.E., K.L. English, and W.J. Kraemer. 2016. *Evidence-Based Practice in Exercise Science: The Six-Step Approach*. Champaign, IL: Human Kinetics.

Armstrong, L.E., and W.J. Kraemer, eds. 2016. *ACSM's Research Methods*. Philadelphia, PA Wolters Kluwer.

Ashworth, B., P. Hogben, N. Singh, L. Tulloch, and D.D. Cohen. 2018. "The Athletic Shoulder (Ash) Test: Reliability of a Novel Upper Body Isometric Strength Test in Elite Rugby Players." *BMJ Open Sport Exerc Med* 23: e000365.

Bangsbo, J., F.M. Iaia, and P. Krustrup. 2008. "The Yo-Yo Intermittent Recovery Test: A Useful Tool for Evaluation of Physical Performance in Intermittent Sports." *Sports Med* 38 (1): 37-51. https://doi.org/10.2165/00007256-200838010-00004.

Barker, A.R., and N. Armstrong. 2011. "Exercise Testing Elite Young Athletes." *Med Sport Sci* 56: 106-125. https://doi.org/10.1159/000320642.

Brechue, W.F., J.L. Mayhew, and F.C. Piper. 2005. "Equipment and Running Surface Alter Sprint Performance of College Football Players." *J Strength Cond Res* 19 (4): 821-825. https://doi.org/10.1519/R-16934.1.

Brown, A.W., K.A. Kaiser, and D.B. Allison. 2018. "Issues With Data and Analyses: Errors, Underlying Themes, and Potential Solutions." *Proc Natl Acad Sci U S A* 115 (11): 2563-2570. https://doi.org/10.1073/pnas.1708279115.

Brzycki, M. 1993. "Strength Testing—Predicting a One-Rep Max from Reps-to-Fatigue." *Journal of Physical Education, Recreation & Dance* 64 (1): 88-90. https://doi.org/10.1080/07303084.1993.10606684.

Buchheit, M. 2008. "The 30-15 Intermittent Fitness Test: Accuracy for Individualizing Interval Training of Young Intermittent Sport Players." *J Strength Cond Res* 22 (2): 365-374. https://doi.org/10.1519/JSC.0b013e3181635b2e.

Carter, J.E.L., and B.H. Heath. 1990. *Somatotyping: Development and Applications.* Cambridge, UK: Cambridge University Press.

Casa, D.J., S.A. Anderson, L. Baker, S. Bennett, M.F. Bergeron, D. Connolly, R. Courson, et al. 2012. "The Inter-Association Task Force for Preventing Sudden Death in Collegiate Conditioning Sessions: Best Practices Recommendations." *J Athl Train* 47 (4): 477-80. https://doi.org/10.4085/1062-6050-47.4.08.

Chaabene, H., Y. Negra, R. Bouguezzi, L. Capranica, E. Franchini, O. Prieske, H. Hbacha, and U. Granacher. 2018. "Tests for the Assessment of Sport-Specific Performance in Olympic Combat Sports: A Systematic Review With Practical Recommendations." *Front Physiol* 9: 386. https://doi.org/10.3389/fphys.2018.00386.

Clark, M.A., and S.C. Lucett. 2011. *NASM Essentials of Corrective Exercise Training.* Philadelphia, PA Wolters Kluwer Health/Lippincott Williams & Wilkins.

Cook, G., L. Burton, B.J. Hoogenboom, and M. Voight. 2014. "Functional Movement Screening: The Use of Fundamental Movements as an Assessment of Function—Part 2." *Int J Sports Phys Ther* 9 (4): 549-563.

Cummings, B., and K.J. Finn. 1998. "Estimation of a One Repetition Maximum Bench Press for Untrained Women." *Journal of Strength and Conditioning Research* 12: 262-265.

Dintiman, G., B. Ward, and T. Tellez. 1998. *Sports Speed.* 2nd ed. Champaign, IL: Human Kinetics.

Doan, B.K., R.U. Newton, Y.H. Kwon, and W.J. Kraemer. 2006. "Effects of Physical Conditioning on Intercollegiate Golfer Performance." *J Strength Cond Res* 20 (1): 62-72. https://doi.org/10.1519/R-17725.1.

Draper, N., and G. Whyute. 1997. "Here's a New Running Based Test of Anaerobic Performance for Which You Need Only a Stopwatch and a Calculator." *Peak Performance* 97: 3-5.

Epley, B. 1985. "Poundage Chart." In *Boyd Epley Workout.* Lincoln, NE.

Epting, L.K., K.N. Riggs, J.D. Knowles, and J.J. Hanky. 2011. "Cheers vs. Jeers: Effects of Audience Feedback on Individual Athletic Performance." *North American Journal of Psychology* 13 (2): 299-312.

Fleming, P., and C. Young. 2006. "Sports Surfaces—Impact Assessment Tools." *The Engineering of Sport 6.* New York, NY: Springer.

French, D.N. 2017. *A Cross-Sectional Performance Analysis and Projection of the UFC Athlete.* UFC Performance Institute (Las Vegas, NV).

French, D.N., A.L. Gómez, J.S. Volek, M.R. Rubin, N.A. Ratamess, M.J. Sharman, L.A. Gotshalk, et al. 2004. "Longitudinal Tracking of Muscular Power Changes of NCAA Division I Collegiate Women Gymnasts." *J Strength Cond Res* 18: 101-107.

French, D.N., and L. Torres Ronda, eds. 2022. *NSCA's Essentials of Sport Science.* Champaign, IL: Human Kinetics.

Fukuda, D.H. 2019. *Assessments for Sport and Athletic Performance.* Champaign, IL: Human Kinetics

Gains, G.L., A.N. Swedenhjelm, J.L. Mayhew, H.M. Bird, and J.J. Houser. 2010. "Comparison of Speed and Agility Performance of College Football Players on Field Turf and Natural Grass." *J Strength Cond Res* 24 (10): 2613-7. https://doi.org/10.1519/JSC.0b013e3181eccdf8.

Hadlow, S.M., D. Panchuk, D.L. Mann, M.R. Portus, and B. Abernethy. 2018. "Modified Perceptual Training in Sport: A New Classification Framework." *J Sci Med Sport* 21 (9): 950-958. https://doi.org/10.1016/j.jsams.2018.01.011.

Haff, G.G., and N.T. Triplett, eds. 2016. *Essentials of Strength Training and Conditioning.* 4th ed. Champaign, IL: Human Kinetics.

Heinrich, A., F. Miller, O. Stoll, and R. Canal-Bruland. 2021. "Selection Bias in Social Facilitation Theory? Audience Effects on Elite Biathletes' Performance Are Gender-Specific." *Psychology of Sport & Exercise* 55: 1-8.

Hoeger, W.W.K., S.L. Barette, D.F. Hale, and D.R. Hopkins. 1987. "Relationship Between Repetitions and Selected Percentages of One Repetition Maximum." *Journal of Applied Sports Science Research* 1 (1): 11-13.

Hoeger, W.W.K., D.R. Hopkins, S.L. Barette, and D.F. Hale. 1990. "Relationship between Repetitions and Selected Percentages of One Repetition Maximum: A Comparison between Untrained and Trained Males and Females." *Journal of Applied Sports Science Research* 4 (2): 47-34.

Hoffman, J.R., J. Kang, N.A. Ratamess, M.W. Hoffman, C.P. Tranchina, and A.D. Faigenbaum. 2009. "Examination of a Pre-Exercise, High Energy Supplement on Exercise Performance." *J Int Soc Sports Nutr* 6: 2. https://doi.org/10.1186/1550-2783-6-2.

Hosokawa, Y., W.M. Adams, D.J. Casa, J.K. Vanos, E.R. Cooper, A.J. Grundstein, O. Jay, et al. 2021. "Roundtable on Preseason Heat Safety in Secondary School Athletics: Environmental Monitoring During Activities in the Heat." *J Athl Train.* https://doi.org/10.4085/1062-6050-0067.20.

Janot, J.M., and N.M. Beltz. 2023. *Laboratory Assessment and Exercise Prescription.* Champaign, IL: Human Kinetics

Kraemer, W.J., B.M. Boyd, D.R. Hooper, M.S. Fragala, D.L. Hatfield, C. Dunn-Lewis, B.A. Comstock, et al. 2014. "Epinephrine Preworkout Elevation May Offset Early Morning Melatonin Concentrations to Maintain Maximal Muscular Force and Power in Track Athletes." *J Strength Cond Res* 28 (9): 2604-10. https://doi.org/10.1519/JSC.0000000000000392.

Kraemer, W.J., S.J. Fleck, and M.R. Deschenes. 2021. *Exercise Physiology: Integrating Theory and Application.* 3rd ed. Philadelphia, PA: Wolters Kluwer.

Kraemer, W.J., S.J. Fleck, C.M. Maresh, N.A. Ratamess, S.E. Gordon, K.L. Goetz, E.A. Harman, et al. 1999. "Acute Hormonal Responses to a Single Bout of Heavy Resistance Exercise in Trained Power Lifters and Untrained Men." *Can J Appl Physiol* 24 (6): 524-37. https://doi.org/10.1139/h99-034.

Kraemer, W.J., A.C. Fry, N.A. Ratamess, and D.N. French. 2006. "Strength Testing: Development and Evaluation of Methodology." In *Physiological Assessments of Human*

Performance, edited by P.J. Maud and C. Foster, 119-150. Champaign, IL: Human Kinetics

Kraemer, W.J., K. Hakkinen, N.T. Triplett-Mcbride, A.C. Fry, L.P. Koziris, N.A. Ratamess, J.E. Bauer, et al. 2003. "Physiological Changes With Periodized Resistance Training in Women Tennis Players." *Med Sci Sports Exerc* 35 (1): 157-68. https://doi.org/10.1097/00005768-200301000-00024.

Lander, J. 1985. "Maximum Based on Reps." *Strength & Conditioning Journal* 6: 60-61.

Leger, L.A., and J. Lambert. 1982. "A Maximal Multistage 20-m Shuttle Run Test to Predict VO_2max." *Eur J Appl Physiol Occup Physiol* 49 (1): 1-12. https://doi.org/10.1007/BF00428958.

Leitzelar, B.N., S. Razon, U. Tokac, S. Dieringer, C. Book, and L.W. Judge. 2016. "Effects of a Supportive Audience on a Handgrip Squeezing Task in Adults." *Int J Exerc Sci* 9 (1): 4-15.

Liguori, G., ed. 2021. *ACSM's Guidelines for Exercise Testing and Prescription*. 11th ed. Philadelphia, PA: Wolter Kluwer/Lippincott Williams & Wilkins.

Mayhew, J., J. Ware, and M. Bemben. 1999. "NFL-225 Test to Predict 1RM Bench Press in NCAA Division I Football Players." *J Strength Cond Res* 13: 130-134.

Mayhew, J.L., T.E. Ball, M.D. Arnold, and J.C. Bowen. 1992. "Relative Muscular Endurance Performance as a Predictor of Bench Press Strength in College Men and Women." *Journal of Strength & Conditioning Research* 6 (4): 200-206.

McHenry, P., and M.J. Nitka, eds. 2022. *NSCA's Guide to High School Strength and Conditioning* Champaign, IL Human Kinetics.

Miller, T., ed. 2012. *NSCA's Guide to Tests & Assessments*. Champaign, IL: Human Kinetics.

Myer, G.D., C.E. Quatman, J. Khoury, E.J. Wall, and T.E. Hewett. 2009. "Youth Versus Adult 'Weightlifting' Injuries Presenting to United States Emergency Rooms: Accidental Versus Nonaccidental Injury Mechanisms." *J Strength Cond Res* 23 (7): 2054-2060. https://doi.org/10.1519/JSC.0b013e3181b86712.

Newton, R., B. Doan, M. Meese, B. Conroy, K. Black, W. Sebstianelli, and W. Kramer. 2002. "Interaction of Wrestling Shoe and Competition Surface: Effects on Coefficient of Friction with Implications for Injury." *Sports Biomech* 1 (2): 157-66. https://doi.org/10.1080/14763140208522794.

Nimphius, S., S.J. Callaghan, T. Spiteri, and R.G. Lockie. 2016. "Change of Direction Deficit: A More Isolated Measure of Change of Direction Performance Than Total 505 Time." *J Strength Cond Res* 30 (11): 3024-3032. https://doi.org/10.1519/JSC.0000000000001421.

Norton, K.I. 2018. "Standards for Anthropometry Assessment." In *Kinanthropometry and Exercise Physiology*, edited by K.I. Norton and R. Eston. New York, NY: Routledge.

NSCA. 2017. "NSCA Strength and Conditioning Professional Standards and Guidelines." *Strength and Conditioning Journal* 39 (6): 1-24.

O'Connor, B., J. Simmons, and P. O'Shea. 1989. *Weight Training Today*. St. Paul, MN: West Publishers.

Parsons, J.T., S.A. Anderson, D.J. Casa, and B. Hainline. 2020. "Preventing Catastrophic Injury and Death in Collegiate Athletes: Interassociation Recommendations Endorsed by 13 Medical and Sports Medicine Organisations." *Br J Sports Med* 54 (4): 208-215. https://doi.org/10.1136/bjsports-2019-101090.

Perna, F.M., K. Coa, R.P. Troiano, H.G. Lawman, C.Y. Wang, Y. Li, R.P. Moser, J.T. Ciccolo, B.A. Comstock, and W.J. Kraemer. 2016. "Muscular Grip Strength Estimates of the U.S. Population From the National Health and Nutrition Examination Survey 2011-2012." *J Strength Cond Res* 30 (3): 867-874. https://doi.org/10.1519/JSC.0000000000001104.

Ratamess, N.A. 2022. *ACSM's Foundations of Strength Training and Conditioning*. Philadelphia, PA: Wolters Kluwer.

Ratamess, N.A., C.M. Chiarello, A.J. Sacco, J.R. Hoffman, A.D. Faigenbaum, R.E. Ross, and J. Kang. 2012. "The Effects of Rest Interval Length Manipulation of the First Upper-Body Resistance Exercise in Sequence on Acute Performance of Subsequent Exercises in Men and Women." *J Strength Cond Res* 26 (11): 2929-38. https://doi.org/10.1519/JSC.0b013e318270fcf0.

Ratamess, N.A., J.R. Hoffman, W.J. Kraemer, R.E. Ross, C.P. Tranchina, S.L. Rashti, N.A. Kelly, J.L. Vingren, J. Kang, and A.D. Faigenbaum. 2013. "Effects of a Competitive Wrestling Season on Body Composition, Endocrine Markers, and Anaerobic Exercise Performance in NCAA Collegiate Wrestlers." *Eur J Appl Physiol* 113 (5): 1157-1168. https://doi.org/10.1007/s00421-012-2520-8.

Ratamess, N.A., J. Kang, T.M. Porfido, C.P. Ismaili, S.N. Selamie, B.D. Williams, J.D. Kuper, J.A. Bush, and A.D. Faigenbaum. 2016. "Acute Resistance Exercise Performance Is Negatively Impacted by Prior Aerobic Endurance Exercise." *J Strength Cond Res* 30 (10): 2667-2681. https://doi.org/10.1519/JSC.0000000000001548.

Ratamess, N.A., W.J. Kraemer, J.S. Volek, M.R. Rubin, A.L. Gomez, D.N. French, M.J. Sharman, et al. 2003. "The Effects of Amino Acid Supplementation on Muscular Performance During Resistance Training Overreaching." *J Strength Cond Res* 17 (2): 250-258. www.ncbi.nlm.nih.gov/pubmed/12741860.

Rhea, M.R., D.M. Landers, B.A. Alvar, and S.M. Arent. 2003. "The Effects of Competition and the Presence of an Audience on Weight Lifting Performance." *J Strength Cond Res* 17 (2): 303-306.

Ross, R.E., N.A. Ratamess, J.R. Hoffman, A.D. Faigenbaum, J. Kang, and A. Chilakos. 2009. "The Effects of Treadmill Sprint Training and Resistance Training on Maximal Running Velocity and Power." *J Strength Cond Res* 23 (2): 385-394. https://doi.org/10.1519/JSC.0b013e3181964a7a.

Sayers, S.P., D.V. Harackiewicz, E.A. Harman, P.N. Frykman, and M.T. Rosenstein. 1999. "Cross-Validation of Three Jump Power Equations." *Med Sci Sports Exerc* 31 (4): 572-577. https://doi.org/10.1097/00005768-199904000-00013.

Schmidt, R.A., and C.A. Wrisberg. 2004. *Motor Learning and Performance.* 3rd ed. Champaign, IL: Human Kinetics.

Sole, C.J., T.J. Suchomel, and M.H. Stone. 2018. "Preliminary Scale of Reference Values for Evaluating Reactive Strength Index-Modified in Male and Female NCAA Division I Athletes." *Sports (Basel)* 6 (4).

Soriano, M.A., P. Jimenez-Reyes, M.R. Rhea, and P.J. Marin. 2015. "The Optimal Load for Maximal Power Production During Lower-Body Resistance Exercises: A Meta-Analysis." *Sports Med* 45 (8): 1191-1205. https://doi.org/10.1007/s40279-015-0341-8.

Soriano, M.A., T.J. Suchomel, and P.J. Marin. 2017. "The Optimal Load for Maximal Power Production During Upper-Body Resistance Exercises: A Meta-Analysis." *Sports Med* 47 (4): 757-768. https://doi.org/10.1007/s40279-016-0626-6.

Suchomel, T.J., C.J. Sole, C.R. Bellon, and M.H. Stone. 2020. "Dynamic Strength Index: Relationships With Common Performance Variables and Contextualization of Training Recommendations." *J Hum Kinet* 74: 59-70. https://doi.org/10.2478/hukin-2020-0014.

Wang, R., J.R. Hoffman, E. Sadres, S. Bartolomei, T.W.D. Muddle, D.H. Fukuda, and J.R. Stout. 2017. "Evaluating Upper-Body Strength and Power from a Single Test: The Ballistic Push-Up." *J Strength Cond Res* 31 (5): 1338-1345. https://doi.org/10.1519/JSC.0000000000001832.

Wathen, D. 1994. "Load Assignment." In *Essentials of Strength Training and Conditioning,* edited by T.R. Baechle, 435-446. Champaign, IL: Human Kinetics.

Zarrouk, N., H. Chtourou, H. Rebai, O. Hammouda, N. Souissi, M. Dogui, and F. Hug. 2012. "Time of Day Effects on Repeated Sprint Ability." *Int J Sports Med* 33 (12): 975-80. https://doi.org/10.1055/s-0032-1312626.

Chapter 4

American College of Sports Medicine. 2002. "American College of Sports Medicine Position Stand: Progression Models in Resistance Training for Healthy Adults." *Med Sci Sports Exerc* 34 (2): 364-380.

American College of Sports Medicine. 2009. "American College of Sports Medicine Position Stand: Progression Models in Resistance Training for Healthy Adults." *Med Sci Sports Exerc* 41 (3): 687-708.

Bickel, C.S., J.M. Cross, and M.M. Bamman. 2011. "Exercise Dosing to Retain Resistance Training Adaptations in Young and Older Adults." *Med Sci Sports Exerc* 43 (7): 1177-1187. https://doi.org/10.1249/MSS.0b013e318207c15d.

Brawner, C.A., S.J. Keteyian, and M. Saval. 2010. "Adaptations to Cardiorespiratory Exercise Training." In *ACSM's Resource Manual for Guidelines for Exercise Testing and Prescription,* 476-488. Philadelphia, PA: Lippincott Williams & Wilkins.

Buckwalter, J.A., and J.A. Martin. 2004. "Sports and Osteoarthritis." *Curr Opin Rheumatol* 16 (5): 634-639. https://doi.org/10.1097/01.bor.0000132647.55056.a9.

Burr, D.B., A.G. Robling, and C.H. Turner. 2002. "Effects of Biomechanical Stress on Bones in Animals." *Bone* 30 (5): 781-786. https://doi.org/10.1016/s8756-3282(02)00707-x.

Casa, D.J., S.A. Anderson, L. Baker, S. Bennett, M.F. Bergeron, D. Connolly, R. Courson, et al. 2012. "The Inter-Association Task Force for Preventing Sudden Death in Collegiate Conditioning Sessions: Best Practices Recommendations." *J Athl Train* 47 (4): 477-80. https://doi.org/10.4085/1062-6050-47.4.08.

Cools, K.S., M.D. Crowder, K.L. Kucera, L.C. Thomas, Y. Hosokawa, D.J. Casa, A. Gasim, S. Lee, and T.M. Schade Willis. 2022. "Sudden Death in High School Athletes: A Case Series Examining the Influence of Sickle Cell Trait." *Pediatr Emerg Care* 38 (2): e497-e500. https://doi.org/10.1097/PEC.0000000000002632.

Damas, F., C.A. Libardi, and C. Ugrinowitsch. 2018. "The Development of Skeletal Muscle Hypertrophy Through Resistance Training: The Role of Muscle Damage and Muscle Protein Synthesis." *Eur J Appl Physiol* 118: 485-500.

Dickerman, R.D., R. Pertusi, and G.H. Smith. 2000. "The Upper Range of Lumbar Spine Bone Mineral Density? An Examination of the Current World Record Holder in the Squat Lift." *Int J Sports Med* 21 (7): 469-470. https://doi.org/10.1055/s-2000-7417.

Fry, A.C. 2004. "The Role of Resistance Exercise Intensity on Muscle Fibre Adaptations." *Sports Med* 34 (10): 663-679. https://doi.org/10.2165/00007256-200434100-00004.

Guadalupe-Grau, A., J. Perez-Gomez, H. Olmedillas, J. Chavarren, C. Dorado, A. Santana, J.A. Serrano-Sanchez, and J.A. Calbet. 2009. "Strength Training Combined With Plyometric Jumps in Adults: Sex Differences in Fat-Bone Axis Adaptations." *J Appl Physiol (1985)* 106 (4): 1100-1111. https://doi.org/10.1152/japplphysiol.91469.2008.

Guth, L.M., and S.M. Roth. 2013. "Genetic Influence on Athletic Performance." *Curr Opin Pediatr* 25 (6): 653-658. https://doi.org/10.1097/MOP.0b013e3283659087.

Haff, G.G., and N.T. Triplett, eds. 2016. *Essentials of Strength Training and Conditioning.* 4th ed. Champaign, IL: Human Kinetics.

Hosokawa, Y., W.M. Adams, D.J. Casa, J.K. Vanos, E.R. Cooper, A.J. Grundstein, O. Jay, et al. 2021. "Roundtable on Preseason Heat Safety in Secondary School Athletics: Environmental Monitoring During Activities in the Heat." *J Athl Train* 56 (4): 362-371. https://doi.org/10.4085/1062-6050-0067.20.

Kjaer, M., H. Langberg, B.F. Miller, R. Boushel, R. Crameri, S. Koskinen, K. Heinemeier, et al. 2005. "Metabolic Activity and Collagen Turnover in Human Tendon in Response to Physical Activity." *J Musculoskelet Neuronal Interact* 5 (1): 41-52.

Kongsgaard, M., S. Reitelseder, T.G. Pedersen, L. Holm, P. Aagaard, M. Kjaer, and S.P. Magnusson. 2007. "Region Specific Patellar Tendon Hypertrophy in Humans Following Resistance Training." *Acta Physiol (Oxf)* 191 (2): 111-121. https://doi.org/10.1111/j.1748-1716.2007.01714.x.

Kraemer, W.J., L.K. Caldwell, E.M. Post, W.H. DuPont, E.R. Martini, N.A. Ratamess, T.K. Szivak, et al. 2020. "Body Composition in Elite Strongman Competitors." *J Strength Cond Res* 34 (12): 3326-3330. https://doi.org/10.1519/JSC.0000000000003763.

Kraemer, W.J., S.J. Fleck, and M.R. Deschenes. 2021. *Exercise Physiology: Integrating Theory and Application*. 3rd ed. Philadelphia, PA: Wolters Kluwer.

Kraemer, W.J., B. Noble, B. Culver, and R.V. Lewis. 1985. "Changes in Plasma Proenkephalin Peptide F and Catecholamine Levels During Graded Exercise in Men." *Proc Natl Acad Sci USA* 82 (18): 6349-6451. https://doi.org/10.1073/pnas.82.18.6349.

Kraemer, W.J., J.F. Patton, S.E. Gordon, E.A. Harman, M.R. Deschenes, K. Reynolds, R.U. Newton, N.T. Triplett, and J.E. Dziados. 1995. "Compatibility of High-Intensity Strength and Endurance Training on Hormonal and Skeletal Muscle Adaptations." *J Appl Physiol* 78 (3): 976-989. https://doi.org/10.1152/jappl.1995.78.3.976.

Kraemer, W.J., N.A. Ratamess, W.C. Hymer, B.C. Nindl, and M.S. Fragala. 2020. "Growth Hormone(s), Testosterone, Insulin-Like Growth Factors, and Cortisol: Roles and Integration for Cellular Development and Growth With Exercise." *Front Endocrinol (Lausanne)* 11: 33. https://doi.org/10.3389/fendo.2020.00033.

Kraemer, W.J., N.A. Ratamess, and B.C. Nindl. 2017. "Recovery Responses of Testosterone, Growth Hormone, and IGF-1 After Resistance Exercise." *J Appl Physiol (1985)* 122 (3): 549-558. https://doi.org/10.1152/japplphysiol.00599.2016.

Kraemer, W.J., N.A. Ratamess, and J.L. Vingren. 2019. "Genetic Contributions to Neuroendocrine Responses to Resistance Training." In *Routledge Handbook of Sport and Exercise Systems Genetics*, edited by J.T. Lightfoot, M.J. Hubal and S.M. Roth, 290-309. New York, NY: Routledge.

Lopiano, D.A., and C. Zotos. 2014. *Athletic Director's Desk Reference*. Champaign, IL: Human Kinetics.

McCrum, C., P. Leow, G. Epro, M. Konig, K. Meijer, and K. Karamanidis. 2018. "Alterations in Leg Extensor Muscle-Tendon Unit Biomechanical Properties With Ageing and Mechanical Loading." *Front Physiol* 9: 150. https://doi.org/10.3389/fphys.2018.00150.

NSCA. 2017. "NSCA Strength and Conditioning Professional Standards and Guidelines." *Strength and Conditioning Journal* 39 (6): 1-24.

Poliquin, C. 1988. "Five Steps to Increasing the Effectiveness of Your Strength Training Program " *NSCA Journal* 10 (3): 34-39.

Puthucheary, Z., J.R. Skipworth, J. Rawal, M. Loosemore, K. Van Someren, and H.E. Montgomery. 2011. "Genetic Influences in Sport and Physical Performance." *Sports Med* 41 (10): 845-859. https://doi.org/10.2165/11593200-000000000-00000.

Ratamess, N.A. 2008. "Adaptations to Anaerobic Training Programs." In *Essentials of Strength Training and Conditioning*, edited by T.R. Baechle and R.W. Earle, 93-119. Champaign, IL: Human KInetics.

Ratamess, N.A. 2022. *ACSM's Foundations of Strength Training and Conditioning*. Philadelphia, PA: Wolters Kluwer.

Rhea, M.R., S.D. Ball, W.T. Phillips, and L.N. Burkett. 2002. "A Comparison of Linear and Daily Undulating Periodized Programs with Equated Volume and Intensity for Strength." *J Strength Cond Res* 16 (2): 250-5.

Szymanski, M.R., S.E. Scarneo-Miller, M.S. Smith, M.L. Bruner, and D.J. Casa. 2020. "Emergency Medical Service Directors' Protocols for Exertional Heat Stroke." *Medicina (Kaunas)* 56 (10). https://doi.org/10.3390/medicina56100494.

Wernbom, M., J. Augustsson, and R. Thomee. 2007. "The Influence of Frequency, Intensity, Volume and Mode of Strength Training on Whole Muscle Cross-Sectional Area in Humans." *Sports Med* 37 (3): 225-264. https://doi.org/10.2165/00007256-200737030-00004.

Yeargin, S.W., Z.Y. Kerr, D.J. Casa, A. Djoko, R. Hayden, J.T. Parsons, and T.P. Dompier. 2016. "Epidemiology of Exertional Heat Illnesses in Youth, High School, and College Football." *Med Sci Sports Exerc* 48 (8): 1523-1529. https://doi.org/10.1249/MSS.0000000000000934.

Chapter 5

Foster, C., J.A. Florhaug, J. Franklin, L. Gottschall, L.A. Hrovatin, S. Parker, P. Doleshal, and C. Dodge. 2001. "A New Approach to Monitoring Exercise Training." *J Strength Cond Res* 15 (1): 109-15.

French, D.N., and L. Torres Ronda, eds. 2022. *NSCA's Essentials of Sport Science*. Champaign, IL: Human Kinetics.

Haff, G.G., and N.T. Triplett, eds. 2016. *Essentials of Strength Training and Conditioning*. 4th ed. Champaign, IL: Human Kinetics.

McGuigan, M. 2017. *Monitoring Training and Performance in Athletes*. Champaign, IL: Human Kinetics.

Ratamess, N.A. 2022. *ACSM's Foundations of Strength Training and Conditioning*. Philadelphia, PA: Wolters Kluwer.

Selye, H. 1976. "Forty Years of Stress Research: Principal Remaining Problems and Misconceptions." *Can Med Assoc J* 115 (1): 53-6.

Chapter 6

Amonette, W.E., K.L. English, and W.J. Kraemer. 2016. *Evidence-Based Practice in Exercise Science: The Six-Step Approach*. Champaign, IL: Human Kinetics.

Antonio, J., A. Leaf, C. Carson, A. Ellenbroek, T. Silver, C. Peacock, P. Bommarito, S. Knafo, and J. Tartar. 2018. "Bone Mineral Density in Competitive Athletes." *J Exerc Nutr* 1: 1-11.

Armstrong, L.E., and W.J. Kraemer, eds. 2016. *ACSM's Research Methods*. Philadelphia, PA: Wolters Kluwer.

Bangsbo, J., F.M. Iaia, and P. Krustrup. 2008. "The Yo-Yo Intermittent Recovery Test: A Useful Tool for Evaluation of Physical Performance in Intermittent Sports." *Sports Med* 38 (1): 37-51. https://doi.org/10.2165/00007256-200838010-00004.

Banister, E.W. 1991. "Modeling Elite Athletic Performance." In *Physiological Testing of Elite Athletes*, edited by J.D. MacDougall, H.A. Wenger and H.J. Green. Champaign, IL: Human Kinetics.

Bartolomei, S., G. Grillone, R. Di Michele, and M. Cortesi. 2021. "A Comparison Between Male and Female

Athletes in Relative Strength and Power Performances." *J Funct Morphol Kinesiol* 6 (1). https://doi.org/10.3390/jfmk6010017.

Bellenger, C.R., J.T. Fuller, R.L. Thomson, K. Davison, E.Y. Robertson, and J.D. Buckley. 2016. "Monitoring Athletic Training Status Through Autonomic Heart Rate Regulation: A Systematic Review and Meta-Analysis." *Sports Med* 46 (10): 1461-1486. https://doi.org/10.1007/s40279-016-0484-2.

Berckmans, K., A.G. Maenhout, L. Matthijs, L. Pieters, B. Castelein, and A.M. Cools. 2017. "The Isokinetic Rotator Cuff Strength Ratios in Overhead Athletes: Assessment and Exercise Effect." *Phys Ther Sport* 27: 65-75. https://doi.org/10.1016/j.ptsp.2017.03.001.

Bourne, M.N., D.A. Opar, M.D. Williams, and A.J. Shield. 2015. "Eccentric Knee Flexor Strength and Risk of Hamstring Injuries in Rugby Union: A Prospective Study." *Am J Sports Med* 43 (11): 2663-2670. https://doi.org/10.1177/0363546515599633.

Brady, C.J., A.J. Harrison, and T.M. Comyns. 2020. "A Review of the Reliability of Biomechanical Variables Produced During the Isometric Mid-Thigh Pull and Isometric Squat and the Reporting of Normative Data." *Sports Biomech* 19 (1): 1-25. https://doi.org/10.1080/14763141.2018.1452968.

Chaabene, H., M. Tabben, B. Mkaouer, E. Franchini, Y. Negra, M. Hammami, S. Amara, R.B. Chaabene, and Y. Hachana. 2015. "Amateur Boxing: Physical and Physiological Attributes." *Sports Med* 45 (3): 337-352. https://doi.org/10.1007/s40279-014-0274-7.

Cummins, C., R. Orr, H. O'Connor, and C. West. 2013. "Global Positioning Systems (GPS) and Microtechnology Sensors in Team Sports: A Systematic Review." *Sports Med* 43 (10): 1025-1042. https://doi.org/10.1007/s40279-013-0069-2.

Dallinga, J.M., A. Benjaminse, and K.A. Lemmink. 2012. "Which Screening Tools Can Predict Injury to the Lower Extremities in Team Sports? A Systematic Review." *Sports Med* 42 (9): 791-815. www.ncbi.nlm.nih.gov/pubmed/22909185.

Dos'Santos, T., C. Thomas, P.A. Jones, and P. Comfort. 2019. "Assessing Asymmetries in Change of Direction Speed Performance: Application of Change of Direction Deficit." *J Strength Cond Res* 33 (11): 2953-2961. https://doi.org/10.1519/JSC.0000000000002438.

Foster, C., J.A. Florhaug, J. Franklin, L. Gottschall, L.A. Hrovatin, S. Parker, P. Doleshal, and C. Dodge. 2001. "A New Approach to Monitoring Exercise Training." *J Strength Cond Res* 15 (1): 109-115.

French, D.N. 2017. *A Cross-Sectional Performance Analysis and Projection of the UFC Athlete.* UFC Performance Institute (Las Vegas, NV).

French, D.N., and L. Torres Ronda, eds. 2022. *NSCA's Essentials of Sport Science.* Champaign, IL: Human Kinetics.

Fukuda, D.H. 2019. *Assessments for Sport and Athletic Performance.* Champaign, IL: Human Kinetics.

Gabbett, T.J. 2016. "The Training-Injury Prevention Paradox: Should Athletes Be Training Smarter and Harder?" *Br J Sports Med* 50 (5): 273-280. https://doi.org/10.1136/bjsports-2015-095788.

Haddad, M., G. Stylianides, L. Djaoui, A. Dellal, and K. Chamari. 2017. "Session-RPE Method for Training Load Monitoring: Validity, Ecological Usefulness, and Influencing Factors." *Front Neurosci* 11: 612.

Haff, G.G., and N.T. Triplett, eds. 2016. *Essentials of Strength Training and Conditioning.* 4th ed. Champaign, IL: Human Kinetics.

Halson, S.L. 2014. "Monitoring Training Load to Understand Fatigue in Athletes." *Sports Med* 44 (Suppl 2): S139-S147. https://doi.org/10.1007/s40279-014-0253-z.

Hedlund, D.P. 2018. "Performance of Future Elite Players at the National Football League Scouting Combine." *J Strength Cond Res* 32 (11): 3112-3118. https://doi.org/10.1519/JSC.0000000000002252.

Hoffman, J. 2006. *Norms for Fitness, Performance, and Health.* Champaign, IL: Human Kinetics.

Johnson, B.L., and J.K. Nelson. 1986. *Practical Measurements for Evaluation in Physical Education.* 4th ed. Minneapolis, MN: MacMillan Publishing.

Kraemer, W.J., L.K. Caldwell, E.M. Post, W.H. DuPont, E.R. Martini, N.A. Ratamess, T.K. Szivak, et al. 2020. "Body Composition in Elite Strongman Competitors." *J Strength Cond Res* 34 (12): 3326-3330. https://doi.org/10.1519/JSC.0000000000003763.

Kraemer, W.J., S.J. Fleck, and M.R. Deschenes. 2021. *Exercise Physiology: Integrating Theory and Application.* 3rd ed. Philadelphia, PA: Wolters Kluwer.

Kraemer, W.J., J.C. Torine, R. Silvestre, D.N. French, N.A. Ratamess, B.A. Spiering, D.L. Hatfield, J.L. Vingren, and J.S. Volek. 2005. "Body Size and Composition of National Football League Players." *J Strength Cond Res* 19 (3): 485-489. https://doi.org/10.1519/18175.1.

McMaster, D.T., N. Gill, J. Cronin, and M. McGuigan. 2014. "A Brief Review of Strength and Ballistic Assessment Methodologies in Sport." *Sports Med* 44 (5): 603-623. https://doi.org/10.1007/s40279-014-0145-2.

Mountjoy, M., J. Sundgot-Borgen, L. Burke, S. Carter, N. Constantini, C. Lebrun, N. Meyer, et al. 2014. "The IOC Consensus Statement: Beyond the Female Athlete Triad—Relative Energy Deficiency in Sport (RED-S)." *Br J Sports Med* 48 (7): 491-497. https://doi.org/10.1136/bjsports-2014-093502.

Nimphius, S., S.J. Callaghan, T. Spiteri, and R.G. Lockie. 2016. "Change of Direction Deficit: A More Isolated Measure of Change of Direction Performance Than Total 505 Time." *J Strength Cond Res* 30 (11): 3024-3032. https://doi.org/10.1519/JSC.0000000000001421.

Opar, D.A., M.D. Williams, R.G. Timmins, J. Hickey, S.J. Duhig, and A.J. Shield. 2015. "Eccentric Hamstring Strength and Hamstring Injury Risk in Australian Footballers." *Med Sci Sports Exerc* 47 (4): 857-65. https://doi.org/10.1249/MSS.0000000000000465.

Padua, D.A., L.J. DiStefano, A.I. Beutler, S.J. de la Motte, M.J. DiStefano, and S.W. Marshall. 2015. "The Landing Error Scoring System as a Screening Tool for an Anterior Cruciate Ligament Injury-Prevention Program in Elite-Youth Soccer Athletes." *J Athl Train* 50 (6): 589-595. https://doi.org/10.4085/1062-6050-50.1.10.

Peterson, M.D. 2012. "Power." In *NSCA's Guide to Tests and Assessments*, 217-252. Champaign, IL: Human Kinetics.

Plisky, P., K. Schwartkopf-Phifer, B. Huebner, M.B. Garner, and G. Bullock. 2021. "Systematic Review and Meta-Analysis of the Y-Balance Test Lower Quarter: Reliability, Discriminant Validity, and Predictive Validity." *Int J Sports Phys Ther* 16 (5): 1190-1209. https://doi.org/10.26603/001c.27634.

Poliquin, C. 1999. "Achieving Structural Balance." *T Nation*. May 14, 1999. www.t-nation.com/training/achieving-structural-balance.

Ransdell, L.B., T. Murray, Y. Gao, P. Jones, and D. Bycura. 2020. "A 4-Year Profile of Game Demands in Elite Women's Division I College Basketball." *J Strength Cond Res* 34 (3): 632-638. https://doi.org/10.1519/JSC.0000000000003425.

Ratamess, N.A. 2022. *ACSM's Foundations of Strength Training and Conditioning*. Philadelphia, PA: Wolters Kluwer.

Ratamess, N.A., J.R. Hoffman, A.D. Faigenbaum, G.T. Mangine, M.J. Falvo, and J. Kang. 2007. "The Combined Effects of Protein Intake and Resistance Training on Serum Osteocalcin Concentrations in Strength and Power Athletes." *J Strength Cond Res* 21 (4): 1197-203. https://doi.org/10.1519/R-21746.1.

Ratamess, N.A., J.R. Hoffman, W.J. Kraemer, R.E. Ross, C.P. Tranchina, S.L. Rashti, N.A. Kelly, J.L. Vingren, J. Kang, and A.D. Faigenbaum. 2013. "Effects of a Competitive Wrestling Season on Body Composition, Endocrine Markers, and Anaerobic Exercise Performance in NCAA Collegiate Wrestlers." *Eur J Appl Physiol* 113 (5): 1157-1168. https://doi.org/10.1007/s00421-012-2520-8.

Rippetoe, M. 2011. *Starting Strength: Basic Barbell Training*. 3rd ed. Wichita Falls, TX: Aasgaard Company.

Ryan, C., A. Uthoff, C. McKenzie, and J. Cronin. 2022. "Traditional and Modified 5-0-5 Change of Direction Test: Normative and Reliability Analysis." *Strength and Conditioning Journal* 44 (4): 23-37.

Sagayama, H., E. Kondo, Y. Tanabe, T. Ohnishi, Y. Yamada, and H. Takahashi. 2020. "Bone Mineral Density in Male Weight-Classified Athletes Is Higher Than That in Male Endurance-Athletes and Non-Athletes." *Clin Nutr ESPEN* 36: 106-110.

Samozino, P., J.B. Morin, F. Hintzy, and A. Belli. 2008. "A Simple Method for Measuring Force, Velocity and Power Output During Squat Jump." *J Biomech* 41 (14): 2940-2945. https://doi.org/10.1016/j.jbiomech.2008.07.028.

Samozino, P., G. Rabita, S. Dorel, J. Slawinski, N. Peyrot, E. Saez de Villarreal, and J.B. Morin. 2016. "A Simple Method for Measuring Power, Force, Velocity Properties, and Mechanical Effectiveness in Sprint Running." *Scand J Med Sci Sports* 26 (6): 648-658. https://doi.org/10.1111/sms.12490.

Sole, C.J., T.J. Suchomel, and M.H. Stone. 2018. "Preliminary Scale of Reference Values for Evaluating Reactive Strength Index-Modified in Male and Female NCAA Division I Athletes." *Sports (Basel)* 6 (4).

Stanforth, D., T. Lu, M.A. Stults-Kolehmainen, B.N. Crim, and P.R. Stanforth. 2016. "Bone Mineral Content and Density Among Female NCAA Division I Athletes Across the Competitive Season and Over a Multi-Year Time Frame." *J Strength Cond Res* 30 (10): 2828-2838. https://doi.org/10.1519/JSC.0000000000000785.

Suchomel, T.J., S. Nimphius, and M.H. Stone. 2016. "The Importance of Muscular Strength in Athletic Performance." *Sports Med* 46 (10): 1419-1449. https://doi.org/10.1007/s40279-016-0486-0.

Thibaudeau, C. 2018. "Destroy Weaknesses." *ThibArmy*. September 27, 2018. https://thibarmy.com/know-your-ratios-destroy-weaknesses.

Wang, R., J.R. Hoffman, E. Sadres, S. Bartolomei, T.W.D. Muddle, D.H. Fukuda, and J.R. Stout. 2017. "Evaluating Upper-Body Strength and Power From a Single Test: The Ballistic Push-Up." *J Strength Cond Res* 31 (5): 1338-1345. https://doi.org/10.1519/JSC.0000000000001832.

Wille, C.M., M.R. Stiffler-Joachim, S.A. Kliethermes, J.L. Sanfilippo, C.S. Tanaka, and B.C. Heiderscheit. 2022. "Preseason Eccentric Strength Is Not Associated With Hamstring Strain Injury: A Prospective Study in Collegiate Athletes." *Med Sci Sports Exerc* 54 (8): 1271-1277. https://doi.org/10.1249/MSS.0000000000002913.

Chapter 7

Afonso, J., J. Olivares-Jabalera, and R. Andrade. 2021. "Time to Move From Mandatory Stretching? We Need to Differentiate 'Can I?' From 'Do I Have To?'." *Front Physiol* 12: 714166. https://doi.org/10.3389/fphys.2021.714166.

Ailioaie, L.M., and G. Litscher. 2021. "Photobiomodulation and Sports: Results of a Narrative Review." *Life (Basel)* 11 (12). https://doi.org/10.3390/life11121339.

Alexander, J., J. Keegan, A. Reedy, and D. Rhodes. 2022. "Effects of Contemporary Cryo-Compression on Post-Training Performance in Elite Academy Footballers." *Biol Sport* 39 (1): 11-17. https://doi.org/10.5114/biolsport.2022.102866.

American College of Sports Medicine. 2009. "American College of Sports Medicine Position Stand: Progression Models in Resistance Training for Healthy Adults." *Med Sci Sports Exerc* 41 (3): 687-708.

American College of Sports Medicine. 2011. "American College of Sports Medicine Position Stand: Quantity and Quality of Exercise for Developing and Maintaining Cardiorespiratory, Musculoskeletal, and Neuromotor Fitness in Apparently Healthy Adults: Guidance for Prescribing Exercise." *Med Sci Sports Exerc* 23 (7): 1334-1359.

Baker, D., and R.U. Newton. 2005. "Acute Effect on Power Output of Alternating an Agonist and Antagonist Muscle

Exercise During Complex Training." *J Strength Cond Res* 19 (1): 202-205. www.ncbi.nlm.nih.gov/pubmed/15705035.

Belenky, G., N.J. Wesensten, D.R. Thorne, M.L. Thomas, H.C. Sing, D.P. Redmond, M.B. Russo, and T.J. Balkin. 2003. "Patterns of Performance Degradation and Restoration During Sleep Restriction and Subsequent Recovery: A Sleep Dose-Response Study." *J Sleep Res* 12 (1): 1-12. https://doi.org/10.1046/j.1365-2869.2003.00337.x.

Belval, L.N., Y. Hosokawa, D.J. Casa, W.M. Adams, L.E. Armstrong, L.B. Baker, L. Burke, et al. 2019. "Practical Hydration Solutions for Sports." *Nutrients* 11 (7). https://doi.org/10.3390/nu11071550.

Bogdanis, G.C., A. Tsoukos, O. Kaloheri, G. Terzis, P. Veligekas, and L.E. Brown. 2019. "Comparison Between Unilateral and Bilateral Plyometric Training on Single- and Double-Leg Jumping Performance and Strength." *J Strength Cond Res* 33 (3): 633-640. https://doi.org/10.1519/JSC.0000000000001962.

Bompa, T.O., and G.G. Haff. 2009. *Periodization: Theory and Methodology of Training*. 5th ed. Champaign, IL: Human Kinetics.

Brooks, G.A. 2020. "The Tortuous Path of Lactate Shuttle Discovery: From Cinders and Boards to the Lab and ICU." *J Sport Health Sci* 9 (5): 446-460. https://doi.org/10.1016/j.jshs.2020.02.006.

Caldwell, L.K., W.J. Kraemer, E.M. Post, J.S. Volek, B.C. Focht, R.U. Newton, K. Hakkinen, and C.M. Maresh. 2022. "Acute Floatation-Rest Improves Perceived Recovery After a High-Intensity Resistance Exercise Stress in Trained Men." *Med Sci Sports Exerc* 54 (8): 1371-1381. https://doi.org/10.1249/MSS.0000000000002906.

Campbell, B.I. 2020. *NSCA's Guide to Sport and Exercise Nutrition*. 2nd ed. Champaign, IL: Human Kinetics.

Cao, S., S.K. Geok, S. Roslan, S. Qian, H. Sun, S.K. Lam, and J. Liu. 2022. "Mindfulness-Based Interventions for the Recovery of Mental Fatigue: A Systematic Review." *Int J Environ Res Public Health* 19 (13). https://doi.org/10.3390/ijerph19137825.

Casa, D.J., J. Almquist, S.A. Anderson, L. Baker, M.F. Bergeron, B. Biagioli, B. Boden, et al. 2013. "The Inter-Association Task Force for Preventing Sudden Death in Secondary School Athletics Programs: Best-Practices Recommendations." *J Athl Train* 48 (4): 546-553. https://doi.org/10.4085/1062-6050-48.4.12.

Casa, D.J., S.A. Anderson, L. Baker, S. Bennett, M.F. Bergeron, D. Connolly, R. Courson, et al. 2012. "The Inter-Association Task Force for Preventing Sudden Death in Collegiate Conditioning Sessions: Best Practices Recommendations." *J Athl Train* 47 (4): 477-480. https://doi.org/10.4085/1062-6050-47.4.08.

Chu, D.A. 1998. *Jumping into Plyometrics*. Champaign, IL: Human Kinetics.

Comfort, P., G.G. Haff, T.J. Suchomel, M.A. Soriano, K.C. Pierce, W.G. Hornsby, E.E. Haff, et al. 2023. "National Strength and Conditioning Association Position Statement on Weightlifting for Sports Performance." *J Strength Cond Res* 37 (6): 1163-1190.

Culav, E.M., C.H. Clark, and M.J. Merrilees. 1999. "Connective Tissues: Matrix Composition and Its Relevance to Physical Therapy." *Phys Ther* 79 (3): 308-319.

Cullen, M.L., G.A. Casazza, and B.A. Davis. 2021. "Passive Recovery Strategies After Exercise: A Narrative Literature Review of the Current Evidence." *Curr Sports Med Rep* 20 (7): 351-358. https://doi.org/10.1249/JSR.0000000000000859.

da Silva, C.A., L. Helal, R.P. da Silva, K.C. Belli, D. Umpierre, and R. Stein. 2018. "Association of Lower Limb Compression Garments During High-Intensity Exercise With Performance and Physiological Responses: A Systematic Review and Meta-Analysis." *Sports Med* 48 (8): 1859-1873. https://doi.org/10.1007/s40279-018-0927-z.

Davies, T., R. Orr, M. Halaki, and D. Hackett. 2016a. "Effect of Training Leading to Repetition Failure on Muscular Strength: A Systematic Review and Meta-Analysis." *Sports Med* 46 (4): 487-502. https://doi.org/10.1007/s40279-015-0451-3.

Davies, T., R. Orr, M. Halaki, and D. Hackett. 2016b. "Erratum To: Effect of Training Leading to Repetition Failure on Muscular Strength: A Systematic Review and Meta-Analysis." *Sports Med* 46 (4): 605-610. https://doi.org/10.1007/s40279-016-0509-x.

Davis, H.L., S. Alabed, and T.J.A. Chico. 2020. "Effect of Sports Massage on Performance and Recovery: A Systematic Review and Meta-Analysis." *BMJ Open Sport Exerc Med* 6 (1): e000614. https://doi.org/10.1136/bmjsem-2019-000614.

de Villarreal, E.S., E. Kellis, W.J. Kraemer, and M. Izquierdo. 2009. "Determining Variables of Plyometric Training for Improving Vertical Jump Height Performance: A Meta-Analysis." *J Strength Cond Res* 23 (2): 495-506. https://doi.org/10.1519/JSC.0b013e318196b7c6.

Delorme, T.L., R.S. Schwab, and A.L. Watkins. 1948. "The Response of the Quadriceps Femoris to Progressive-Resistance Exercises in Poliomyelitic Patients." *J Bone Joint Surg Am* 30A (4): 834-847.

Delorme, T.L., and A.L. Watkins. 1948. "Technics of Progressive Resistance Exercise." *Arch Phys Med Rehabil* 29 (5): 263-273. Accessed May. www.ncbi.nlm.nih.gov/pubmed/18860422.

Delorme, T.L., F.E. West, and W.J. Shriber. 1950. "Influence of Progressive Resistance Exercises on Knee Function Following Femoral Fractures." *J Bone Joint Surg Am* 32 A (4): 910-924.

Drillera, M.W., and C.K. Argusbc. 2016. "Flotation Restricted Environmental Stimulation Therapy and Napping on Mood State and Muscle Soreness in Elite Athletes: A Novel Recovery Strategy?" *Performance Enhancement & Health* 5 (2): 60-65.

DuPont, W.H., B.J. Meuris, V.H. Hardesty, E.C. Barnhart, L.H. Tompkins, M.J.P. Golden, C.J. Usher, et al. 2017. "The Effects Combining Cryocompression Therapy Following an Acute Bout of Resistance Exercise on Performance and Recovery." *J Sports Sci Med* 16 (3): 333-342.

Earp, J.E., D.L. Hatfield, A. Sherman, E.C. Lee, and W.J. Kraemer. 2019. "Cold-Water Immersion Blunts and Delays Increases in Circulating Testosterone and Cytokines Post-Resistance Exercise." *Eur J Appl Physiol* 119 (8): 1901-1907. https://doi.org/10.1007/s00421-019-04178-7.

Earp, J.E., and W.J. Kraemer. 2010. "Medicine Ball Training Implications for Rotational Power Sports." *Strength and Conditioning Journal* 32 (4): 20-25.

Ebben, W.P. 2006. *NSCA Performance Journal* 6: 12-16.

Ferlito, J.V., M.V. Ferlito, E.C.P. Leal-Junior, S.S. Tomazoni, and T. De Marchi. 2022. "Comparison Between Cryotherapy and Photobiomodulation in Muscle Recovery: A Systematic Review and Meta-Analysis." *Lasers Med Sci* 37 (3): 1375-1388. https://doi.org/10.1007/s10103-021-03442-7.

Fleck, S.J., and W.J. Kraemer. 1997. *Designing Resistance Training Programs*. 2nd ed. Champaign, IL: Human Kinetics.

Fleck, S.J., and W.J. Kraemer. 2014. *Designing Resistance Training Programs*. 4th ed. Champaign, IL: Human Kinetics.

French, D.N., and L. Torres Ronda, eds. 2022. *NSCA's Essentials of Sport Science*. Champaign, IL: Human Kinetics.

Fry, A.C., W.J. Kraemer, F. van Borselen, J.M. Lynch, J.L. Marsit, E.P. Roy, N.T. Triplett, and H.G. Knuttgen. 1994. "Performance Decrements With High-Intensity Resistance Exercise Overtraining." *Med Sci Sports Exerc* 26 (9): 1165-1173.

Haugen, T., S. Seiler, O. Sandbakk, and E. Tonnessen. 2019. "The Training and Development of Elite Sprint Performance: An Integration of Scientific and Best Practice Literature." *Sports Med Open* 5 (1): 44. https://doi.org/10.1186/s40798-019-0221-0.

Issurin, V.B. 2008. *Block Periodization: Breakthrough in Sport Training*. Edited by M.A. Yessis. Ultimate Athlete Concepts.

Jones, K., B. P., G. Hunter, and G. Fleisig. 2001. "The Effects of Varying Resistance-Training Loads on Intermediate- and High-Velocity-Specific Adaptations." *J Strength Cond Res* 15: 349-356.

Kim, K., J.C. Monroe, T.P. Gavin, and B.T. Roseguini. 2020. "Local Heat Therapy to Accelerate Recovery After Exercise-Induced Muscle Damage." *Exerc Sport Sci Rev* 48 (4): 163-169. https://doi.org/10.1249/JES.0000000000000230.

Kim, K., B.A. Reid, C.A. Casey, B.E. Bender, B. Ro, Q. Song, A.J. Trewin, et al. 2020. "Effects of Repeated Local Heat Therapy on Skeletal Muscle Structure and Function in Humans." *J Appl Physiol* 128 (3): 483-492. https://doi.org/10.1152/japplphysiol.00701.2019.

Kim, T.Y., and J.H. Kim. 2021. "Performance Enhancement through Meditation in Athletes: Insights From a Systematic Review of Randomized Controlled Trials." *Explore (NY)* 17 (5): 403-409. https://doi.org/10.1016/j.explore.2021.02.003.

Knuttgen, H.G., and W.J. Kraemer. 1987. "Terminology and Measurement in Exercise Performance." *J Appl Sport Sci Res* 1 (1): 1-10.

Konrad, A., M. Nakamura, and D.G. Behm. 2022. "The Effects of Foam Rolling Training on Performance Parameters: A Systematic Review and Meta-Analysis Including Controlled and Randomized Controlled Trials." *Int J Environ Res Public Health* 19 (18). https://doi.org/10.3390/ijerph191811638.

Kraemer, W.J. 1997. "A Series of Studies—the Physiological Basis for Strength Training in American Football: Fact Over Philosophy." *J Strength Cond Res* 11 (3): 131-142.

Kraemer, W.J., J.A. Bush, J.A. Bauer, N.T. Triplett-McBride, N.J. Paxton, A. Clemson, L.P. Koriris, L.C. Mangino, A.C. Fry, and R.U. Newton. 1996. "Influence of Compression Garments on Vertical Jump Performances in NCAA I Volleyball Players." *J Strength Cond Res* 10 (3): 180-183.

Kraemer, W.J., J.A. Bush, R.B. Wickham, C.R. Denegar, A.L. Gomez, L.A. Gotshalk, N.D. Duncan, J.S. Volek, M. Putukian, and W.J. Sebastianelli. 2001. "Influence of Compression Therapy on Symptoms Following Soft Tissue Injury From Maximal Eccentric Exercise." *J Orthop Sports Phys Ther* 31 (6): 282-90. https://doi.org/10.2519/jospt.2001.31.6.282.

Kraemer, W.J., S.D. Flanagan, B.A. Comstock, M.S. Fragala, J.E. Earp, C. Dunn-Lewis, J.Y. Ho, et al. 2010. "Effects of a Whole Body Compression Garment on Markers of Recovery After a Heavy Resistance Workout in Men and Women." *J Strength Cond Res* 24 (3): 804-814. https://doi.org/10.1519/JSC.0b013e3181d33025.

Kraemer, W.J., and S. Fleck. 2007. *Optimizing Strength Training: Designing Nonlinear Periodization Workouts*. Champaign, IL: Human Kinetics.

Kraemer, W.J., S.J. Fleck, and M.R. Deschenes. 2021. *Exercise Physiology: Integrating Theory and Application*. 3rd ed. Philadelphia, PA: Wolters Kluwer.

Kraemer, W.J., S.J. Fleck, J.E. Dziados, E.A. Harman, L.J. Marchitelli, S.E. Gordon, R. Mello, P.N. Frykman, L.P. Koziris, and N.T. Triplett. 1993. "Changes in Hormonal Concentrations After Different Heavy-Resistance Exercise Protocols in Women." *J Appl Physiol* 75 (2): 594-604. https://doi.org/10.1152/jappl.1993.75.2.594.

Kraemer, W.J., K. Hakkinen, N.T. Triplett-Mcbride, A.C. Fry, L.P. Koziris, N.A. Ratamess, J.E. Bauer, et al. 2003. "Physiological Changes With Periodized Resistance Training in Women Tennis Players." *Med Sci Sports Exerc* 35 (1): 157-168. https://doi.org/10.1097/00005768-200301000-00024.

Kraemer, W.J., D.R. Hooper, B.R. Kupchak, C. Saenz, L.E. Brown, J.L. Vingren, H.Y. Luk, et al. 2016. "The Effects of a Roundtrip Trans-American Jet Travel on Physiological Stress, Neuromuscular Performance, and Recovery." *J Appl Physiol (1985)* 121 (2): 438-448. https://doi.org/10.1152/japplphysiol.00429.2016.

Kraemer, W.J., L. Marchitelli, S.E. Gordon, E. Harman, J.E. Dziados, R. Mello, P. Frykman, D. McCurry, and S.J. Fleck. 1990. "Hormonal and Growth Factor Responses to

Heavy Resistance Exercise Protocols." *J Appl Physiol* 69 (4): 1442-1450. https://doi.org/10.1152/jappl.1990.69.4.1442.

Kraemer, W.J., N. Ratamess, A.C. Fry, T. Triplett-McBride, L.P. Koziris, J.A. Bauer, J.M. Lynch, and S.J. Fleck. 2000. "Influence of Resistance Training Volume and Periodization on Physiological and Performance Adaptations in Collegiate Women Tennis Players." *Am J Sports Med* 28 (5): 626-633. https://doi.org/10.1177/03635465000280050201.

Kraemer, W.J., and N.A. Ratamess. 2004. "Fundamentals of Resistance Training: Progression and Exercise Prescription." *Med Sci Sports Exerc* 36 (4): 674-688. https://doi.org/10.1249/01.mss.0000121945.36635.61.

Loose, L.F., J. Manuel, M. Karst, L.K. Schmidt, and F. Beissner. 2021. "Flotation Restricted Environmental Stimulation Therapy for Chronic Pain: A Randomized Clinical Trial." *JAMA Netw Open* 4 (5): e219627. https://doi.org/10.1001/jamanetworkopen.2021.9627.

Matveyev, L. 1965. *Periodisation of Sports Training*. Moscow, Russia: Fizkultura i Sport.

Mazzetti, S.A., W.J. Kraemer, J.S. Volek, N.D. Duncan, N.A. Ratamess, A.L. Gomez, R.U. Newton, K. Hakkinen, and S.J. Fleck. 2000. "The Influence of Direct Supervision of Resistance Training on Strength Performance." *Med Sci Sports Exerc* 32 (6): 1175-1184. https://doi.org/10.1097/00005768-200006000-00023.

McGuigan, M., ed. 2017. *Developing Power*. Edited by National Strength and Conditioning Association. Champaign, IL: Human Kinetics.

Medvedyev, A.S. 1986. *A System of Multi-Year Training in Weightlifting*. Moscow, Russia: Fizkultura i Sport.

Michalski, T., T. Król, P. Michalik, M. Rutkowska, M. Dąbrowska-Galas, D. Ziaja, and M. Kuszewski. 2022. "Does the Self-Myofascial Release Affect the Activity of Selected Lower Limb Muscles of Soccer Players?" *Journal of Human Kinetics* 83: 49-57 https://doi.org/10.2478/hukin-2022-0050.

Nelson, A.G., N.M. Driscoll, D.K. Landin, M.A. Young, and I.C. Schexnayder. 2005. "Acute Effects of Passive Muscle Stretching on Sprint Performance." *J Sports Sci* 23 (5): 449-454. https://doi.org/10.1080/02640410410001730205.

Nelson, A.G., J. Kokkonen, and D.A. Arnall. 2005. "Acute Muscle Stretching Inhibits Muscle Strength Endurance Performance." *J Strength Cond Res* 19 (2): 338-343. https://doi.org/10.1519/R-15894.1.

NSCA. 1993. "Position Statement: Explosive/Plyometric Exercises." *NSCA Journal* 15 (3): 16.

Nygaard Falch, H., H. Guldteig Raedergard, and R. van den Tillaar. 2019. "Effect of Different Physical Training Forms on Change of Direction Ability: A Systematic Review and Meta-Analysis." *Sports Med Open* 5 (1): 53. https://doi.org/10.1186/s40798-019-0223-y.

Pernigoni, M., D. Conte, J. Calleja-Gonzalez, G. Boccia, M. Romagnoli, and D. Ferioli. 2022. "The Application of Recovery Strategies in Basketball: A Worldwide Survey." *Front Physiol* 13: 887507. https://doi.org/10.3389/fphys.2022.887507.

Petrofsky, J.S., I.A. Khowailed, H. Lee, L. Berk, G.S. Bains, S. Akerkar, J. Shah, F. Al-Dabbak, and M.S. Laymon. 2015. "Cold vs. Heat After Exercise—Is There a Clear Winner for Muscle Soreness." *J Strength Cond Res* 29 (11): 3245-3252. https://doi.org/10.1519/JSC.0000000000001127.

Plisk, S.S., and M.H. Stone. 2003. "Periodization Strategies." *Strength and Conditioning Journal* 25 (6): 19-37.

Pohl, A., F. Schunemann, K. Bersiner, and S. Gehlert. 2021. "The Impact of Vegan and Vegetarian Diets on Physical Performance and Molecular Signaling in Skeletal Muscle." *Nutrients* 13 (11). https://doi.org/10.3390/nu13113884.

Poliquin, C. 1988. "Five Steps to Increasing the Effectiveness of Your Strength Training Program." *NSCA Journal* 10 (3): 34-39.

Poole, D.C., H.B. Rossiter, G.A. Brooks, and L.B. Gladden. 2021. "The Anaerobic Threshold: 50+ Years of Controversy." *J Physiol* 599 (3): 737-767. https://doi.org/10.1113/JP279963.

Ratamess, N.A. 2022. *ACSM's Foundations of Strength Training and Conditioning*. Philadelphia, PA: Wolters Kluwer.

Ratamess, N.A., C.M. Chiarello, A.J. Sacco, J.R. Hoffman, A.D. Faigenbaum, R.E. Ross, and J. Kang. 2012a. "The Effects of Rest Interval Length Manipulation of the First Upper-Body Resistance Exercise in Sequence on Acute Performance of Subsequent Exercises in Men and Women." *J Strength Cond Res* 26 (11): 2929-2938. https://doi.org/10.1519/JSC.0b013e318270fcf0.

Ratamess, N.A., C.M. Chiarello, A.J. Sacco, J.R. Hoffman, A.D. Faigenbaum, R.E. Ross, and J. Kang. 2012b. "The Effects of Rest Interval Length on Acute Bench Press Performance: The Influence of Gender and Muscle Strength." *J Strength Cond Res* 26 (7): 1817-1826. https://doi.org/10.1519/JSC.0b013e31825bb492.

Ratamess, N.A., M.J. Falvo, G.T. Mangine, J.R. Hoffman, A.D. Faigenbaum, and J. Kang. 2007. "The Effect of Rest Interval Length on Metabolic Responses to the Bench Press Exercise." *Eur J Appl Physiol* 100 (1): 1-17. https://doi.org/10.1007/s00421-007-0394-y.

Rhea, M.R., S.D. Ball, W.T. Phillips, and L.N. Burkett. 2002. "A Comparison of Linear and Daily Undulating Periodized Programs With Equated Volume and Intensity for Strength." *J Strength Cond Res* 16 (2): 250-255.

Rippetoe, M., and A. Baker. 2017. *Practical Programming for Strength Training*. 3rd ed. Wichita Falls, TX: Aasgaard Company.

Robergs, R.A., F. Ghiasvand, and D. Parker. 2004. "Biochemistry of Exercise-Induced Metabolic Acidosis." *Am J Physiol Regul Integr Comp Physiol* 287 (3): R502-R516. https://doi.org/10.1152/ajpregu.00114.2004.

Sakamoto, A., and P.J. Sinclair. 2006. "Effect of Movement Velocity on the Relationship Between Training Load and the Number of Repetitions of Bench Press." *J Strength Cond Res* 20 (3): 523-527. https://doi.org/10.1519/16794.1.

Selye, H. 1950. "Stress and the General Adaptation Syndrome." *Br Med J* 1 (4667): 1383-1392. https://doi.org/10.1136/bmj.1.4667.1383.

Selye, H. 1976. "Forty Years of Stress Research: Principal Remaining Problems and Misconceptions." *Can Med Assoc J* 115 (1): 53-56.

Shaw, M.P., V. Andersen, A.H. Saeterbakken, G. Paulsen, L.E. Samnoy, and T.E.J. Solstad. 2022. "Contemporary Training Practices of Norwegian Powerlifters." *J Strength Cond Res* 36 (9): 2544-2551. https://doi.org/10.1519/JSC.0000000000003584.

Shimano, T., W.J. Kraemer, B.A. Spiering, J.S. Volek, D.L. Hatfield, R. Silvestre, J.L. Vingren, et al. 2006. "Relationship Between the Number of Repetitions and Selected Percentages of One Repetition Maximum in Free Weight Exercises in Trained and Untrained Men." *J Strength Cond Res* 20 (4): 819-823. https://doi.org/10.1519/R-18195.1.

Shrier, I. 2004. "Does Stretching Improve Performance? A Systematic and Critical Review of the Literature." *Clin J Sport Med* 14 (5): 267-73. https://doi.org/10.1097/00042752-200409000-00004.

Shrier, I., and M. McHugh. 2012. "Does Static Stretching Reduce Maximal Muscle Performance? A Review." *Clin J Sport Med* 22 (5): 450-451. https://doi.org/10.1097/JSM.0b013e31826a08ee.

Simmons, L. 2007. *Westside Barbell Book of Methods*. Westside Barbell.

Spreuwenberg, L.P., W.J. Kraemer, B.A. Spiering, J.S. Volek, D.L. Hatfield, R. Silvestre, J.L Vingren, M.S. Fragala, K. Häkkinen, R.U. Newton, C.M. Maresh, and S.J. Fleck. 2006. "Influence of exercise order in a resistance-training exercise session." *Journal of Strength Cond Research* 20 (1): 141-4.

Sriwongtong, M., J. Goldman, Y. Kobayashi, and A.W. Gottschalk. 2020. "Does Massage Help Athletes After Exercise?" *Ochsner J* 20 (2): 121-122. https://doi.org/10.31486/toj.20.0008.

Statuta, S., and K. Pugh. 2019. "Training Room Procedures

Statuta, S., and K. Pugh. 2019. "Training Room Procedures and Use of Therapeutic Modalities in Athletes." *Clin Sports Med* 38 (4): 619-638. https://doi.org/10.1016/j.csm.2019.06.006.

Stone, M.H., H. O'Bryant, and J. Garhammer. 1981. "A Hypothetical Model for Strength Training." *J Sports Med Phys Fitness* 21 (4): 342-351.

Stone, M.H., H. O'Bryant, J. Garhammer, J. McMillan, and R. Rozenek. 1982. "A Theoretical Model of Strength Training." *National Strength and Conditioning Association Journal* 4 (4): 36-39.

Todd, J.S., J.P. Shurley, and T.C. Todd. 2012. "Thomas L. Delorme and the Science of Progressive Resistance Exercise." *J Strength Cond Res* 26 (11): 2913-2923. https://doi.org/10.1519/JSC.0b013e31825adcb4.

Torres, E.M., W.J. Kraemer, J.L. Vingren, J.S. Volek, D.L. Hatfield, B.A. Spiering, J.Y. Ho, et al. 2008. "Effects of Stretching on Upper-Body Muscular Performance." *J Strength Cond Res* 22 (4): 1279-1285. https://doi.org/10.1519/JSC.0b013e31816eb501.

Verkhoshansky, Y.V. 1977. *Fundamentals of Special Strength-Training in Sport*. Moscow, Russia: Fizkultura i Sport.

Verkhoshansky, Y.V., and M.C. Siff. 2009. *Supertraining*. 6th ed. Quebec, Canada: Dokumen.

Volek, J.S., D.J. Freidenreich, C. Saenz, L.J. Kunces, B.C. Creighton, J.M. Bartley, P.M. Davitt, et al. 2016. "Metabolic Characteristics of Keto-Adapted Ultra-Endurance Runners." *Metabolism* 65 (3): 100-110. https://doi.org/10.1016/j.metabol.2015.10.028.

Volek, J.S., and S.D. Phinney. 2012. *The Art and Science of Low Carbohydrate Performance*. Dublin, OH: Beyond Obesity.

Wang, Y., H. Lu, S. Li, Y. Zhang, F. Yan, Y. Huang, X. Chen, A. Yang, L. Han, and Y. Ma. 2022. "Effect of Cold and Heat Therapies on Pain Relief in Patients With Delayed Onset Muscle Soreness: A Network Meta-Analysis." *J Rehabil Med* 54: jrm00258. https://doi.org/10.2340/jrm.v53.331.

Wax, B., C.M. Kerksick, A.R. Jagim, J.J. Mayo, B.C. Lyons, and R.B. Kreider. 2021. "Creatine for Exercise and Sports Performance, With Recovery Considerations for Healthy Populations." *Nutrients* 13 (6). https://doi.org/10.3390/nu13061915.

Weakley, J., B. Mann, H. McLaren, S. Shaun; Scott, and A. T.G.R. 2021. "Velocity-Based Training: From Theory to Application." *Strength and Conditioning Journal* 43 (2): 31-49.

Wiewelhove, T., A. Doweling, C. Schneider, L. Hottenrott, T. Meyer, M. Kellmann, M. Pfeiffer, and A. Ferrauti. 2019. "A Meta-Analysis of the Effects of Foam Rolling on Performance and Recovery." *Front Physiol* 10: 376. https://doi.org/10.3389/fphys.2019.00376.

Wilk, M., M. Krzysztofk, and M. Bialas. 2020. "The Influence of Compressive Gear on Maximal Load Lifted in Competitive Powerlifting." *Biology of Sport* 37 (4): 437-441.

Zatsiorsky, V.M., W.J. Kraemer, and A.C. Fry. 2020. *Science and Practice of Strength Training*. 3rd ed. Champaign, IL: Human Kinetics

Zourdos, M.C., A. Klemp, C. Dolan, J.M. Quiles, K.A. Schau, E. Jo, E. Helms, et al. 2016. "Novel Resistance Training-Specific RPE Scale Measuring Repetitions in Reserve." *Journal of Strength and Conditioning Research* 30 (1): 267-275.

Chapter 8

Berryman, J.W. 1995. *Out of Many, One: A History of the American College of Sports Medicine*. Champaign, IL: Human Kinetics.

Coleman, B.J. 2012. "Identifying the 'Players' in Sports Analytics Research." *Interfaces* 42 (2): 109-118.

Delorme, T.L., and A.L. Watkins. 1951. *Progressive Resistance Exercise: Technic and Medical Application*. Norwalk, CT: Appleton-Century-Crofts.

English, K.L., J.J. Bloomberg, A.P. Mulavara, and L.L. Ploutz-Snyder. 2019. "Exercise Countermeasures to Neuromuscular Deconditioning in Spaceflight." *Compr Physiol* 10 (1): 171-196. https://doi.org/10.1002/cphy.c190005.

English, K.L., M. Downs, E. Goetchius, R. Buxton, J.W. Ryder, R. Ploutz-Snyder, M. Guilliams, J.M. Scott, and

L.L. Ploutz-Snyder. 2020. "High Intensity Training During Spaceflight: Results From the NASA Sprint Study." *NPJ Microgravity* 6: 21. https://doi.org/10.1038/s41526-020-00111-x.

Guttmann, A. 1988. "The Cold War and the Olympics." *International Journal: Canada's Journal of Global Policy Analysis* 43 (4): 554-568.

Henriksen, K., R. Schinke, K. Moesch, S. McCann, W.D. Parham, C.H. Larsen, and P. Terry. 2020. "Consensus Statement on Improving the Mental Health of High Performance Athletes." *International Journal of Sport and Exercise Psychology* 18 (5): 553-560.

Hoffman, J.R., N.A. Ratamess, M. Klatt, A.D. Faigenbaum, R.E. Ross, N.M. Tranchina, R.C. McCurley, J. Kang, and W.J. Kraemer. 2009. "Comparison Between Different Off-Season Resistance Training Programs in Division III American College Football Players." *J Strength Cond Res* 23 (1): 11-19. https://doi.org/10.1519/jsc.0b013e3181876a78.

Hudy, A. 2014. *Power Positions: Championship Prescriptions for Ultimate Sports Performance*. Dubuque, IA: Kendall Hunt Publishing

Kraemer, W.J. 1983. "Detraining the 'Bulked up' Athlete." *National Strength and Conditioning Association Journal* 5 (2): 10-12.

Kraemer, W.J. 1997. "A Series of Studies—the Physiological Basis for Strength Training in American Football: Fact Over Philosophy." *J Strength Cond Res* 11 (3): 131-142.

Kraemer, W.J., and S. Fleck. 2007. *Optimizing Strength Training: Designing Nonlinear Periodization Workouts*. Champaign, IL: Human Kinetics.

Kraemer, W.J., S.J. Fleck, J.E. Dziados, E.A. Harman, L.J. Marchitelli, S.E. Gordon, R. Mello, P.N. Frykman, L.P. Koziris, and N.T. Triplett. 1993. "Changes in Hormonal Concentrations After Different Heavy-Resistance Exercise Protocols in Women." *J Appl Physiol* 75 (2): 594-604. https://doi.org/10.1152/jappl.1993.75.2.594.

Kraemer, W.J., K. Hakkinen, N.T. Triplett-Mcbride, A.C. Fry, L.P. Koziris, N.A. Ratamess, J.E. Bauer, et al. 2003. "Physiological Changes with Periodized Resistance Training in Women Tennis Players." *Med Sci Sports Exerc* 35 (1): 157-168. https://doi.org/10.1097/00005768-200301000-00024.

Kraemer, W.J., L. Marchitelli, S.E. Gordon, E. Harman, J.E. Dziados, R. Mello, P. Frykman, D. McCurry, and S.J. Fleck. 1990. "Hormonal and Growth Factor Responses to Heavy Resistance Exercise Protocols." *J Appl Physiol* 69 (4): 1442-1450. https://doi.org/10.1152/jappl.1990.69.4.1442.

Kraemer, W.J., S.A. Mazzetti, B.C. Nindl, L.A. Gotshalk, J.S. Volek, J.A. Bush, J.O. Marx, et al. 2001. "Effect of Resistance Training on Women's Strength/Power and Occupational Performances." *Med Sci Sports Exerc* 33 (6): 1011-1025. https://doi.org/10.1097/00005768-200106000-00022.

Kraemer, W.J., and M. Nitka. 2022. "Development of the High School Sports Performance Program: Simple, Safe, and Successful." *Strength and Conditioning Journal* 44 (2): 131-133.

Kraemer, W.J., B.J. Noble, M.J. Clark, and B.W. Culver. 1987. "Physiologic Responses to Heavy-Resistance Exercise With Very Short Rest Periods." *Int J Sports Med* 8 (4): 247-252. https://doi.org/10.1055/s-2008-1025663.

Kraemer, W.J., J.F. Patton, S.E. Gordon, E.A. Harman, M.R. Deschenes, K. Reynolds, R.U. Newton, N.T. Triplett, and J.E. Dziados. 1995. "Compatibility of High-Intensity Strength and Endurance Training on Hormonal and Skeletal Muscle Adaptations." *J Appl Physiol* 78 (3): 976-989. https://doi.org/10.1152/jappl.1995.78.3.976.

Kraemer, W.J., N. Ratamess, A.C. Fry, T. Triplett-McBride, L.P. Koziris, J.A. Bauer, J.M. Lynch, and S.J. Fleck. 2000. "Influence of Resistance Training Volume and Periodization on Physiological and Performance Adaptations in Collegiate Women Tennis Players." *Am J Sports Med* 28 (5): 626-633. https://doi.org/10.1177/03635465000280050201.

Kraemer, W.J., N.A. Ratamess, W.C. Hymer, B.C. Nindl, and M.S. Fragala. 2020. "Growth Hormone(s), Testosterone, Insulin-Like Growth Factors, and Cortisol: Roles and Integration for Cellular Development and Growth With Exercise." *Front Endocrinol (Lausanne)* 11: 33. https://doi.org/10.3389/fendo.2020.00033.

Massengale, J.D., and R.A. Swanson, eds. 1996. *The History of Exercise and Sport Science*. Champaign, IL: Human Kinetics.

McKight, K., K. Bernes, T. Gunn, D. Chorney, D. Orr, and A. Bardick. 2009. "Life After Sport: Athletic Career Transition and Transferable Skills." *Journal of Excellence* (13): 63-77.

McQuilkin, S.A., and R.A. Smith. 2005. *The History of the National Strength and Conditioning Association, 1978-2000*. Colorado Springs, CO: National Strength and Conditioning Association.

Means, R.K., and A.E. Nolte. 1987. "Fifty Years of Health Education in AAHPERD: A Chronology, 1937-1987." *Health Education* 18 (1): 22-36.

Shurley, J.P., J. Todd, and T. Todd. 2019. *Strength Coaching in America: A History of the Innovation That Transformed Sports*. Austin, TX: University of Texas Press.

Tipton, C.M., ed. 2014. *History of Exercise Physiology*. Champaign, IL: Human Kinetics.

Todd, J.S., J.P. Shurley, and T.C. Todd. 2012. "Thomas L. Delorme and the Science of Progressive Resistance Exercise." *J Strength Cond Res* 26 (11): 2913-2923. https://doi.org/10.1519/JSC.0b013e31825adcb4.

Ward, B., and M. Engel. 2015. *Building the Perfect Star: Changing the Trajectory of Sports and the People in Them*. Olathe, KS: Bob Snodgrass and Ascend Books.

Weldon, A., M.J. Duncan, A. Turner, D. LaPlaca, J. Sampaio, and C.J. Christie. 2022. "Practices of Strength and Conditioning Coaches: A Snapshot From Different Sports, Countries, and Expertise Levels." *J Strength Cond Res* 36 (5): 1335-1344. https://doi.org/10.1519/JSC.0000000000003773.

Weldon, A., M.J. Duncan, A. Turner, R.G. Lockie, and I. Loturco. 2022. "Practices of Strength and Conditioning Coaches in Professional Sports: A Systematic Review." *Biol Sport* 39 (3): 715-726. https://doi.org/10.5114/biolsport.2022.107480.

Wikipedia. 2023. "Shape America." Last Modified July 25, 2023. https://en.wikipedia.org/wiki/SHAPE_America.

Wylleman, P., D. Alfermann, and D. Lavallee. 2004. "Career Transitions in Sport: European Perspectives." *Psychology of Sport and Exercise* 5: 7-20.

Index

A
absolute loading 76
academic research 231-232
acceleration, training for 218-219
accounting, importance of 126-127
acid-base balance 223-224
active rest 191
acute exercise response 109-111
adaptations to training 111-123
ADP (air displacement plethysmography) 69
aerobic endurance
    exercise prescription 186, 201
    needs analysis and 46
    testing 77-81, 169-171
aerobic system 110-111
agility
    needs analysis and 49
    testing 92-94, 178
    training for 220-222
air displacement plethysmography (ADP) 69
alleles 112
American College of Sports Medicine 102, 231
American football, sample needs analysis 39
AMS (athlete management) systems 125, 135
anaerobic capacity, testing 81, 89-91, 176
analytic research 159
analytics. *See* sport data analytics
androgen receptor 118
annual audit 147-148
anthropometry
    definition 33
    testing 65-70, 159-162
articular cartilage 117
artificial intelligence 238
assessments. *See* testing and assessments
athlete(s)
    development. *See* player development
    post-career transition 2, 245-246
    reports for 148-149
    responsibilities 135-137
    training status of 49, 120
athlete composite 4, 21, 23, 156
athlete management (AMS) systems 125, 135
athleticism, definition 11

ATP–phosphocreatine (ATP–PC) system 110
auditing workouts 143-148

B
balance
    needs analysis and 48
    testing 94-96, 178-179
balance error scoring system (BESS) 96
ballistic resistance exercise 214
beep tests 78-79, 169-170
BESS (balance error scoring system) 96
bioelectrical impedance analysis (BIA) 69-70
biological demands of sport 42-43
biomarkers 142, 179-180
biomechanics
    data collection 142
    demands of sport 40-42
block periodization 226
BMD (bone mineral density) 116-117, 161-162
bodily proportions 35-38
Bod Pod 69
body composition
    definition 33
    needs analysis and 47
    testing 65-70, 159-162
body density, definition 69
body fat percentages 159-161
body weight measurement 66
Bompa, Tudor 225, 226
Bondarchuk, Anatoliy 225
bone biomarkers 117
bone mineral density (BMD) 116-117, 161-162
bone modeling 116
bottom-up model of player development 234-235, 240
broad jump 86
buffering capacity 42, 110, 223-224

C
candidate genes 112
cardiac output 111
cardiovascular (CV) system 8
    exercise response 111, 119-120
    monitoring 171-173
Carroll College 241-242
cartilage 117-118

Casa, Douglas 103
Center for Sports Medicine 27-28, 233-234
certification of professionals 5, 55
change-of-direction (COD) ability
    definition 49
    testing 92-94, 178
    training for 220-222
classical linear periodization 224-225
clothing, for testing 63
CMJ (countermovement jump) 84-86, 187-188
coaches. *See* sport coaches
COD. *See* change-of-direction (COD) ability
cold-water immersion 198-199
colleges. *See* universities/colleges
communication
    in player development team 25-26
    virtual 237-238
competence of professionals 55, 130
competition variables 140
compression garments 198
computer competencies 130-131
concentric force–velocity relationship 44
conjugate periodization 225
connective tissue (CT) 116
Cooper 12-minute walk or run 78
coordination 48
Counsilman, James Edward "Doc" 232
countermovement jump (CMJ) 84-86, 187-188
credentials of professionals 5, 55
cryotherapies 198-199
CT (connective tissue) 116
CV system. *See* cardiovascular (CV) system
cytokines 111

D
data
    accounting 126-127
    analysis. *See* sport data analytics (SDA)
    entry of 132, 142-148, 156-157
    ethical considerations 2
    graphing 134-135
    interpreting 158-180
    metric selection 128-129, 137-139
    privacy issues 2

data *(continued)*
  quality of 2, 132-133, 142-143
  statistics 133-134
  technology and 128-129
  from testing and assessment 56-57
  types of 139
  visualizations 135, 136
databases 156-157
deceleration, training for 219-220
decision-making, in player development 26-27
Delorme, Thomas 189, 244
depth jump 85
descriptive research 159
descriptive statistics 133
diet of the athlete 141, 195-196, 197
disruptors 25, 106-107, 108, 129-130, 139-140
documentation
  of data entry 143
  policy manuals 103
  reports to coaches and athletes 148-149
  training logs 126, 137, 138
dry float 199
dual-energy X-ray absorptiometry (DXA) 68
duties, assigning 128
dynamic balance 48
dynamic flexibility 46, 222
dynamic maximal strength 163-164
dynamic stretching 195
dynapenia 11

E
EAPI (Epley Athletic Performance Index) 31-33
early specialization 13
Edgren side step test 94, 95
8-week mesocycle program 242, 243
endocrine system 8, 109-110, 118
endurance. *See* aerobic endurance; muscular endurance
energy systems 42-43, 110
environment
  conditions during testing 63
  as training factor 50
Epic Performance Index 24
epigenetics 112
Epley, Boyd 239
Epley Athletic Performance Index (EAPI) 31-33
equipment, for testing 62-63
errors, in testing 60, 157-158
Eskridge, Chris 24
essential body fat 160
evidence-based practice
  in search for norms 159

steps of 27
use of 155, 156
exercise(s)
  choice of 188, 202-206
  competence levels 135
  sequence of 206
exercise deficit disorder 11
exercise periodization 122
experimental research 159
explosive strength 45
external loads 52, 177-178

F
facility, as training factor 49
fascicles 116
fast-twitch (FT) muscle fibers 101, 102, 109, 114-115
female triad 162
Fick equation 46
fight-or-flight 109, 110, 239
505 COD test 92-93
flexibility
  needs analysis and 46-47
  testing 81-83, 173, 174
  training for 201, 222-223
flexible nonlinear periodization 107-108, 226, 244-245
flotation therapies 199-200
FMS (functional movement screen) 83, 84
foam rolling 195, 201, 223
footwear, for testing 63
force
  motor unit recruitment 101-102
  relationship to velocity 44, 212
  testing 86, 166-167
force plates 86, 176
40-yard dash 91
Fry, Andrew 190
FT (fast-twitch) muscle fibers 101, 102, 109, 114-115
functional movement screen (FMS) 83, 84
functional overreaching 105
functional strength 45

G
general adaptation syndrome (GAS) 184
general-to-specific model of progression 120-122
genes/genetics 6, 9-10, 23, 111
girth measurement 67
global positioning systems (GPS) 91, 177
glycolysis 110
goals, as training factor 49
GPS (global positioning systems) 91, 177
graphs 134-135
gross motor coordination 48
growth factors 113

H
Haff, Greg 224, 225, 226
Hagen, Josh 235
health
  biomarkers 142
  in needs analysis 49
  long-term 2, 3, 245-246
health-related fitness components
  in needs analysis 43-47
  testing 65-83
heart rate (HR) 171-173
heart rate variability (HRV) 141, 171-173
heat therapy 198-199
height measurement 66
Henneman's size principle 8, 101-102
heritability. *See* genes/genetics
hexagon test 94
high-intensity endurance 45, 74
high-performance management model 27
high school
  athletes 17-18
  model for player development 236-237
hormones. *See* endocrine system
HR (heart rate) 171-173
HRV (heart rate variability) 141, 171-173
Hudy, Andrea 226, 244, 245
hydration 196
hypertrophy 47, 115-116, 216-218

I
ICCR (interclass correlation) 60
immune system 111
IMT (integrative neuromuscular training) 15
individualization
  of programs 30, 183-184
  of recovery strategies 191, 192
inferential statistics 133
inflammation 111
injury
  data collection 141-142
  element of sport evaluation 42
  in intermediate stage of programming
  player development and 2
  as training factor 49
instrument calibrations 63
integrative neuromuscular training (IMT) 15
intensity 206-207
interclass correlation (ICCR) 60
intermittent fitness test 81
internal loads 52
inter-rater reliability 59-60
intraplayer analysis 158

isokinetic strength testing 45, 73-74
isometric strength tests 73, 164-166
Issurin, Vladimir 225
Jordan, Henry Bryce 234
jump training 85-86, 187-188

K

kinesiological demands of sport 40-42
knowledge
    sources of 152
    types of 152-153
Knuttgen, Howard 234
Korey Stringer Institute 4, 103, 237
KPIs 50-51
Kraemer, William J. 27-28, 188, 226, 234, 241-242, 244, 246

L

lactate threshold (LT) 81
landing error scoring system (LESS) 96
landing tests 95-96
lean body mass (LBM) 161
LESS (landing error scoring system) 96
light therapy 198-199
line drill 91
long-term athletic development (LTAD)
    definition 13
    models of 13-17
    pillars of 14
long-term health 2, 3
lower cross syndrome 82
LT (lactate threshold) 81
LTAD. *See* long-term athletic development (LTAD)

M

machine learning 238
Marotti, Mickey 235
Martin, Jerry 1, 226, 234, 240, 244
massage 195
Matveyev, Leo 225
maximal isometric force 45
maximal oxygen uptake ($\dot{V}O_2$max) 46, 77, 169, 171
maximal strength testing 70, 162, 163-164
mechanotransduction 114
medicine ball (MB) throws 89
meditation 200
mesocycle audit 146-147
metabolic circuit 239-240
metabolic demands of sport 42-43
metrics, choosing 128-129, 137-139
mindfulness 200
mobility
    assessing 83
    definition 15
modified sit-and-reach test 82

monitoring
    importance of 123, 125-127, 140, 240
    technology for 128-129, 140
motor skills, effect of strength training on 17
motor unit
    definition 8
    recruitment 101-102, 103, 109
multiple-joint exercises 203
multistage 20-meter shuttle run—beep test 78-79
muscle fibers 101, 102, 109, 110, 114-115
muscular endurance
    needs analysis and 45-46
    testing 74-77, 167-169
    training for 217-218
muscular strength. *See* strength
muscular system 8
Muskego High School 236-237
mutable characteristics 6-7, 9-10, 23, 24, 31, 33
myofascial release 195, 223

N

National Strength and Conditioning Association (NSCA)
    history 7, 28, 231, 232
    position stand on plyometrics 187
NCAA 232
needs analysis
    definition 38
    health-related fitness components 43-50
    necessity of 38-39
    profiling and benchmarking 50-52
    samples 39-40
    sport evaluation 40-43
nervous system 8, 109, 113-114
Newman, Tom 23, 240
Nitka, Mike 236-237
non-essential fat 160
nonfunctional overreaching 105
nonlinear periodization 107-108, 226, 244-245
nonmutable characteristics 6-7, 9, 23, 24, 31, 33
norms 158
NSCA. *See* National Strength and Conditioning Association (NSCA)
nutrition 141, 195-196, 197

O

Ohio State University 235-236
Olympic training centers 27-28, 193, 230-231
1.5-mile run 78
120-yard dash 92

one-repetition maximum (1RM)
    importance of 3
    strength testing 70-71
one-step vertical jump test 85
overload 113-117, 119, 200-201
over-recovery 191
overspeed training 218

P

PACER (progressive aerobic endurance run) test 78-79, 169-170
parasympathetic nervous system 109
peak height velocity 15
Penn State 27-28, 190, 234, 244
perceived exertion 141
performance
    factors affecting 8-9
    pursuing peak performance 104
periodization 106-108, 122, 224-226
physical education in schools 11
physiological adaptations to training 111-123
physiological athlete composite 22
physiological demands of sport 42-43
physiologically-based KPIs 51-52
physique types 34-35
planned functional overreaching 105
player development
    advanced models 233-238
    challenges in 229
    classic model 232-233
    decision-making 26-27
    high school model 236-237
    history and 27-28, 230-231
    multidisciplinary model 27-28
    programming 184-190
    science in 153-155
    virtual models 237-238
player development team
    communication 25-26
    creating 4-6, 25
    decision-making 26-27
    qualifications of each member 55-56, 130
    roles within 151-152
    skills of members 130
    units in 28-31
plyometric training 16-17, 186-188, 215-216
PNF (proprioceptive neuromuscular facilitation) stretching 195, 223
policy manuals 103
Poliquin, Charles 167, 226
polymorphisms 112
position matching 52-53
posture, assessing 83
postworkout audit 146

power
    assessing 83, 86, 173-175
    in needs analysis 47-48
    training for 213-216
power endurance 76
power–velocity relationship 44
preworkout audit 144-146
pro agility test 93-94
professional expertise 4-6, 30
programmed drills 222
program variables 104-106, 184
progressive aerobic endurance run (PACER) test 78-79, 169-170
progressive overload 114, 200-201
pronator distortion syndrome 82
proportions, bodily 35-37, 38
proprioceptive neuromuscular facilitation (PNF) stretching 195, 223
pulsatility 118
punching force 167

Q
quickness drills 222

R
range of motion (ROM) 46, 82, 173, 174
rate of force development (RFD)
    definition 47
    testing 83, 86-87, 165-166
RD (registered dietitian) 29
reaction time
    needs analysis and 48
    testing 96-98
reactive drills 222
recovery
    programming for 105-106, 190-194
    tracking 140
registered dietitian (RD) 29
relative energy deficiency in sport (RED-S) 162
relative muscular strength 44
reliability of tests 59-60, 157
relative loading 76
repeated 40s test 90-91
repetitions 145, 207
repetitions in reserve (RIR) 213
resistance training
    program variables 105, 188-190
    for youth 16-17
resisted speed training 218-219
respiratory system 8
response time 96-98
rest
    recovery days 190-191
    short periods of 239, 240
    sleep 141, 193
    within workout 189-190, 211-212
reverse periodization 224

RFD. See rate of force development (RFD)
rhabdomyolysis 239, 240
Rhea, Matthew 226
RIR (repetitions in reserve) 213
ROM (range of motion) 46, 82, 173, 174
running-based anaerobic sprint test 90

S
Saenz, Cathy 197
safety
    prioritizing 102-103, 240
    and virtual model of player development 237
SAID principle 105
schedule, as training factor 50
scientific method 153-154
scientific process 154-155
SDA. See sport data analytics (SDA)
SEBT (star excursion balance test) 95
self-myofascial release 195, 223
session RPE 141, 179
shoulder elevation test 82
shuttle tests 78-79, 90, 169-170, 176
Simmons, Louie 225
single-joint exercises 203
single-leg squat 95
size principle 8, 101
SJ (squat jump) 85-86, 187-188
skeletal system 7
skill-based KPIs 51
skill-related fitness components
    assessing 83
    in needs analysis 47-49
skills, of player development team 130
skinfold assessments 69
sleep 141, 193
slow-twitch (ST) muscle fibers 101, 105, 109, 114
software
    cost of 2
    education on 131-132
    for graphing 135
somatotyping
    body composition assessment 70
    definition 34
Soviet Union
    cold war with 230
    methodologies from 184, 224-225
specialization in one sport 12
specificity 201
speed
    needs analysis and 48-49
    testing 91-92, 176-177
    training for 218-219
speed strength 45, 47
speed zone 45
split routine 206

sport analytic professionals 29
sport coaches
    reports for 148-149
    responsibilities 137
    role in player development team 30-31
sport composite 6
sport data analytics (SDA)
    as complement to coaching 53, 238
    issues and challenges 2-3, 238
    KPIs and 51
    sport analytic professionals 29
sport demands 37
sport nutrition 29
sport performance professionals 28
sport psychologists 29-30
sports adrenal medulla 118
sport sampling 12
sport science professionals 28-29
sports medicine 29
sport sociologists 30
sport specialization 12
sport-specific tests 98
squat jump (SJ) 85-86, 187-188
ST (slow-twitch) muscle fibers 101, 105, 109, 114
star excursion balance test (SEBT) 95
starting strength 47
static balance 48
static flexibility 46, 222
static stretching 195
statistics 133-134, 157
stimulus-response-adaptation cycle 103-104
Stone, Meg 229
strategy-based KPIs 51
strength
    needs analysis and 43-44
    ratios 167, 168
    testing 70-74, 162-167
    training 3-4, 201-213, 241-242
strength and conditioning professionals 28, 232
strength endurance 45
stretching 194-195
stretch-shortening cycle 186-187, 195
strength-to-mass ratio 44
stroboscopic visual training 48
stroke volume 111
submaximal muscular endurance 45, 74
supplements 196
sympathetic nervous system 109
synergistic adaptation 14

T
talent identification
    assessments for 65
    nonmutable characteristics and 33-34

team cohesion 141
technology
    computer competencies 130-131
    databases 156-157
    decisions based on 238
    GPS 91, 177
    metric selection 128-129
    rollout of 132
    software 131-133, 135
    staff training 131-133
temporal component of sport 41
tendons 117
10-yard dash 91
testing and assessments
    additive errors 60
    audience effects 62
    choice of tests 64
    clothing and footwear 63
    environmental conditions 63
    equipment 62-63
    logistics 61
    mistakes made 64
    number of testers 62
    order of tests 61-62
    preparing for 57-58
    protocols 58
    reliability 59-60
    risk reduction 57
    standards for 56-57
    surfaces for tests 63
    time of day 63-64
    validity 58-59
test–retest reliability 60
30-15 intermittent fitness test 81
three-cone drill 94, 222

three Cs 55-56
300-yard shuttle 90, 176
top-down model of player development 234
total-body workouts 206
training factors 49-50
training impulse (TRIMP) 172-173
training load 65, 179, 208-211
training log 126, 137, 138
training specificity 8
training status 49, 120
trait analysis 24
TRIMP (training impulse) 172-173
trunk rotation test 82
T-test 93
type I (slow-twitch) muscle fibers 101, 105, 109, 114
type II (fast-twitch) muscle fibers 101, 102, 109, 114-115

U
underwater weighing 68-69
University of Connecticut 4, 103, 226, 234-235, 237, 244-245
universities/colleges
    academic research 231-232
    college athletes 18
    player development in 233
upper cross syndrome 82

V
validity of tests 58-59
variables. *See* competition variables; program variables
variation
    as element of program design 201
    importance of 184
    methods 224-226
velocity 44, 200, 207, 212-213
velocity-based training 208
Verkhoshansky, Yuri 187, 225, 226
vertical jump, testing 83-86
virtual models for player development 237-238
volleyball, sample needs analysis 40
volume load 211
$\dot{V}O_2$max (maximal oxygen uptake) 46, 77, 169, 171

W
Ward, Bob 232
weight measurement 66
wet float 199
Wingate anaerobic power test 89-90, 176
workout(s)
    auditing 143-148
    logging. *See* training log

Y
Yale University 197, 240, 242, 245
Y balance test (YBT) 95, 96
young athletes, development of 9-18
youth physical development (YPD) model 15
Yo-Yo intermittent recovery tests 79-80, 169-170, 171

Z
Zatsiorsky, Vladimir M. 225

About the Authors

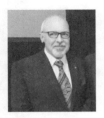

William J. Kraemer, PhD, CSCS,*D, FNSCA, FACSM, acts as the senior advisor for sport performance and sport sciences at The Ohio State University and is a member of the performance innovation team for the university's department of athletics. Although retired as a full professor, he still works as an adjunct professor as a research scientist in the department of human sciences at The Ohio State University, continuing his research and writing. He is a professor emeritus in the department of kinesiology at the University of Connecticut and holds an adjunct professorship in the Exercise Medicine Research Institute at Edith Cowan University in Perth, Australia. He has held full professorships at Pennsylvania State University, Ball State University, and the University of Connecticut as well as appointments at their medical schools. In 2016, he received an honorary doctorate from the University of Jyvaskyla in Finland for the worldwide impact of his research.

Dr. Kraemer has published 12 books and over 500 peer-reviewed papers in the scientific literature and a multitude of other educational publications. He is a fellow in several organizations, including the American College of Sports Medicine (ACSM), National Strength and Conditioning Association (NSCA), International Society of Sports Nutrition (ISSN), and American Nutrition Association (ANA), and he is a member of the American Physiological Society. He is a past president of the NSCA and has served on the board of trustees for the ACSM and has been a chapter president and honor award winner. Dr. Kraemer has received many other awards, including the NSCA's Lifetime Achievement Award, and the Outstanding Sport Scientist award was named in his honor in 2006. He was ranked as the top sport scientist in the world for over two decades. The University of Jyvaskyla's University Medal was awarded to him in 2009 as the first non-Finnish recipient of this award. In 2020, he was honored with one of the highest awards by the ACSM: the Citation Award.

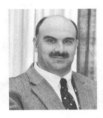

Nicholas A. Ratamess, PhD, CSCS,*D, FNSCA, is a professor in the department of kinesiology and health sciences at The College of New Jersey. His major research interest is examining physiological responses and adaptations to strength training and conditioning and sports supplementation. Dr. Ratamess has authored or coauthored more than 205 scientific investigations, educational articles, review papers, chapters, and books. He is currently the editor in chief of the NSCA's *Journal of Strength and Conditioning Research*. He also coauthored four position stands from the ACSM and the NSCA regarding progression models in resistance training and anabolic androgenic steroids and growth hormone use in athletes. Dr. Ratamess is a certified strength and conditioning specialist with distinction (CSCS,*D) and a fellow of the NSCA.

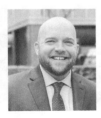

Thomas H. Newman, MS, CSCS, is a seasoned professional in human performance who currently holds the role of lead performance specialist at the Center for Sports Performance Research at Mass General Brigham Hospital. Having accumulated 15 years of valuable experience across both the private and college sectors, Newman brings a deep understanding and practical knowledge to his role. His academic background includes a BA from the University of Rhode Island and an MS from the University of Southern Connecticut, equipping him with a robust theoretical foundation. Newman's professional journey led him to Yale University, where he was named the first-ever director of sports performance and innovation. There, he oversaw all 32 varsity programs, leading the teams to unprecedented success, both on and off the field. Before his tenure at Yale, Newman exhibited his entrepreneurial prowess as the CEO of Athletic Standard, a tech startup with the mission of developing a global digital platform for athlete development and talent identification. Recognized by the NSCA with the certified strength and conditioning specialist (CSCS) credential, Newman's commitment to his field is evident. His combination of academic knowledge, hands-on experience, and entrepreneurial spirit positions him as a respected figure in human performance.

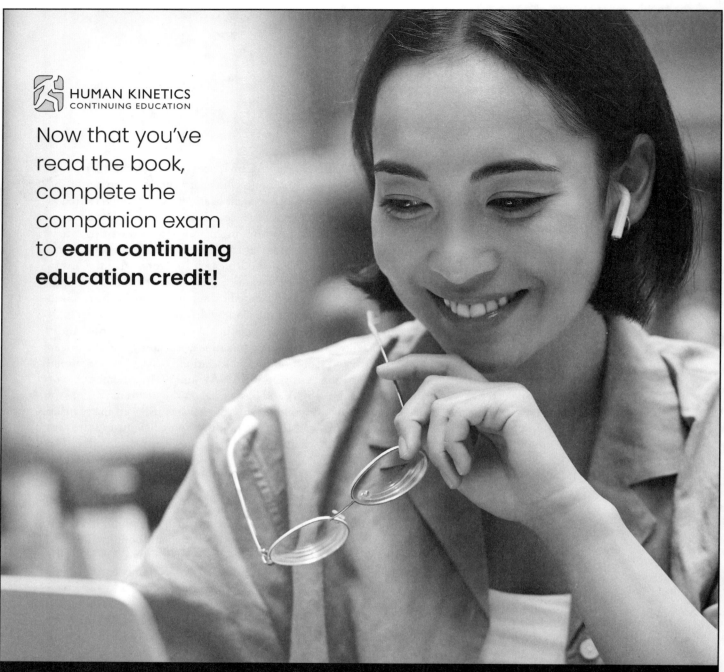

HUMAN KINETICS
CONTINUING EDUCATION

Now that you've read the book, complete the companion exam to **earn continuing education credit!**

Find your CE exam here:
US & International: US.HumanKinetics.com/collections/Continuing-Education
Canada: Canada.HumanKinetics.com/collections/Continuing-Education

Subscribe to our newsletters today!

US

Canada

Get exclusive offers and stay apprised of CE opportunities.